THE SOCIETAL BURDEN OF CHILD ABUSE

Long-Term Mental Health and Behavioral Consequences

THE SOCIETAL BURDEN OF CHILD ABUSE

Long-Term Mental Health and Behavioral Consequences

Edited by

Lisa Albers Prock, MD

APPLE ACADEMIC PRESS

Apple Academic Press Inc.	Apple Academic Press Inc.
3333 Mistwell Crescent	9 Spinnaker Way
Oakville, ON L6L 0A2	Waretown, NJ 08758
Canada	USA

Exclusive worldwide distribution by CRC Press, a member of Taylor & Francis Group

International Standard Book Number-13: 978-1-77188-244-6 (Hardcover)

International Standard Book Number-13: 978-1-77188-246-0 (ebook)

Library and Archives Canada Cataloguing in Publication

The societal burden of child abuse : long-term mental health and behavioral consequences / edited by Lisa Albers Prock, MD.

Includes bibliographical references and index.
ISBN 978-1-77188-244-6 (bound)
1. Child abuse--Social aspects. 2. Child abuse--Psychological aspects. 3. Psychic trauma in children. 4. Behavior disorders in children. 5. Abused children--Mental health. I. Prock, Lisa Albers, editor

HV6626.5.S62 2015 362.76 C2015-903269-5

Library of Congress Cataloging-in-Publication Data

The societal burden of child abuse : long-term mental health and behavioral consequences / editor, Lisa Albers Prock, MD.

pages cm
Includes bibliographical references and index.
ISBN 978-1-77188-244-6 (alk. paper)
1. Child abuse--Psychological aspects. 2. Abused children--Mental health. 3. Psychic trauma in children. 4. Heath behavior. 5. Criminal behavior. 6. Criminal psychology. I. Prock, Lisa Albers.

RC569.5.C55S67 2015 362.76--dc23 2015016808

Apple Academic Press also publishes its books in a variety of electronic formats. Some content that appears in print may not be available in electronic format. For information about Apple Academic Press products, visit our website at **www.appleacademicpress.com** and the CRC Press website at **www.crcpress.com**

MIX
Paper from responsible sources
FSC www.fsc.org FSC® C013056

Printed and bound in Great Britain by
TJ International Ltd, Padstow, Cornwall

ABOUT THE EDITOR

LISA ALBERS PROCK, MD

Dr. Lisa Albers Prock is a Developmental Behavioral Pediatrician at Children's Hospital (Boston) and Harvard Medical School. She attended college at the University of Chicago, medical school at Columbia University, and received a Master's Degree in Public Health from the Harvard School of Public Health. Board Certified in General Pediatrics and Developmental Behavioral Pediatrics, she currently is Clinical Director of Developmental and Behavioral Pediatrics and Consultant to the Walker School, a residential school serving children in foster care. Dr. Prock has combined her clinical interests in child development and international health with advocacy for children in medical, residential, and educational settings since 1991. She has worked in Cambodia teaching pediatrics and studying tuberculosis epidemiology; and in Eastern Europe visiting children with severe neurodevelopmental challenges in orphanages. She has co-authored numerous original publications and articles for families. She is a also nonprofit board member for organizations and has received numerous local and national awards for her work with children and families.

CONTENTS

ACKNOWLEDGMENT AND HOW TO CITE

The editor and publisher thank each of the authors who contributed to this book. The chapters in this book were previously published elsewhere. To cite the work contained in this book and to view the individual permissions, please refer to the citation at the beginning of each chapter. Each chapter was read individually and carefully selected by the editor; the result is a book that provides a comprehensive perspective on child abuse's long-term mental health and behavioral consequences, which place a heavy burden on both individuals and society. The chapters included examine the following topics:

- The article by Collin-Vézina and her colleagues was selected because it offers a good overview of the topic (used in chapters 1 and 6), as well as a sound summary conclusion (used in chapter 17).
- The articles included in chapters 2 through 5 were chosen because they offer insight into the society-wide costs of child abuse, including prevalence, sexual offending later in life, delinquency, and adult aggression.
- Chapters 6 through 12 contain articles selected because of their studies of the connections between child abuse and health. Included in these articles is research into cognitive development, suicide, smoking, and sleep.
- The articles selected for chapters 13 through 16 provide fascinating insight into the ways in which child abuse may have impact on the genetic level. The twin study by York and his colleagues (chapter 16) is particularly insightful.

LIST OF CONTRIBUTORS

Steven H. Aggen

Virginia Institute for Psychiatric and Behavioral Genetics, Virginia Commonwealth University, Richmond, Virginia, United States of America; Department of Psychiatry, Virginia Commonwealth University, Richmond, Virginia, United States of America

Sonia A. Alemagno

Department of Health Policy and Management, College of Public Health, Kent State University, Kent, Ohio, United States of America

Ananda B. Amstadter

Virginia Institute for Psychiatric and Behavioral Genetics, Virginia Commonwealth University, Richmond, Virginia, United States of America; Department of Psychiatry, Virginia Commonwealth University, Richmond, Virginia, United States of America

Mark A. Bellis

Professor of Public Health, Centre for Public Health, Liverpool John Moores University, 15-21 Webster Street, Liverpool L3 2ET, UK

Madhav P. Bhatta

Department of Biostatistics, Environmental Health Sciences and Epidemiology, College of Public Health, Kent State University, Kent, Ohio, United States of America

Sabrina Bleich

Rehabilitation and Organization Division, Baden-Wuerttemberg Registered Hospital Association, Association of Hospitals, Rehabilitation- and Care Establishments, Birkenwaldstraße 151, Stuttgart, 70191, Germany

Emily A. Blood

Harvard Medical School, Boston, Massachusetts, USA, Clinical Research Center, Children's Hospital Boston, Boston, Massachusetts, USA

Nada Borghol

Sackler Program for Epigenetics & Developmental Psychobiology, McGill University, 3655 Promenade Sir William Osler, Montreal H3G 1Y6, QC, Canada; Department of Pharmacology and Therapeutics, McGill University, 3655 Promenade Sir William Osler, Montreal H3G 1Y6, QC, Canada

Jenni Brumelle

Department of Human and Molecular Genetics, Virginia Commonwealth University, Richmond, Virginia, United States of America; Department of Pathology, Virginia Commonwealth University, Richmond, Virginia, United States of America

Bryan Buss

Centers for Disease Control and Prevention, Atlanta, Georgia

Betsy L. Cadwell

Centers for Disease Control and Prevention, Atlanta, Georgia

Valeria Carola
European Molecular Biology Laboratory (EMBL), Mouse Biology Unit, Monterotondo, Italy

Daniel P. Chapman
Division of Population Health, National Center for Chronic Disease Prevention and Health Promotion, Centers for Disease Control and Prevention, 4770 Buford Highway NE, Mailstop K-67, Atlanta, GA, 30041, USA

Delphine Collin-Vézina
School of Social Work, McGill University, 3506 University Street, room 321A, Montreal (QC), Canada H3A 2A7.

P. Courtet
INSERM U1061, Montpellier, France; University of Montpellier 1, Montpellier, France; Department of Emergency Psychiatry, University Hospital of Montpellier, Montpellier, France

Janet B. Croft
National Center for Chronic Disease Prevention and Health Promotion, Division of Adult and Community Health, Centers for Disease Control and Prevention, Atlanta, GA, USA

Carlos A. Cuevas
Office of Juvenile Justice and Delinquency Prevention

Isabelle Daigneault
Psychology Department, Université de Montréal, P.O. Box 6128, Downtown Station, Montréal QC, Canada H3C 3J7.

Satvinder Dhingra
Office of Public Health Preparedness and Response, Office of Science and Public Health Practice, Centers for Disease Control and Prevention, Atlanta, GA, USA

K. Dieben
Department of Mental Health and Psychiatry, University Hospitals of Geneva, Geneva, Switzerland

Theo A. H. Doreleijers
VU University Medical Center, Amsterdam and Department of Criminal Justice, Leiden University, The Netherlands

Shanta R. Dube
National Center for Chronic Disease Prevention and Health Promotion, Office of Smoking and Health, Atlanta, GA, USA

Lindon J. Eaves
Department of Human and Molecular Genetics, Virginia Commonwealth University, Richmond, Virginia, United States of America; Virginia Institute for Psychiatric and Behavioral Genetics, Virginia Commonwealth University, Richmond, Virginia, United States of America; Department of Psychiatry, Virginia Commonwealth University, Richmond, Virginia, United States of America

Valerie J. Edwards
National Center for Chronic Disease Prevention and Health Promotion, Division of Adult and Community Health, Centers for Disease Control and Prevention, Atlanta, GA, USA

Byron Egeland
Institute of Child Development, University of Minnesota, Minneapolis, Minnesota, USA

Michelle Bosquet Enlow
Department of Psychiatry, Children's Hospital Boston, Boston, Massachusetts, USA, Harvard Medical School, Boston, Massachusetts, USA

Jörg M. Fegert
Department of Child and Adolescent Psychiatry and Psychotherapy, University of Ulm, Steinhoevelstr. 5, Ulm, 89075, Germany

Andrea Ferreira-Gonzalez
Department of Pathology, Virginia Commonwealth University, Richmond, Virginia, United States of America

David Finkelhor
Office of Juvenile Justice and Delinquency Prevention

Giovanni Frazzetto
European Molecular Biology Laboratory (EMBL), Mouse Biology Unit, Monterotondo, Italy

Cornelius Gross
European Molecular Biology Laboratory (EMBL), Mouse Biology Unit, Monterotondo, Italy

S. Guillaume
INSERM U1061, Montpellier, France; University of Montpellier 1, Montpellier, France; Department of Emergency Psychiatry, University Hospital of Montpellier, Montpellier, France

Susanne Habetha
IGSF Institute for Health System Research GmbH, Schauenburgerstr, 116, 24118, Kiel, Germany

Sherry Hamby
Office of Juvenile Justice and Delinquency Prevention

Dominic Harrison
Director of Public Health, National Health Service, Guide Business Centre, School Lane, Blackburn, Lancashire BB1 2QH, UK

Martine Hébert
Sexology Department, Université du Québec à Montréal, P.O. Box 8888, Downtown Station, Montréal QC, Canada H3C 3P8.

Clyde Hertzman
Human Early Learning Partnership, University of British Columbia, Suite 440, 2206 East Mall, Vancouver V6T 1Z3, BC, Canada

Karen Hughes
Reader in Behavioural Epidemiology, Centre for Public Health, Liverpool John Moores University, 15-21 Webster Street, Liverpool L3 2ET, UK

P. Huguelet
Department of Mental Health and Psychiatry, University Hospitals of Geneva, Geneva, Switzerland

Colleen Jackson-Cook
Department of Human and Molecular Genetics, Virginia Commonwealth University, Richmond, Virginia, United States of America; Department of Pathology, Virginia Commonwealth University, Richmond, Virginia, United States of America

Eric Jefferis
Department of Social and Behavioral Sciences, College of Public Health, Kent State University, Kent, Ohio, United States of America

Kimberly H. Jones
Neodiagnostix, Inc, Rockville, Maryland, United States of America; Department of Pathology, Virginia Commonwealth University, Richmond, Virginia, United States of America

Jane Juusola
Department of Pathology, Virginia Commonwealth University, Richmond, Virginia, United States of America

Angela Kavadas
Department of Social and Behavioral Sciences, College of Public Health, Kent State University, Kent, Ohio, United States of America

Kenneth S. Kendler
Department of Human and Molecular Genetics, Virginia Commonwealth University, Richmond, Virginia, United States of America; Virginia Institute for Psychiatric and Behavioral Genetics, Virginia Commonwealth University, Richmond, Virginia, United States of America; Department of Psychiatry, Virginia Commonwealth University, Richmond, Virginia, United States of America

Nicola Leckenby
Research Assistant, Centre for Public Health, Liverpool John Moores University, 15-21 Webster Street, Liverpool L3 2ET, UK

Laura E. W. Leenarts
VU University Medical Center, Amsterdam, The Netherlands

Giorgio Di Lorenzo
Department of Neurosciences, University of Rome Tor Vergata, Rome, Italy

Helen Lowey
Consultant in Public Health, Centre for Public Health, Liverpool John Moores University, 15-21 Webster Street, Liverpool L3 2ET, UK

Yong Liu
Division of Population Health, National Center for Chronic Disease Prevention and Health Promotion, Centers for Disease Control and Prevention, 4770 Buford Highway NE, Mailstop K-67, Atlanta, GA, 30041, USA

A. Malafosse
Department of Psychiatry, University of Geneva, Chêne-Bourg, Switzerland; Department of Medical Genetic and Laboratories, University Hospitals of Geneva, Geneva, Switzerland

David Mannino
University of Kentucky College of Public Health, Lexington, Kentucky

Patrick O. McGowan
Centre for Environmental Epigenetics and Development, Toronto, ON, Canada; Department of Biological Sciences, University of Toronto, Scarborough, ON, Canada; Cell and Systems Biology, University of Toronto, Toronto, ON, Canada

Lela McKnight-Eily
National Center for Chronic Disease Prevention and Health Promotion, Division of Adult and Community Health, Centers for Disease Control and Prevention, Atlanta, GA, USA

Larkin S. McReynolds
Columbia University Medical Center, New York City, USA

D. Mouthon
Department of Medical Genetic and Laboratories, University Hospitals of Geneva, Geneva, Switzerland

R. Nicastro
Department of Mental Health and Psychiatry, University Hospitals of Geneva, Geneva, Switzerland

E. Olié
INSERM U1061, Montpellier, France; University of Montpellier 1, Montpellier, France; Department of Emergency Psychiatry, University Hospital of Montpellier, Montpellier, France

A. Paoloni-Giacobino
Department of Medical Genetic and Laboratories, University Hospitals of Geneva, Geneva, Switzerland

Jane J. Pappas
Sackler Program for Epigenetics & Developmental Psychobiology, McGill University, 3655 Promenade Sir William Osler, Montreal H3G 1Y6, QC, Canada; Department of Pharmacology and Therapeutics, McGill University, 3655 Promenade Sir William Osler, Montreal H3G 1Y6, QC, Canada

Marcus Pembrey
Clinical and Molecular Genetics Unit, UCL Institute of Child Health, 30 Guilford Street, London WC1N 1EH, UK

Snehal M. Pinto Pereira
MRC Centre of Epidemiology for Child Health/ Centre for Paediatric Epidemiology and Biostatistics, UCL Institute of Child Health, 30 Guilford Street, London WC1N 1EH, UK

N. Perroud
Department of Psychiatry, University of Geneva, Chêne-Bourg, Switzerland

Geraldine S. Perry
Division of Population Health, National Center for Chronic Disease Prevention and Health Promotion, Centers for Disease Control and Prevention, 4770 Buford Highway NE

Chris Power
MRC Centre of Epidemiology for Child Health/ Centre for Paediatric Epidemiology and Biostatistics, UCL Institute of Child Health, 30 Guilford Street, London WC1N 1EH, UK

P. Prada
Department of Mental Health and Psychiatry, University Hospitals of Geneva, Geneva, Switzerland

Angela Witt Prehn
Walden University, Minneapolis, MN, USA

Letitia R. Presley-Cantrell
Division of Population Health, National Center for Chronic Disease Prevention and Health Promotion, Centers for Disease Control and Prevention, 4770 Buford Highway NE, Mailstop K-67, Atlanta, GA, 30041, USA

Luca Proietti
Department of Neurosciences, University of Rome Tor Vergata, Rome, Italy

Sandra Rasmussen
Walden University, Minneapolis, MN, USA; Williamsville Wellness, Hanover, VA, USA

Thomas Safranek
Nebraska Department of Health and Human Services, Lincoln, Nebraska

A. Salzmann
Department of Psychiatry, University of Geneva, Chêne-Bourg, Switzerland

Peggy Shaffer-King
Department of Social and Behavioral Sciences, College of Public Health, Kent State University, Kent, Ohio, United States of America

Anne Shattuck
Office of Juvenile Justice and Delinquency Prevention

Alberto Siracusano
Department of Neurosciences, University of Rome Tor Vergata, Rome, Italy

Ewa Sokolowska
European Molecular Biology Laboratory (EMBL), Mouse Biology Unit, Monterotondo, Italy

C. Stouder
Department of Medical Genetic and Laboratories, University Hospitals of Geneva, Geneva, Switzerland

Tara W. Strine
Office of Public Health Preparedness and Response, Office of Science and Public Health Practice, Centers for Disease Control and Prevention, Atlanta, GA, USA; Office of Surveillance, Epidemiology, and Laboratory Services, Centers for Disease Control and Prevention, 2500 Century Pkwy Mailstop E-97, Atlanta, GA, 30345, USA

Matthew Suderman
Sackler Program for Epigenetics & Developmental Psychobiology, McGill University, 3655 Promenade Sir William Osler, Montreal H3G 1Y6, QC, Canada; Department of Pharmacology and Therapeutics, McGill University, 3655 Promenade Sir William Osler, Montreal H3G 1Y6, QC, Canada; McGill Centre for Bioinformatics, McGill University, 3649 Promenade Sir William Osler, Montreal H3G 0B1, QC, Canada

Moshe Szyf
Sackler Program for Epigenetics & Developmental Psychobiology, McGill University, 3655 Promenade Sir William Osler, Montreal H3G 1Y6, QC, Canada; Department of Pharmacology and Therapeutics, McGill University, 3655 Promenade Sir William Osler, Montreal H3G 1Y6, QC, Canada

Alfonso Troisi
Department of Neurosciences, University of Rome Tor Vergata, Rome, Italy

Heather Turner
Office of Juvenile Justice and Delinquency Prevention

Robert R. J. M. Vermeiren
Curium University Medical Center, Leiden and VU University Medical Center, Amsterdam, The Netherlands

Morton Wagenfeld
Walden University, Minneapolis, MN, USA; Western Michigan University, Kalamazoo, MI, USA

Gail A. Wasserman
Columbia University Medical Center, New York City, USA

Jörg Weidenhammer
IGSF Institute for Health System Research GmbH, Schauenburgerstr, 116, 24118, Kiel, Germany

Anne G. Wheaton
Division of Population Health, National Center for Chronic Disease Prevention and Health Promotion, Centers for Disease Control and Prevention, 4770 Buford Highway NE, Mailstop K-67, Atlanta, GA, 30041, USA

Robert O. Wright
Harvard Medical School, Boston, Massachusetts, USA; Department of Medicine, Children's Hospital Boston, Boston, Massachusetts, USA; Department of Environmental Health, Harvard School of Public Health, Boston, Massachusetts, USA

Rosalind J. Wright
Harvard Medical School, Boston, Massachusetts, USA; Department of Environmental Health, Harvard School of Public Health, Boston, Massachusetts, USA; Channing Laboratory, Department of Medicine, Brigham & Women's Hospital, Boston, Massachusetts, USA

Kristin Yeoman
Epidemic Intelligence Service Officer assigned to Nebraska Department of Health and Human Services

Timothy P. York
Department of Human and Molecular Genetics, Virginia Commonwealth University, Richmond, Virginia, United States of America; Virginia Institute for Psychiatric and Behavioral Genetics, Virginia Commonwealth University, Richmond, Virginia, United States of America

INTRODUCTION

The immediate acute impact of child abuse to the individual, which may range from bruises, broken bones or even death, is hard to deny. However, the long-term impact is more difficult to access. Other aspects of childhood abuse besides physical abuse, including sexual abuse, emotional abuse, or neglect, are also often harder to observe. All types of abuse and neglect, however, contribute to society's health-care and child-welfare needs and expenses. There are additional costs to society as well, which are substantial. Emerging evidence demonstrates a range of biological changes at a cellular level that may precipitate additional challenges for affected individuals that have enormous societal implications including:

- increased risk of homelessness in childhood/adolescence
- increased risk of negative behaviors contributing to delinquency and/or further involvement with the legal system
- increased risk of negative health behaviors in adulthood (for example smoking; poor sleep hygiene)
- increased risk of mental issues and suicide

The articles included in this compendium contain recent research into the various consequences of child abuse. Together they present a multifaceted perspective of a serious societal problem.

—*Lisa Albers Prock, M.D.*

Although child sexual abuse (CSA) is recognized as a serious violation of human well-being and of the law, no community has yet developed mechanisms that ensure that none of their youth will be sexually abused. CSA is, sadly, an international problem of great magnitude that can affect children of all ages, sexes, races, ethnicities, and socioeconomic classes. In chapters 1, 6, and 17, Collin-Vézina et al. provide a brief overview of a few lessons we can draw from CSA scholarly research. Their overview, with which this volume begins and concludes, focuses on the prevalence of CSA, the associated mental health outcomes, and the preventive strategies to prevent CSA from happening in the first place.

Traumatization in childhood can result in lifelong health impairment and may have a negative impact on other areas of life such as education, social contacts, and employment as well. Despite the frequent occurrence of traumatization, which is reflected in a 14.5 percent prevalence rate of severe child abuse and neglect, the economic burden of the consequences is hardly known. In chapter 2, Habetha et al. offer a prevalence-based cost-of-illness study to show how impairment of the individual is reflected in economic trauma follow-up costs borne by society as a whole in Germany. They then compare the results with Australian, Canadian, and American costs, based on purchasing power parity. They conclude that creating a reliable cost data basis can pave the way for long-term cost savings.

In chapter 3, Leenarts, et al. examine the contributions of demographic characteristics, mental health problems, and interpersonal trauma history to juvenile sexual offending, and the degree to which juvenile sexual offenders differ from nonsexual interpersonal offenders. Their results are based on secondary analysis of a large dataset (n= 2920) of psychiatric assessments of juveniles (in the United States). T-test and chi-square analyses compared demographic, offense, and diagnostic characteristics of juvenile sexual offenders and nonsexual interpersonal offenders. Logistic regression examined the relationship between type of trauma exposure and sex offender status, adjusting for other significant demographic and diagnostic contributors. Their results show that compared to juvenile nonsexual interpersonal offenders, sexual offenders were significantly less likely to be female, to be African American, or to meet criteria for a substance use disorder; juvenile sexual offenders were significantly more likely to have a lifetime history of a suicide attempt and a history of sexual victimization. A set of demographic and diagnostic characteristics contributed significantly to juvenile sexual offending, as did self-reported history of sexual trauma. The authors' findings indicate that juvenile sexual offenders in some aspects differ from nonsexual interpersonal offenders; sexual victimization plays an important role in explaining some sexually abusive behavior. Further research is needed to identify interventions that are effective for these youth.

The association between delinquency and victimization is a common focus in juvenile justice research. Some observers have found that victimization and delinquency largely overlap, with most victims engaging in delinquency and most delinquents being victimized at some point in their lives. The literature in the bullying and peer victimization field paints a different picture. It points to three distinct groups of children: in addition to the children who are both victims and offenders (often referred to as bully-victims or, as in this bulletin, delinquent-victims), a second group are primarily victims, and a third group are primarily offenders. In chapter 4, Cuevas et al. explain the contrast in this way: many studies have relied simply on measures of association between delinquency and victimization (e.g., correlation or regression analyses). When researchers look beyond the association between delinquency and victimization (even when that association is strong), they are likely to find groups of children who are primarily victims or primarily offenders. Research has not fully explored how large these groups are and how their characteristics and experiences differ.

Previous research has reported that a functional polymorphism in the monoamine oxidase A (MAOA) gene promoter can moderate the association between early life adversity and increased risk for violence and antisocial behavior. In chapter 5, Frazzetto et al. offer a study of a combined population of psychiatric outpatients and healthy volunteers, in which they tested the hypothesis that MAOA genotype moderates the association between early traumatic life events experienced during the first 15 years of life and the display of physical aggression during adulthood, as assessed by the Aggression Questionnaire. An ANOVA model including gender, exposure to early trauma, and MAOA genotype as between-subjects factors showed significant interaction effects. Physical aggression scores were higher in men who had experienced early traumatic life events and who carried the low MAOA activity allele. Frazzeto and colleagues repeated the analysis in the subgroup of healthy volunteers to exclude the observed GxE interactions being due to the inclusion of psychiatric patients in their sample that would not be generalizable to the population at large. The results for the subgroup of healthy volunteers were identical to those for the entire sample. Their results support the hypothesis that, when combined with exposure to early traumatic life events, low MAOA activity is a significant risk factor for aggressive behavior during adulthood and suggest that the use of dimensional measures focusing on behavioral aspects of aggression may increase the likelihood of detecting significant gene-by-environment interactions in studies of MAOA-related aggression.

Childhood trauma exposure has also been associated with deficits in cognitive functioning. The influence of timing of exposure on the magnitude and persistence of deficits is not well understood. The impact of exposure in early development has been especially under-investigated. In chapter 7, Enlow et al. examine the impact of interpersonal trauma exposure (IPT) in the first years of life on childhood cognitive functioning. They found that IPT was significantly associated with decreased cognitive scores at all time points, even after controlling for sociodemographic factors, maternal IQ, birth complications, birth weight, and cognitive stimulation in the home. IPT in the first 2 years appeared to be especially detrimental. On average, compared with children not exposed to IPT in the first 2 years, exposed children scored one-half SD lower across cognitive assessments. They conclude that IPT in early life may have adverse effects on cognitive development, and that IPT during the first 2 years may have particular impact, with effects persisting at least into later childhood.

Other studies suggest strong links between adverse childhood experiences and poor adult health and social outcomes. However, the use of such studies in non-US populations is relatively scarce. Bellis et al. discuss in chapter 8 a retrospective cross-sectional survey of 1500 residents and 67 substance users aged 18–70 years in a relatively deprived and ethnically diverse UK population. They found that increasing ACEs were strongly related to adverse behavioral, health, and social outcomes, which included smoking, heavy drinking, incarceration, and morbid obesity. They also had greater risk of poor educational and employment outcomes; low mental wellbeing and life satisfaction; recent violence involvement; recent inpatient hospital care and chronic health conditions. Higher ACEs were also associated with having caused or been unintentionally pregnant before 18 years of age and having been born to a mother who was less than 20 years old. The authors conclude that ACEs contribute to poor life-course health and social outcomes in a UK population. That ACEs are linked to involvement in violence, early unplanned pregnancy, incarceration, and unemployment suggests a cyclic effect where those with higher ACE counts have higher risks of exposing their own children to ACEs.

Smoking is still another public health risk; the prevalence of smoking among adults in Nebraska is 18.4%. Studies indicate that maltreatment of children alters their brain development, possibly increasing risk for tobacco use. Previous studies have documented associations between childhood maltreatment and adult health behaviors, demonstrating the influence of adverse experiences on tobacco use. In chapter 9, Yeoman et al. examine prevalence and associations between adverse childhood experiences and smoking among Nebraskans, using the 2011 Nebraska Behavioral Risk Factor Surveillance System (Adverse Childhood Experience module) data, defining adverse childhood experience exposures as physical, sexual, and verbal abuse (i.e., direct exposures), and household dysfunction associated with mental illness, substance abuse, divorce, domestic violence, and living with persons with incarceration histories (i.e., environmental exposures). The authors estimated prevalence of exposures, taking into account the complex survey design. They used logistic regression with predicted margins to estimate adjusted relative risk for smoking by direct or environmental exposure. The study found that approximately 51% of Nebraskans experienced one or more adverse childhood events; 7% experienced five or more. Prevalence of environmental exposures (42%) was significantly higher than that of direct exposures (31%). Prevalence of individual exposures ranged from 6% (incarceration of a household member) to 25% (verbal abuse). Adjusted relative risks of smoking for direct and environmental exposures were 1.5 and 1.8, respectively. The authors conclude that the prevalence of adverse childhood experiences is high among Nebraskans, and these exposures are associated with smoking. They call for state-specific strategies to monitor adverse events among children and provide interventions to help to decrease the smoking rate in this population.

Research suggests that ACEs have a long-term impact on the behavioral, emotional, and cognitive development of children. These disruptions can lead to adoption of unhealthy coping behaviors throughout the lifespan. In chapter 10, Strine et al. examine psychological distress as a potential mediator of sex-specific associations between adverse childhood experiences and adult smoking. They use data from 7,210 Kaiser-Permanente members in San Diego California collected between April and October 1997, finding that among women, psychological distress mediated a significant portion of the association between ACEs and smoking (21% for emotional abuse, 16% for physical abuse, 15% for physical neglect, 10% for parental separation or divorce). Among men, the associations between ACEs and smoking were not significant. These findings suggest that for women, current smoking cessation strategies may benefit from understanding the potential role of childhood trauma.

Although adverse childhood experiences has been demonstrated to be adversely associated with a variety of health outcomes in adulthood, their specific association with sleep among adults has not been examined. To better address this issue, Chapman et al. in chapter 11 examine the relationship between eight self-reported ACEs and frequent insufficient sleep among community-dwelling adults residing in five U.S. states in 2009. To assess whether ACEs were associated with frequent insufficient sleep (respondent did not get sufficient rest or sleep ≥14 days in past 30 days) in adulthood, they analyzed ACE data collected in the 2009 Behavioral Risk Factor Surveillance System, a random-digit-dialed telephone survey in Arkansas, Louisiana, New Mexico, Tennessee, and Washington. ACEs included physical abuse, sexual abuse, verbal abuse, household mental illness, incarcerated household members, household substance abuse, parental separation/divorce, and witnessing domestic violence before age 18. Smoking status and frequent mental distress (FMD) (≥14 days in past 30 days when self-perceived mental health was not good) were assessed as potential mediators in multivariate logistic regression analyses of frequent insufficient sleep by ACEs adjusted for race/ethnicity, gender, education, and body mass index. Overall, 28.8% of 25,810 respondents reported frequent insufficient sleep, 18.8% were current smokers, 10.8% reported frequent mental distress, 59.5% percent reported ≥1 ACE, and 8.7% reported ≥ 5 ACEs. Each ACE was associated with frequent insufficient sleep in multivariate analyses. Odds of frequent insufficient sleep were 2.5 (95% CI, 2.1-3.1) times higher in persons with ≥5 ACEs compared to those with no ACEs. Most relationships were modestly attenuated by smoking and FMD, but remained significant. The authors conclude that childhood exposures to eight indicators of child maltreatment and household dysfunction were significantly associated with frequent insufficient sleep during adulthood in this population. ACEs could be potential indicators promoting further investigation of sleep insufficiency, along with consideration of family dynamics, smoking, and academic achievement

In chapter 12, Bhatta et al. assess the influence of multiple adverse life experiences (sexual abuse, homelessness, running away, and substance abuse in the family) on suicide ideation and suicide attempt among adolescents at an urban juvenile detention facility in the United States. The study sample included a total of 3,156 adolescents processed at a juvenile detention facility in an urban area in Ohio between 2003 and 2007. The participants, interacting anonymously with a voice-enabled computer, self-administered a questionnaire with 100 items related to health risk behaviors. Overall 19.0% reported ever having thought about suicide (suicide ideation) and 11.9% reported ever having attempted suicide (suicide attempt). In the multivariable logistic regression analysis those reporting sexual abuse (Odds Ratio = 2.75; 95% confidence interval = 2.08–3.63) and homelessness (1.51; 1.17–1.94) were associated with increased odds of suicide ideation, while sexual abuse (3.01; 2.22–4.08), homelessness (1.49; 1.12–1.98), and running away from home (1.38; 1.06–1.81) were associated with increased odds of a suicide attempt. Those experiencing all four adverse events were 7.81 times more likely (2.41–25.37) to report having ever attempted suicide than those who experienced none of the adverse events. Considering the high prevalence of adverse life experiences and their association with suicidal behaviors in detained adolescents, these factors should not only be included in the suicide screening tools at the intake and during detention, but should also be used for the intervention programming for suicide prevention.

Childhood abuse is associated with later psychopathology, including conduct disorder, antisocial personality disorder, anxiety and depression as well as a heightened risk of health and social problems. However, the neurobiological mechanisms by which childhood adversity increases vulnerability to psychopathology remain poorly understood. There is likely to be a complex interaction between environmental experiences (such as abuse) and individual differences in risk versus protective genes, which influences the neurobiological circuitry underpinning psychological and emotional development. Neuroendocrine studies indicate an association between early adversity and atypical development of the hypothalamic-pituitary-adrenal (HPA) axis stress response, which may predispose to psychiatric vulnerability in adulthood. Brain imaging research in children and adults is providing evidence of several structural and functional brain differences associated with early adversity. Structural differences have been reported in the corpus callosum, cerebellum and prefrontal cortex. Functional differences have been reported in regions implicated in emotional and behavioural regulation, including the amygdala and anterior cingulate cortex. These differences at the neurobiological level may represent adaptations to early experiences of heightened stress that lead to an increased risk of psychopathology. In chapter 13, McCrory et al. consider the clinical implications of current and future neurobiological and genetic research.

Childhood abuse is associated with increased adult disease risk, suggesting that processes acting over the long-term, such as epigenetic regulation of gene activity, may be involved. DNA methylation is a critical mechanism in epigenetic regulation. Suderman et al. aimed to establish in chapter 14 whether childhood abuse was associated with adult DNA methylation profiles. In 40 males from the 1958 British Birth Cohort, they compared genome-wide promoter DNA methylation in blood taken at 45 years for those with, versus those without, childhood abuse (n=12 vs 28). We analysed the promoter methylation of over 20,000 genes and 489 microRNAs, using MeDIP (methylated DNA immunoprecipitation) in triplicate. They found 997 differentially methylated gene promoters (311 hypermethylated and 686 hypomethylated) in association with childhood abuse and these promoters were enriched for genes involved in key cell signaling pathways related to transcriptional regulation and development. Using bisulfite-pyrosequencing, abuse-associated methylation (MeDIP) at the metalloproteinase gene, *PM20D1*, was validated and then replicated in an additional 27 males. Abuse-associated methylation was observed in 39 microRNAs; in 6 of these, the hypermethylated state was consistent with the hypomethylation of their downstream gene targets. Although distributed across the genome, the differentially methylated promoters associated with child abuse clustered in genome regions of at least one megabase. The observations for child abuse showed little overlap with methylation patterns associated with socioeconomic position. The authors conclude that the observed genome-wide methylation profiles in adult DNA associated with childhood abuse justify the further exploration of epigenetic regulation as a mediating mechanism for long-term health outcomes.

Childhood adversity can have life-long consequences for the response to stressful events later in life. Abuse and severe neglect are well-known risk factors for post-traumatic stress disorder (PTSD), at least in part via changes in neural systems mediating the endocrine response to stress. Determining the biological signatures of risk for stress-related mental disorders such as PTSD is important for identifying homogenous subgroups and improving treatment options. The review by McGowan in chapter 15 focuses on epigenetic regulation in early life by adversity and parental care—prime mediators of offspring neurodevelopment—in order to address several questions: (1) what have studies of humans and analogous animal models taught us about molecular mechanisms underlying changes in stress-sensitive physiological systems in response to early life trauma? (2) What are the considerations for studies relating early adversity and PTSD risk, going forward? The author summarizes studies in animals and humans that address the epigenetic response to early adversity in the brain and in peripheral tissues. In so doing, the McGowan describes work on the glucocorticoid receptor and other well-characterized genes within the stress response pathway. He then turns to genomic studies to illustrate the use of increasingly powerful high-throughput approaches to the study of epigenomic mechanisms.

Childhood sexual abuse (CSA) is a traumatic life event associated with an increased lifetime risk for psychopathology/morbidity. The long-term biological consequences of CSA-elicited stress on chromosomal stability in adults are unknown. The primary aim of York and colleagues' study in chapter 16 is to determine if the rate of acquired chromosomal changes, measured using the cytokinesis-block micronucleus assay on stimulated peripheral blood lymphocytes, differs in adult female monozygotic twins discordant for CSA. Monozygotic twin pairs discordant for CSA were identified from a larger population-based sample of female adult twins for whom the experience of CSA was assessed by self-report (51 individuals including a reference sample). Micronuclei (MN) contain chromatin from structurally normal or abnormal chromosomes that are excluded from the daughter nuclei during cell division and serve as a biomarker to assess acquired chromosomal instability. The authors found that female twins exposed to CSA exhibited a 1.63-fold average increase in their frequency of MN compared to their nonexposed genetically identical cotwins (Paired t-test, $t_{16} = 2.65$, $P = 0.017$). No additional effects of familial factors were detected after controlling for the effect of CSA exposure. A significant interaction between CSA history and age was observed, suggesting that the biological effects of CSA on MN formation may be cumulative. These data support a direct link between CSA exposure and MN formation measured in adults that is not attributable to genetic or environmental factors shared by siblings. Further research is warranted to understand the biological basis for the observed increase in acquired chromosomal findings in people exposed to CSA and to determine if acquired somatic chromosomal abnormalities/somatic clonal mosaicism might mediate the adult pathology associated with CSA.

OVERVIEW OF THE TOPIC

CHAPTER 1

Lessons Learned from Child Sexual Abuse Research: Prevalence, Outcomes, and Preventive Strategies

DELPHINE COLLIN-VÉZINA, ISABELLE DAIGNEAULT, AND MARTINE HÉBERT

1.1 INTRODUCTION

Although only recently acknowledged as a concerning social problem, child sexual abuse (CSA) is, in our day, at the forefront of worldwide social policies and practices. Four decades of research has certainly contributed to better our knowledge on the experiences of victims of CSA. With more than 20,000 research papers on CSA listed under the most renowned research databases, child and adolescent mental health practitioners, researchers and decision-makers may find it challenging to keep up with this rapidly increasing literature. In response to this need, the aim of the current paper is to provide a brief overview on CSA to heighten awareness of practitioners on this utmost important and widespread social problem. The content of this paper was first presented at the annual symposium of the *Centre for Child Protection*, headed by the Institute of Psychology at the Pontifical Gregorian University and scholars of the University of Ulm, to a group of religious leaders responding to the sexual abuse of minors around the world, including Argentina, Ecuador, Germany, Ghana, India, Indonesia, Italy and Kenya. Upon invitation, this current publication is a unique opportunity to highlight a few of the main lessons we have learned from the scholarly literature on CSA, with a focus on its prevalence, mental health outcomes and preventive strategies.

1.2 MAGNITUDE: HOW PREVALENT IS CSA?

Until recently, there was much disagreement as to what should be included in the definition of CSA [1]. In some definitions, only contact abuse was included, such as penetration, fondling, kissing, and touching [2]. Noncontact sexual abuse, such as exhibitionism and voyeurism, were not always considered abusive. Nowadays, the field is evolving towards a more inclusive understanding of CSA that is broadly defined as any sexual activity perpetrated against a minor by threat, force, intimidation, or manipulation. The array of sexual activities thus includes fondling, inviting a child to touch or be touched sexually, intercourse, rape, incest, sodomy, exhibitionism, involving a child in prostitution or pornography, or online child luring by cyberpredators [3,4]. CSA experiences vary greatly over multiple dimensions including, but not limited to: duration, frequency, intrusiveness of acts perpetrated, and relationship with perpetrator. Although sexual activity between children has long been thought to be harmless, child on child CSA experiences, such as those involving siblings, is increasingly being recognized as detrimental for the emotional well-being of children as adult on child CSA [5-7]. While adult-to-child interactions in which the purpose is sexual gratification are considered abusive, sexual behaviours between children are less clear-cut as there is no universal definition of sexual abuse that differentiates it from normal sex play and exploration [8]. Although a 2- to 5-year age difference between children was first suggested as necessary to consider sexual behaviours between siblings to be incest [9], this criterion is being questioned as studies have shown this age difference to be much lower in many substantiated cases of child-to-child abuse [10]. This formulation of CSA is in keeping with the recommendations from the 1999 World Health Organization Consultation on Child Abuse

Prevention, where CSA is defined as any activity of a sexual nature 'between a child and an adult or another child who by age or development is in a relationship of responsibility, trust or power, the activity being intended to gratify or satisfy the needs of the other person'. That said, some definitional issues have not yet been resolved in the field. First, much disparity exists regarding age for sexual consent, or age for sexual maturity, which has an influence on the extent to which statutory sex offenses are considered CSA. Sexual activities that involve a person below a statutorily designated age fall under the large umbrella of CSA; however, the age of consent varies greatly across countries, from as young as 12 or 13 (e.g. Tonga, Spain) to 17 or 18 years of age (e.g. some states in the US, Australia). In virtually all European jurisdictions, sexual relations are legal from age 16 onwards, but some countries have set the age for sexual consent at 14 or 15 [11]. In other words, when no coercion or force is used, cases that involve sexual activities between an adult and, for example, a 14-year-old teenager, will be either perceived as a consensual sexual relationship or criminalized and defined as sexual abuse, depending on the legal statutorily designated age of the country where the event occurred. In Canada, a bill was recently adopted to change the age of consent from 14 to 16, a premiere in Canada's history, which emphasizes the impact governmental decisions can have on definitional issues of CSA in societies over time [12]. Second, although coerced sexual activities that occur in dating or romantic relationships is recognized as a form of sexual violence by the World Health Association (see for example a WHO multicountry study from Garcia-Moreno and colleagues [13]), the extent to which this form of interpersonal violence is socially recognized and acknowledged in different legislations around the world is unclear.

In that vein, the exact extent of the problem of CSA is difficult to approximate given the lack of consensus on the definition used in research inquiries, as well as the differences in the data collection systems across areas [14]. For example, in their review of the current rates of CSA across 55 studies from 24 countries, Barth and colleagues [15] found much heterogeneity in studies they reviewed and concluded that rates of CSA for females ranged from 8 to 31% and from 3 to 17% for males. Though, despite these methodological challenges, recent systematic reviews and meta-analyses that included studies conducted worldwide across hundreds of different age-cohort samples have consistently shown an alarming rate of CSA, with averages of 18-20% for females and of 8-10% for males [16], with the lowest rates for both girls (11.3%) and boys (4.1%) found in Asia, and highest rates found for girls in Australia (21.5%) and for boys in Africa (19.3%) [17]. Research findings do, however, clearly demonstrate a major lack of congruence between the low number of official reports of CSA to authorities, and the high rates of CSA that youth and adults self-report retrospectively. Indeed, the recent comprehensive meta-analysis conducted by Stoltenborgh and colleagues [17] that combined estimations of CSA in 217 studies published between 1980 and 2008, showed the rates of CSA to be more than 30 times greater in studies relying on self-reports (127 by 1000) than in official-report inquiries, such as those based on data from child protection services and the police (4/1000). In other words, while 1 out of 8 people report having experienced CSA, official incidence estimates center around only 1 per 250 children.

This discrepancy can be explained by the different steps that CSA cases go through before they are substantiated, and thus counted in official-report inquiries. First, victims of CSA or their confidants have to disclose their suspicions to the authorities. Many reports of child abuse are never passed on. In fact, the majority of studies highlight the fact that many victims continue to be unrecognized [3]. A review of CSA studies by Finkelhor [2] found that across all studies, only about half of victims had disclosed the abuse to anyone. This problem is often referred to as the phenomenon of the “tip of the iceberg” [18], where only a fraction of CSA situations are visible and a much higher proportion remain undetected. Disclosure is a delicate and sensitive process that is influenced by several factors, including implicit or explicit pressure for secrecy, feelings of responsibility or blame, feelings of shame or embarrassment, or fear of negative consequences [2,19,20]. Ethnic and religious cultures may also influence the way by which the process of disclosure is experienced and can act as either facilitators or barriers to the telling and reporting of CSA [21], which may explain variations of CSA rates across geographical areas [17]. Moreover, mandatory reporting regulations that have been adopted over the past decades in several countries, which imply that professionals are obliged to bring their suspicions of CSA to the attention of the authorities, can also impact the official counts of CSA in different countries [22]. In jurisdictions that have chosen not to enact mandatory reporting, including New Zealand, the United Kingdom, and Germany, a large discrepancy between adult self-reports of CSA and official data is to be expected as more cases may not be divulged to the authorities than in countries where reporting is mandatory. Second, based upon the initial disclosure or reporting, cases are screened in or out for further investigation by child protection workers or the police. Not all sexual abuse cases are considered to fall under the jurisdiction of child protection services, such as those that were assessed to involve no imminent risk to the child with regards to his/her security and development. For instance, cases where the alleged perpetrator is not the child's caregiver may be less likely to be retained for investigation as it may not be under child welfare responsibilities to investigate these cases [23]. Finally, in light of evidence gathered in the course of the investigation process, cases are deemed substantiated or not by child protection workers and the police. When the child's testimony is deemed unreliable or when the proof is perceived as questionable, cases may be considered unfounded and will, as a result, not be counted towards official data. Indeed, there is some evidence that police are less likely to charge sexual offenses than any other type of violent crime [24]. Other factors, such as the victim's gender, may also influence substantiation decisions as demonstrated in a recent American study that showed, using the National Survey of Child and Adolescent Well-Being, that workers were less likely to substantiate cases involving male victims [25]. As improper interviewing techniques may hamper the capacity of victims to report accurately the abusive experience they were subjected to, promoting and sustaining best-practice interviewer techniques, notably among police officers, should be prioritized [26]. Considering the impact that all these different layers of influence have on cutting down the number of CSA cases that are known to and substantiated by the authorities, victims identified in official-report inquiries are therefore believed to represent only a small fraction of the true occurrence. For all these reasons, relying on official reports to determine the magnitude of CSA is a method that carries a constant error of underestimation. In other words, children that are identified are only those that were able to disclose, were believed, reported to, and followed up by proper authorities, and those cases that presented enough evidence to be substantiated as CSA. In terms of risk factors, being female is considered a major risk factor for CSA as girls are about two times more likely to be victims than males [16,17]. Several authors do, however, point out that there is a strong likelihood that boys are more frequently abused than the ratio of reported cases would suggest given their probable reluctance to report the abuse [27]. A recent Canadian population-based study confirmed this assumption by showing that among CSA survivors, 16% of female victims had never disclosed the abuse, whereas this proportion rose to 30% for male victims [28]. With respect to age, children who are most vulnerable to CSA are in the school-aged and adolescent stages of development, though about a quarter of CSA survivors report they were first abused before the age of 6 [3]. In addition, girls are considered to be at high risk for CSA starting at an earlier age and lasting longer, while boys' victimisation peaks later and for a briefer period of time. The presence of disability is also considered a risk factor for CSA and other forms of maltreatment as the impairments may heighten the vulnerability of the child [29]. Aside, the absence of one or both parents or the presence of a stepfather, parental conflicts, family adversity, substance abuse and social isolation have also been linked to a higher risk for CSA [30]. In terms of the presupposed impact of socioeconomic status and ethnic background, the existing literature has many weaknesses and obvious contradictions. Overall, while low family or neighborhood socioeconomic status is a great risk factor for physical abuse and neglect [31,32], its impact on CSA is not as proven. On one hand, CSA could appear to occur more frequently among underprivileged families because of the disproportionate number of CSA cases reported to child protective services that come from lower socioeconomic classes [3]. In that vein, some populations of children have been overrepresented in research that focuses on vulnerable populations, such as Black American children from low socioeconomic status families, which may create an erroneous belief that race and ethnicity are risk factors for CSA [33]. On the other hand, some recent population-based studies are showing that, amongst other factors, living in poverty is a predictive factor for children to be subjected to both physical and sexual abusive experiences [34,35].

REFERENCES

1. Olafson E: Child sexual abuse: Demography, impact, and interventions. J Child Adolesc Trauma 2011, 4:8–21.
2. Finkelhor D: Current information on the scope and nature of child sexual abuse. Sexual Abuse of Children 1994, 4:31–53.
3. Putnam FW: Ten-year research update review: Child sexual abuse. J Am Acad Child Adolesc Psychiatry 2003, 42:269–278.
4. Wolak J, Finkelhor D, Mitchell KJ, Ybarra M: Online "predators" and their victims: Myths, realities, and implications for prevention and treatment. Am Psychol 2008, 63:111–128.
5. Ballantine MW: Sibling incest dynamics: Therapeutic themes and clinical challenges. Clin Soc Work J 2012, 40:56–65.
6. Cyr M, Wright J, McDuff P, Perron A: Intrafamilial sexual abuse: Brothersister incest does not differ from father-daughter or stepfather-daughter incest. Child Abuse Negl 2002, 26:957–973.
7. Cyr M, McDuff P, Collin-Vézina D, Hébert M: Les agressions sexuelles commises par un membre de la fratrie: En quoi diffèrent-elles de celles commises par d'autres mineurs? Les cahiers de Plaidoyer-Victime Antenne sur la Victimologie 2012, 8:29–35.
8. Caffaro JV, Conn-Caffaro A: Treating sibling abuse families. Aggress Violent Beh 2005, 10:604–623.
9. Gilbert CM: Sibling incest: A descriptive study of family dynamics. J Child Adolesc Psychiatry, Ment Health Nurs 1992, 5:5–9.
10. Carlson BE, Maciol K, Schneider J: Sibling incest: Reports of forty-one survivors. J Child Sex Abus 2006, 15:19–34.
11. Graupner H: Sexual consent: The criminal law in Europe and overseas. Arch Sex Behav 2000, 29:415–461.
12. Wong JP: Age of consent to sexual activity in Canada: Background to proposed new legislation on 'age of protection'. Can J Hum Sex 2006, 15:163–169.
13. Garcia-Moreno C, Jansen HA, Ellsberg M, Heise L, Watts CH: Prevalence of intimate partner violence: findings from the WHO multi-country study on women's health and domestic violence. Lancet 2006, 368:1260–1269.
14. Johnson RJ: Advances in understanding and treating childhood sexual abuse: Implications for research and policy. Fam Community Health 2008, 31(Suppl1):S24–S34.
15. Barth J, Bermetz L, Heim E, Trelle S, Tonia T: The current prevalence of child sexual abuse worldwide: A systematic review and meta-analysis. Int J Public Health 2012, 58:469–483.

16. Pereda N, Guilera G, Forns M, Gòmez-Benito J: The international epidemiology of child sexual abuse: A continuation of Finkelhor (1994). Child Abuse Negl 2009, 33:331–342.
17. Stoltenborgh M, van IJzendoorn MH, Euser EM, Bakermans-Kranenburg MJ: A global perspective on child sexual abuse: Meta-analysis of prevalence around the world. Child Maltreat 2011, 16:79–101.
18. MacMillan HL, Jamieson E, Walsh CA: Reported contact with child protection services among those reporting child physical and sexual abuse: Results from a community survey. Child Abuse Negl 2003, 27:1397–1408.
19. Goodman-Brown TB, Edelstein RS, Goodman GS, Jones DPH, Gordon DS: Why children tell: A model of children's disclosure of sexual abuse. Child Abuse Negl 2003, 27:525–540.
20. Paine ML, Hansen DJ: Factors influencing children to self-disclose sexual abuse. Clin Psychol Rev 2002, 22:271–295.
21. Fontes LA, Plummer C: Cultural issues in disclosure of child sexual abuse. J Child Sex Abus 2010, 19:491–518.
22. Matthews B, Kenny MC: Mandatory reporting legislation in the United States, Canada, and Australia: A cross-jurisdictional review of key features, differences, and issues. Child Maltreat 2008, 13:50–63.
23. Jones LM, Finkelhor D, Kopiec K: Why is sexual abuse declining? A survey of state child protection administrators. Child Abuse Negl 2001, 25:1139–1158.
24. Kong R, Johnson H, Beattie S, Cardillo A: Sexual offences in Canada. Juristat: Canadian Centre for Justice Statistics 2003, 23:1–28.
25. Maikovich AK, Koenen KC, Jaffe SR: Posttraumatic stress symptoms and trajectories in child sexual abuse victims: An analysis of sex differences using the National Survey of Child and Adolescent Well-Being. J Abnorm Child Psychol 2009, 37:727–737.
26. Powell MA, Wright R, Clark S: Improving the competency of police officers in conducting investigative interviews with children. Police Prac Res: An Int J 2010, 11:211–226.
27. O'Leary PJ, Barber J: Gender differences in silencing following childhood sexual abuse. J Child Sex Abus 2008, 17:133–143.
28. Hébert M, Tourigny M, Cyr M, McDuff P, Joly J: Prevalence of childhood sexual abuse and timing of disclosure in a representative sample of adults from the province of Quebec. Can J Psychiatry 2009, 54:631–636.
29. Horner-Johnson W, Drum CE: Prevalence of Maltreatment of People with Intellectual Disabilities: A Review of Recently Published Research. Ment Retard Dev Disabil Res Rev 2006, 12:57–69.
30. Wolfe VV: Child sexual abuse. In Assessment of childhood disorders. 4th edition. Edited by Mash EJ, Barkley RA. New York, NY: Guilford; 2007:685–748.
31. Coulton CJ, Crampton DS, Irwin M, Spilsbury JC, Korbin JE: How neighborhoods influence child maltreatment: A review of the literature and alternative pathways. Child Abuse Negl 2007, 31:1117–1142.
32. Sedlak A, Mettenburg J, Basena M, Petta I, McPherson K, Green A, Li S: Fourth national incidence study of child abuse and neglect (NIS-4): Report to Congress.

Washington D.C: US Department of Health and Human Services, Administration for Children and Families; 2010.

33. Kenny M, McEachern A: Prevalence and characteristics of childhood sexual abuse in multiethnic college students. J Child Sex Abus 2000, 9:57–70.
34. MacMillan HL, Tanaka M, Duku E, Vaillancourt T, Boyle MH: Child physical and sexual abuse in a community sample of young adults: Results from the Ontario Child Health Survey. Child Abuse Negl 2013, 37:14–21.
35. Hussey JM, Chang JJ, Kotch JB: Child maltreatment in the United States: Prevalence, risk factors, and adolescent health consequences. Pediatrics 2006, 118:933–942.

This article is continued on page 95.

PART I

THE SOCIETAL EFFECTS OF EARLY TRAUMA

CHAPTER 2

A Prevalence-Based Approach to Societal Costs Occurring in Consequence of Child Abuse and Neglect

SUSANNE HABETHA, SABRINA BLEICH, JÖRG WEIDENHAMMER, AND JÖRG M FEGERT

2.1 BACKGROUND

2.1.1 CHILDHOOD TRAUMATIZATION

Traumatization of children (the United Nations Convention on the Rights of the Child defines a "child" as "a human being below the age of 18 years") occurs in many ways. Due to their often very pronounced after-effects, sexual, physical and emotional abuse in the home environment play a central role. For example, Maercker et al. [1] describe a Post-Traumatic Stress Disorder after sexualized violence in more than one third of the cases and Steil and Straube [2] in up to 80% of the cases. Close relationship with the offender, repetitions and combinations of various forms of abuse significantly contribute to this strong impact on the individual [3-6].

All in all, childhood traumatization is not a rare event. In two German studies on juveniles and young adults, 25.5% of the male and 17.7% of the female participants [7], or a total of 22.5% of the investigated juveniles [8] had already experienced at least one traumatic event. The most common types of traumatic events were violent attacks, accidents and witnessing trauma. Child neglect – mostly subdivided into physical and emotional neglect – also belongs to the most common types of traumatization [4,9,10].

A recent representative population survey in Germany [10] has shown that emotional abuse concerned 14.9%, physical abuse 12.0% and sexual abuse 12.5% of the respondents, where 14.5% were affected by "severe/extreme" abuse or neglect, respectively. In a somewhat older investigation by Wetzels [6], 38.8% of the participants had experienced physical violence by the parents more often than rarely, while 4.7% were severely affected. Contact sexual abuse before the age of 18 was indicated by 6.5% of the respondents (3.2% of men and 9.6% of women). A share of 8.9% of the participants had witnessed violence between the parents more than rarely.

A characteristic feature of childhood traumatization is that children are often affected by several types of traumatization. This has been shown for Germany [6,10] and in large population studies for Canada [11] and the USA [12,13]. The rate of children who were affected by at least two types of traumatization is presented with 40% in a German study [10] and with one quarter in a US-American study [13].

2.1.2 CONSEQUENCES OF CHILDHOOD TRAUMATIZATION

The consequences of childhood traumatization (hereinafter referred to as trauma-related disorders) are–apart from acute injuries and reactions–additionally mirrored in restricted social, emotional and physical development, which are associated with an increased risk of mental disorders, alcohol- and drug abuse as well as physical diseases in adulthood [14]. The "Final Report of the Independent Commissioner for Accounting for Child Sexual Abuse, Dr. Christine Bergmann" [15] published in May 2011 clearly demonstrates – especially by the integrated statements of the people concerned

– how severely childhood traumatization can affect later life. With regard to the consequences of abuse, somatic complaints were reported starting at a rate of 50%, followed by relationship- and partnership problems, a row of symptoms typical of post-traumatic stress, performance impairment in connection with poorer school results, problems in professional education, occupational disability, etc., problems with self-esteem, self-hatred and self-disgust up to problems with corporeality and sexuality in even more than one-fifth of the persons concerned.

Besides Post-Traumatic Stress Disorder (PTSD)–a trauma-related disorder by definition–increased risks after childhood traumatization have been shown and connections proven, respectively, in the following selected mental illnesses in retrospective and partly also prospective studies: depressive disorders [7,9,12,13,16-19], anxiety disorders [7,12,16,17,20], addictions [7,12,13,16-18,21,22], somatoform disorders [7,9,23-28], personality disorders [12,18,29-31] and conduct disorder [12,16,17,29]. The same applies to the following somatic diseases: overweight [3,13,19,32,33], diabetes mellitus [13,32,34,35], hypertension [36,37] and ischemic heart diseases [13,38-41]. The strength of the association between traumatization and trauma-related disorder reported in the aforementioned studies varies due to different approaches and methodologies.

Trauma-related disorders are thus by no means limited to the time of traumatization; they often accompany patients throughout their lives, with the time lag to the trauma being highly variable. While PTSD is defined over a close time connection of several weeks or months [42], trauma-related disorders such as depression, anxiety disorders, addiction or obesity can occur even in adulthood, i.e., years to decades after traumatization [3]. The far-reaching consequences of trauma-associated developmental disorders [43,44] and the multifaceted manifestation of trauma-related disorders, which affect various areas of life such as education, social contacts and working ability, are also mirrored in the high comorbidity rates that have been proven comprehensively for mental and somatic disorders in large studies [5,7,12,13,45-47].

However, childhood traumatization can by no means be regarded as the sole cause of the development of diseases or disorders [43]. Traumatization represents one of several variables in a biopsychosocial model, which measurably increases the risk of suffering from a certain disease or disorder. The extent of this risk increase varies depending on the type and severity of traumatization, individual conditions (e.g. gender) and the influence of external risk- and protective factors [2,23,48-50].

2.1.3 COSTS OF CHILDHOOD TRAUMATIZATION

Up to now, there are only few sources examining the cost side of childhood traumatization and the relevant social- and health policy questions. The total societal costs incurring due to childhood traumatization (hereinafter referred to as trauma follow-up costs) are unknown. A few studies from English-speaking countries have attempted to give at least approximate estimates of trauma follow-up costs. Authors of a cost-benefit analysis by the *National Center of Early Assistance (NZFH, Nationales Zentrum Frühe Hilfen)* [51] express concern that national studies on trauma follow-up costs are neither available nor feasible in Germany due to the non-availability of data.

What all studies known to the authors have in common is great uncertainty and incompleteness of the available data – starting from the prevalence of traumatization over the definition of cost areas to the calculation and allocation of costs. The variability of individual progressions between complete resilience and lifelong trauma-related disorders must be estimated as well, since they directly determine the long-term follow-up costs. By means of their conservative calculation methodology, studies on trauma follow-up costs explain in detail that the results of this puzzle are throughout underestimating [52-58]. In summary, underestimation is most notably explained by the insufficient availability of relevant data, which leaves certain cost areas partially or completely out of consideration, and by the uncertainty with regard to trauma prevalence, the dark figure of which (estimated number of unknown cases) can at best be taken into consideration but approximately.

One US-American study estimates societal costs related to reported cases of child abuse and neglect at USD 103.8 billion per year – without taking intangible costs into consideration [54]. For Australia, trauma follow-up costs have been calculated for the year 2007 in the amount of approximately AUD 4.0 billion on the basis of a population survey and in the amount of AUD 10.7 billion on the basis of prevalence information from literature [53]. In Canada, the annual amount is around CAD 15.7 billion–calculated as "a minimum cost to society" [55]. In the US state of Michigan, two consecutive cost-benefit studies refer to costs in the amount of USD 823 million for the year 1992 [56] and USD 1.8 billion for the year 2002 [57]. A cost-benefit study conducted in the state of New York quotes USD 9.0 million per year for "catastrophic maltreatment" [58].

Sources about federal costs in Germany are not known to the authors. The objectives of the present study are to estimate societal trauma-follow up costs (including direct and indirect costs) in Germany for the first time and to compare the results to costs in Australia, Canada and the USA.

2.2 METHODS

2.2.1 DERIVATION OF THE TOTAL TRAUMA FOLLOW-UP COSTS

This prevalence-based cost-of-illness study is performed from the societal perspective. This perspective comprises not only individual costs, but most of all costs borne by society, caused by expenses in cost sectors such as health insurance, social service or losses in added value. The costs include those directly linked to traumatization as well as short- and long-term costs occurring due to aftereffects (indirect costs). The insufficiency of the available data did not allow for any estimation of opportunity costs. In order to estimate annual trauma follow-up costs in Germany, already published, aggregated data was used. The cost derivation follows a bottom-up approach based on the following formula:

Number of "A" units x costs per unit "A" = Total cost of "A" units.

In this context, unit "A" represents a case of (former) child abuse and/or neglect, respectively, where trauma-related disorders incur additional, economical costs for a lifetime.

Prevalence data for the determination of the number of "A" units were taken from the most recent survey on the prevalence of child abuse and

TABLE 1. Characteristics of the German prevalence study [10].

	Study characteristics
Study type	Retrospective population survey
Objective	Prevalence of child maltreatment (physical, emotional, sexual) and neglect (physical, emotional) in Germany
Sample	Random sample
	Representative of the German population
	Sample size: 2,504
	Females: 53.2%, males 46.8%
	Age: 14–90 years, mean value: 50.6 years
Methods	Assessment of child maltreatment and neglect through the Childhood Trauma Questionnaire (German version)

neglect in Germany [10]. The survey provides up-to-date results on a good quality level, main features are summarized in Table 1.

The costs per unit "A" were obtained from the "Expertise on Cost-Benefit of Early Assistance" ("*Expertise Kosten und Nutzen Früher Hilfen*") by Meier-Gräwe and Wagenknecht [51]. To the knowledge of the authors, it is the first study of direct and indirect trauma follow-up costs in Germany that comprises a long lifespan up to the age of 67 years and which has been done in a very detailed and comprehensive way with respect to modeling costs. Study characteristics are shown in Table 2. Due to the large uncertainties resulting from the lack of reliable data, Meier-Gräwe and Wagenknecht have chosen a case-by-case approach for their cost-benefit-analysis. The result is four case scenarios for the representation of trauma follow-up costs, two "cheaper", moderate cases and two "expensive", pessimistic ones.

In order to account for uncertainty, sensitivity analysis was performed by estimating a frame of trauma follow-up costs, based on the two different scenario types. Because of the great uncertainty of the information base and the lack of alternative resources, this cost-of-illness study

TABLE 2. Characteristics of the German cost study [51].

	Study characteristics
Study type	Cost-benefit-analysis
Objective	Assessment of cost and benefit of an Early Family Assistance Program
Methods	One prevention scenario versus four scenarios under the assumption of early child endangerment (child abuse and neglect fall within this definition)
	Case scenarios based on literature and expert knowledge
	Costs modeled on the basis of available data, supplemented by literature
Cost year	2008
Cost types	Healthcare services, social services, educational services and losses in productivity (due to low professional qualification, unemployment and occupational disability)
Direct Costs	Different types of educational family/parent support and foster care
Indirect Costs	Treatment of trauma-related disorders, educational services and productivity losses

follows a conservative approach. In order to abide by this principle and to create a coherent age range several adjustments had to be applied to prevalence and to cost data.

At first, the prevalence rate [10] was transferred to the German population utilizing population data from the German Federal Statistical Office [59]. From the given age groups the range of 15 to 64 years was the one that conformed best with the age ranges of the prevalence rate (≥ 14 years) and cost data (3 to 67 years). The exclusion of individuals aged 65 years and more is not expected to have any relevant influence on the prevalence rate, because only physical neglect was associated with a slightly higher risk in elderly persons (OR 1.03) [10].

Secondly, due to the individually different histories after traumatization, it cannot be assumed that all traumatized persons will suffer lifelong aftereffects [23,50], in particular not in an extent that would incur further costs in the dimension described later. Therefore, only the prevalence of "severe/extreme" cases as defined by the CTQ[10] was considered.

Yet even for the group of "severely/extremely" affected, it is not clear to what extent the consequences of trauma are reflected as measurable costs. Since one of the few available German studies [4] estimates the frequency of permanently impaired children among severely affected cases in child protection centers to be 21% (including cases of developmental retardation and learning disability), the authors have decided to use this 21% rate for derivation.

Furthermore, the case costs were adjusted for the age range of 15 to 64 years as defined by population data. As a consequence, the matters of expense in the years below and above that age range were deducted. This step was made on the assumption that costs are homogeneously distributed throughout the highest age group (51 to 67 years), whereas in the age group of 13 to 16 years the single matter of expense is considered in relation to the corresponding age.

Finally, the case costs were converted into annual costs by dividing them by the age range of 50 years (15 up to including 64 years). The case scenarios are presented on the 2008 cost level [51]. Consequently, total trauma follow-up costs are quoted in Euro for the year 2008. Since other years' cost figures are not included, no discounting was applied.

2.2.2 CALCULATION OF INTERNATIONAL COMPARATIVE VALUES

For a comparison of German costs with results from other countries, three prevalence-based cost studies from Australia [53], the USA [52] and Canada [55] were selected. These studies contain detailed descriptions of the calculation procedures and data resources so that the results can be better assessed. The study characteristics are presented in Table 3.

Comparison is made on the basis of purchasing power parity. While the German cost study [51] calculates prices of the year 2008, the international studies refer to the years 1993 [52], 1998 [55] and 2007 [53], respectively. Therefore, in a first step the foreign currencies were converted into Euro using the respective year's purchasing power parity and were adjusted for inflation in a second step. These two steps were applied both to total trauma follow-up costs as presented in literature and to per capita

TABLE 3. Characteristics of the Cost Studies used for International Comparison.

Annual Costs* (million)	Population	Costing Methodology	Cost Types
Australia [53]:AUD 3,947**	One-year prevalence in 0-17-year-olds: 3.7% (based on a population survey on physical and sexual abuse)	Short- and long-term costs of physical, emotional and psychological, sexual abuse, neglect and witness of (or knowledge of) family violence by a combination of top-down and bottom-up methods	Health, Additional educational assistance, Productivity losses of child abuse survivors and due to premature death, Crime, Government expenditures on care and protection, Deadweight losses
Canada [55]:CAD 15,706	Lifetime prevalence in 15-64-year-olds: 30% total, 14.6% severe (based on a population survey on physical and sexual abuse); Lifetime prevalence in 0-14-year-olds: 6.89% (based on the number of investigated cases of physical, emotional, sexual abuse or neglect)	Short- and long-term costs of physical, emotional, sexual abuse, neglect and witnessing violence by a combination of top-down and bottom-up methods	Judicial, Social Services, Education, Health, Employment, Personal
USA [52]:USD 7,300	Number of 0-17-year-old abuse victims (sexual, emotional and physical) in the year 1990: 794,000 (based on a national study of recognized child abuse and neglect); equal to 1,24% of that age group [own calculation]	Short- and long-term costs of physical, sexual and emotional abuse by a combination of top-down and bottom-up methods	Productivity, Medical Care/Ambulance, Mental Health Care, Police/Fire Services, Social/Victim Services, Property Loss/Damage

*Excluding intangible costs.
**From the three presented results the "best estimate" was chosen for comparison.

costs, which were obtained by dividing the total costs by the respective country's population in the respective cost year. The conversion and adjustment rates are shown in Table 4.

Additionally, the international costs were calculated as notional total costs for Germany by multiplying per capita costs of the respective

TABLE 4. Rates used for Purchasing Power Parity Conversion and Inflation Adjustment.

	Year	PPP* Euro [60], own calculation]	Inflation[61]
Australia	2007	1.719532906	0.98
Canada	1998	1.202424923	0.85
USA	1993	0.99786743	0.78
Germany	2008	1	1

*PPP: Purchasing Power Parity.

country by the German population. These figures serve as a complementary way of illustrating the results, in order to point out the cost dimension of traumatization in relation to other societal expenses.

By means of these methods, differences between the individual countries with regard to purchasing power, population size and currency shall be balanced, so that results can be compared in the form of single figures on one level.

2.3 RESULTS

2.3.1 TOTAL TRAUMA FOLLOW-UP COSTS

The prevalence rate of at least one form of child abuse or neglect classified as "severe/extreme" is 14.5% [10]. This 14.5% share transferred to the German population aged between 15 and 64 years (54.1 million in the year 2008 [59]), the number of people concerned would be 7.8 million.

On the basis of the indications available in literature, only a 21% share of the 7.8 million individuals affected by "severe/extreme" child abuse or neglect has been included in the derivation of costs. This percentage equals 1.6 million (or 3.0% of the population aged 15 to 64 years), which represent the number of units "A".

The costs of the moderate scenarios average to EUR 432,951 (mean value of EUR 424,005 and EUR 441,896) for the age range of three to

67-year-olds; of the pessimistic scenarios, the average costs are EUR 1,159,294 (mean value of EUR 1,243,002 and EUR 1,075,585) for the age range of six to 67-year-olds [51]. By adjusting the costs for the age range of 15 to 64 years, average costs are reduced to a total of EUR 335,421 (mean value of EUR 326,745 and EUR 344,096) in the moderate scenario and to EUR 904,375 (mean value of EUR 870,579 and EUR 938,169) in the pessimistic scenario. The resulting average annual costs, related to a period of 50 years, amount to EUR 6,708 per unit "A" in the moderate scenario and to EUR 18,087 in the pessimistic scenario.

Substituting the variables of the above described formula by figures of the cost margin's lower bound (moderate scenario):

$$1{,}648{,}389 \times 6{,}708\text{Euro} = 11{,}057{,}396{,}330\text{Euro}, \tag{1}$$

the resulting total annual costs amount to EUR 11.1 billion, which incur as follow-up costs of child abuse and neglect, respectively, for German society. In other words, the annual per capita trauma follow-up costs would amount to EUR 134.84 (German population 2008: 82,002,400 [59]).

Applying the costs of the pessimistic scenario to the formula:

$$1{,}648{,}389 \times 18{,}087\text{Euro} = 29{,}814{,}419{,}711\text{Euro}, \tag{2}$$

the upper bound of the annual trauma follow-up cost frame is EUR 29.8 billion in total or EUR 363.58 per capita.

2.3.2 INTERNATIONAL COMPARATIVE VALUES

The international, comparative values of per capita trauma follow-up costs (without intangible costs) are EUR 106.20 according to the Australian, EUR 22.14 according to the US-American, and EUR 368.16 according to the Canadian calculation each year (cf. Table 5). As notional total annual costs for the German society, these values would amount to EUR 8.7 billion (Australian calculation), EUR 1.8 billion (US-American calculation), and EUR 30.2 billion (Canadian calculation), respectively.

TABLE 5. Conversion of International Cost Values into Euro in the Year 2008.

	Original total annual costs in national currency	Total annual costs in Euro, different cost years	Total annual costs in Euro, 2008	Per capita costs* in Euro, different cost years	Per capita costs* in Euro, 2008
Australia, without intangible costs [53]	3,947,000,000	2,295,390,793	2,249,482,977	108.37	106.20
ustralia, including intangible costs [53]	10,691,000,000	6,217,386,108	6,093,038,386	293.54	287.67
USA, without intangible costs [52]	7,300,000,000	7,315,601,034	5,706,168,807	28.38	22.14
USA, including intangible costs [52]	56,000,000,000	56,119,679,168	43,773,349,751	217.70	169.81
Canada, without intangible costs [55]	15,705,910,047	13,061,863,365	11,102,583,860	433.13	368.16

*Australian population in the year 2007: 21,180,632 [62], Canadian population in the year 1998: 30,157,082 [63], US-American population in the year 1993: 257,783,000 [64]. Calculation was made – to the extent possible – prior to rounding of values..

The German lower bound in the amount of EUR 11.1 billion per year is close to the Australian result, while the Canadian study has returned costs very close to the German upper bound. The US-American study is somewhat out of scope with about one sixth of the German lower bound costs.

The Australian and US-American studies additionally quote intangible costs, whereby results are increased to EUR 287.67 and EUR 169.81, respectively, per capita (EUR 23.6 billion and EUR 13.9 billion total costs).

2.4 DISCUSSION

2.4.1 TOTAL TRAUMA FOLLOW-UP COSTS

The objective of the present study was to estimate trauma follow-up costs for Germany. A margin of total annual trauma follow-up costs was calculated in the amount of EUR 11.1 billion for the lower bound and EUR 29.8 billion for the upper bound, respectively. The correspondence of the Australian result with Germany's lower bound should be considered with utmost caution, since both cost studies are based on completely different methods and also include different cost areas. In contrast to the Australian study [53], the German cost calculation [51] does not take crime and deadweight losses into consideration, whereas the areas health, education, productivity and social services have been considered equally.

In both studies, prevalence is based on a population survey with similar results for the lifetime prevalence of physical and sexual abuse (17.8% in Australia [53] and approximately 15.9% in Germany [10, own calculation]). However, the Australian study uses only the one-year prevalence of 0 to 17- year-olds and does not include emotional abuse or neglect. Thus, the number of people concerned is much lower in the Australian study, whereas the total costs per person must lie close to those of Germany's upper bound: the upper bound costs (EUR 18,087) multiplied by Australia's prevalence (3.7% of Germany's population aged 0–15 years: 412.147, age range as presented by the German Federal Statistical Office [59]) would yield – with EUR 7.5 billion–a result quite close to the Australian one.

The Canadian result [55] is very close to the German upper bound, but relies on higher prevalence rates (cf. Table 3), which have been used for cost calculation in a sophisticated way. Canadian costs comprise expenses related to the legal system, social services, education, health, employment and personal costs, with the employment sector being the most expensive one, accounting for 72% of the total costs (CAD 11.3 billion of a total of CAD 15.7 billion). Other than in the Australian and US-American studies, Canada has based their cost calculation in the employment sector on a large population survey, which combined information on income with physical and sexual abuse in the respondents' history (*Ontario Health Survey Mental Health Supplement (OHSUP)*).

With a loss of productivity of over 70% in the moderate case scenarios and over 50% in the pessimistic ones, the German cost-benefit-analysis [51] ranks close to the Canadian result. Since costs are oriented towards individual life courses in both countries – in Canada on the basis of a population survey and in Germany on the basis of individual case scenarios– this result could in fact point in the right direction, namely to regarding productivity losses as the main cost driver of societal trauma follow-up costs. The other two studies [52,53] rely on less specific, aggregated data. In Australia [53], losses of productivity rank far behind the other areas, while an approximate proportion of almost 30% can be derivated for the United States [52].

The total costs in the United States [52] are considerably lower than those in other countries, even though the cost sectors taken into consideration largely correspond. However, on the one hand, child neglect is not included for methodological reasons, and on the other hand, the number of child abuse victims is not determined on the basis of a population survey, but official information sources are used [65]. Despite the attempt to calculate institutionally unknown cases, the dark figure remains largely unconsidered. There is naturally no precise information regarding the magnitude of this dark figure. Wetzels [6] indicates an optimistic estimate at the ratio of one to ten. This estimate projected on the US-American study would yield a result of EUR 18 billion instead of EUR 1.8 billion and thus above the Australian costs and within the German cost frame.

The two results from Australia [53] and the United States [52], which contain intangible costs, cannot be compared with the German result (without intangible costs). In the Australian study, intangible costs make up for 1.7 times, in the US-American study even 6.7 times of the tangible costs. In spite of this large difference it can be stated on the transnational level that intangible costs as a measure for personally experienced burden considerably exceed the actual expenses in the form of tangible costs in any case.

Generally, the comparison of the four aforementioned results of trauma follow-up costs is limited due to the time lag of altogether fifteen years between the individual studies, which have certainly influenced prices, services and their utilization. Additionally, national service organization and funding structures, e.g. of the health care systems, are fundamentally different [66]. These variations presumably influence the availability and the assessment of costs and their assignment to various sectors, so that differences in costs are to be expected a priori due to structural conditions.

The calculated amount of trauma follow-up costs clearly has economic relevance, constituting 0.44% (lower bound) and 1.20% (upper bound) of Germany's 2008 Gross Domestic Product (EUR 2,489.4 billion) [67]. The figures have an additional relevance due to the fact that with early and effective intervention or prevention, they reveal a considerable saving potential [9,51,56-58].

Basically, trauma follow-up costs were determined by following a conservative approach. This is reflected in several details, for example in the restriction to a 21% share of only severely affected cases [4,10]. Results of risk- and resilience research lie around this value for the share of traumatized individuals with long-term consequences caused by trauma-related disorders [50,68].

Moreover, total costs have only been taken into account for the age group from 15 up to including 64 years. Consequently, direct costs are only considered to a small extent and indirect costs of older ages remain completely excluded. With existing trauma-related disorders, it can be assumed that the age-related, increasing instability of life situation leads to further health problems, which again incur additional costs in higher age. In general, trauma-related disorders do not tend to decrease in higher age [1,69], but elderly people are often severely impaired due to e.g., insufficient specialized care [15].

Last but not least it should be noted that types of traumatization other than sexual, physical and emotional abuse and neglect are left unconsidered in the present study, so that no statements can be made on their prevalence or on follow-up costs. However, it appears reasonable to limit the derivation of trauma follow-up costs to child abuse and neglect, since other current data are not available and international cost studies [52-58] refer to these types of traumatization exclusively or predominantly, so that results can be better compared with each other.

When trying to estimate whether the true costs may tend towards the lower or the upper bound one has to keep in mind that the cost scenarios are based on early childhood traumatization, whereas the prevalence data include the entire childhood and adolescence as defined by the CTQ. Since trauma-related disorders tend to be more severe the earlier traumatization was experienced [2,70], this discrepancy leads in the direction of the lower bound.

The international comparison supports both the lower and the upper bound of the cost margin–depending on the respective study. Due to methodological differences the results have to be interpreted rather as crude reference points, though. Despite all limitations, the comparison shows that the cost margin calculated for Germany is well associated with other countries' results.

2.4.2 LIMITATIONS

Limitations associated with the use of already existing data are particularly given by the fact that these data have been collected with different objectives and are not well-matched. The question arises, in particular, to what extent the cost scenarios – determined under the assumption of child endangerment [51]–can be projected on the number of traumatized individuals identified in epidemiologic studies [4,10]. While various age limits of the investigated populations can be approximated, it cannot be stated with certainty whether the cost scenarios described by Meier-Gräwe and Wagenknecht [51] are based on the same kind of traumatization as the determination of prevalence by Häuser et al. [10].

The prevalence of traumatization has been determined by Häuser et al. [10] retrospectively, which may represent yet another source of error – due to blurred or imprecise memories. However, several studies of this kind illustrate the fact very well that the number of errors is to be estimated rather low and of conservative type, in other words, that the results tend to underestimate reality [3,5,11,20,45,71,72].

Another significant uncertainty lies in the cost data themselves. The authors of the cost study explain in detail that due to the lack of data, several parts had to be completed by expert knowledge and international literature [51]. The complete case scenarios are thus but a construct, which has been developed as close to reality as possible with the help of various information sources.

The problem of low availability and unsatisfactory quality of the data with regard to the estimation of trauma follow-up costs does not only exist in Germany but it is criticized in all cost studies [52-58]. Consequently, results are consistently presented as fragmentary and underestimating. Since it can therefore be assumed that all cost studies deviate from reality in the same direction–with the extent of deviation being unclear – a comparison is possible and reasonable. Nevertheless, it can only be valued as a comparison of cost dimensions, not of amounts calculated precisely to the cent, solely due to the different methodologies. In view of the generally weak data, it should be noted that by using more precise procedures, only the illusion of higher precision could be created. This is not the intention of the authors.

2.4.3 PERSPECTIVE

Realizing numerous questions and imponderabilities in the assessment of results, creating a reliable data basis must be of highest priority in Germany, in order to answer the question how expensive it is not to provide sufficient and timely assistance to traumatized children and juveniles. The gathering of reliable cost data seems to be a highly challenging task in the light of an extremely fragmentary information basis. Serious efforts should therefore be undertaken to collect reliable data, in the first place. Only on the basis of results that are accepted by all sides due to their validity can steps be ground in order to sustainably improve the status quo of prevention and post-traumatic care.

Starting points for the improvement of care and thus assumingly also for long-term cost savings are indicated in numerous literature sources, which, for example demand a stronger interconnectedness of the respective institutions [15,73-77] or a more specific qualification in the medical community [15,78-81]. Fiscally responsible decision-making, though, should rely on the economic evaluation of any intervention or prevention program [82].

2.5 CONCLUSIONS

Total costs of EUR 11.1 billion or EUR 29.8 billion, respectively, for the consequences of childhood traumatization by various types of severe child abuse as well as neglect are undoubtedly relevant for German economy. Considering the paucity of data, especially of cost data, the result cannot be seen without restrictions. Therefore serious efforts should be undertaken to generate reliable data, in the first place.

Besides the question of personal suffering, political decision-makers should pay much more attention to the economic perspective of childhood traumatization and its comprehensive dimension of long-term consequences. By improving trauma-related care and prevention, the societal economic burden might be reduced.

REFERENCES

1. Maercker A, Forstmeier S, Wagner B, Brähler E, Glaesmer H: Posttraumatische Belastungsstörungen in Deutschland. Ergebnisse einer gesamtdeutschen epidemiologischen Untersuchung. Nervenarzt 2008, 79:577-586.
2. Steil R, Straube ER: Posttraumatische Belastungsstörung bei Kindern und Jugendlichen.Z Klin Psychol Psychother 2002, 31:1-13.
3. Gilbert R, Widom CS, Browne K, Fergusson D, Webb E, Janson S: Burden and consequences of child maltreatment in high-income countries. Lancet 2009, 373:68-81.
4. Thyen U, Kirchhofer F, Wattam C: Gewalterfahrung in der Kindheit – Risiken und gesundheitliche Folgen. Gesundheitswesen 2000, 62:311-319.
5. Kessler RC, Sonnega A, Bromet E, Hughes M, Nelson CB: Posttraumatic Stress Disorder in the National Comorbidity Survey. Arch Gen Psychiatry 1995, 52:1048-1060.
6. Wetzels P: Gewalterfahrungen in der Kindheit. Sexueller Mißbrauch, körperliche Mißhandlung und deren langfristige Konsequenzen. Baden Baden: Nomos. [Criminological Research Institute of Lower Saxony (Series Editor)Interdisziplinäre Beiträge zur kriminologischen Forschung, vol 8.]; 1997.

7. Perkonigg A, Kessler RC, Storz S, Wittchen H-U: Traumatic events and post-traumatic stress disorder in the community: prevalence, risk factors and comorbidity. Acta Psychiatr Scand 2000, 101:46-59.
8. Essau CA, Conradt J, Petermann F: Häufigkeit der Posttraumatischen Belastungsstörung bei Jugendlichen: Ergebnisse der Bremer Jugendstudie. Z Kinder Jugendpsychiatr Psychother 1999, 27:37-45.
9. Felitti VJ, Anda RF: The relationship of adverse childhood experiences to adult medical disease, psychiatric disorders, and sexual behavior: implications for healthcare. In The Impact of Early Life Trauma on Health and Disease: The Hidden Epidemic. 1st edition. Edited by Lanius RA, Vermetten E, Pain C. New York: Cambridge University Press; 2010:77-87.
10. Häuser W, Schmutzer G, Brähler E, Glaesmer H: Misshandlungen in Kindheit und Jugend: Ergebnisse einer Umfrage in einer repräsentativen Stichprobe der deutschen Bevölkerung. Dtsch Arztebl Int 2011, 108:287-294.
11. MacMillan HL, Fleming JE, Trocmé N, Boyle MH, Wong M, Racine YA, Beardslee WR, Offord DR: Prevalence of child physical and sexual abuse in the community. Results from the Ontario health supplement. JAMA 1997, 278:131-135.
12. Kessler R, Davis CG, Kendler KS: Childhood adversity and adult psychiatric disorder in the US National Comorbidity Survey. Psychol Med 1997, 27:1101-1119.
13. Felitti VJ, Anda RF, Nordenberg D, Williamson DF, Spitz AM, Edwards V, Koss MP, Marks JS: Relationship of childhood abuse and household dysfunction to many of the leading causes of death in adults. The adverse childhood experiences study (ACE). Am J Prev Med 1998, 14:245-258.
14. Putnam FW: The impact of trauma on child development. Juv Fam Ct J 2006, 57:1-11.
15. Geschäftsstelle der Unabhängigen Beauftragten zur Aufarbeitung des sexuellen Kindesmissbrauchs: Abschlussbericht der Unabhängigen Beauftragten zur Aufarbeitung des sexuellen Kindesmissbrauchs, Dr. Christine Bergmann. Berlin; 2011.
16. Nelson EC, Heath AC, Madden PAF, Cooper ML, Dinwiddie SH, Bucholz KK, Glowinski A, McLaughlin T, Dunne MP, Statham DJ, Martin NG: Association between self-reported childhood sexual abuse and adverse psychosocial outcomes. Arch Gen Psychiatry 2002, 59:139-145.
17. Fergusson DM, Horwood LJ, Lynskey MT: Childhood sexual abuse and psychiatric disorder in young adulthood: II. Psychiatric outcomes of childhood sexual abuse. J Am Acad Child Adolesc Psychiatry 1996, 34:1365-1374.
18. Silverman AB, Reinherz HZ, Giaconia RM: The long-term sequelae of child and adolescent abuse: a longitudinal community study. Child Abuse Negl 1996, 20:709-723.
19. Rohde P, Ichikawa L, Simon GE, Judmann EJ, Linde JA, Jeffery RW, Operskalski BA: Associations of child sexual and physical abuse with obesity and depression in middle-aged women. Child Abuse Negl 2008, 32:878-887
20. Goodwin RD, Fergusson DM, Horwood LJ: Childhood abuse and familial violence and the risk of panic attacks and panic disorder in young adulthood. Psychol Med 2005, 35:881-890.
21. Schäfer M, Schnack B, Soyka M: Sexueller und körperlicher Mißbrauch während früher Kindheit oder Adoleszenz bei späterer Drogenabhängigkeit. PPmP Psychother Psychosom med Psychol 2000, 50:38-50.

22. European Monitoring Centre for Drugs and Drug Addiction (EMCDDA): Preventing later substance use disorders in at-risk children and adolescents: a review of the theory and evidence base of indicated prevention. In Thematic papers. Luxembourg: Office for Official Publications of the European Communities; 2009.
23. Egle UT, Hoffmann SO, Steffens M: Psychosoziale Risiko- und Schutzfaktoren in Kindheit und Jugend als Prädisposition für psychische Störungen im Erwachsenenalter. Nervenarzt 1997, 68:683-695.
24. Waldinger RJ, Schulz MS, Barsky AJ, Ahern DK: Mapping the road from childhood trauma to adult somatization: the role of attachment. Psychosom Med 2006, 68:129-135.
25. Sansone RA, Wiederman MW, Sansone LA: Adult somatic preoccupation and its relationship to childhood trauma. Violence Vict 2001, 16:39-47.
26. Sansone RA, Gaither GA, Sansone LA: Childhood trauma and adult somatic preoccupation by body area among women in an internal medicine setting: a pilot study. Int J Psychiatry Med 2001, 31:147-154.
27. Walker EA, Katon WJ, Roy-Byrne PP, Jemelka RP, Russo J: Histories of sexual victimization in patients with irritable bowel syndrome or inflammatory bowel disease. Am J Psychiatry 1993, 150:1502-1506.
28. Barsky AJ, Wool C, Barnett MC, Cleary PD: Histories of childhood trauma in adult hypochondriacal patients. Am J Psychiatry 1994, 151:397-401.
29. Spataro J, Mullen PE, Burgess PM, Wells DL, Moss SA: Impact of child sexual abuse on mental health. Br J Psychiatry 2004, 184:416-421.
30. Kopp D, Spitzer C, Kuwert P, Barnow S, Orlob S, Lüth H, Freyberger HJ, Dudeck M: Psychische Störungen und Kindheitstraumata bei Strafgefangenen mit antisozialer Persönlichkeitsstörung. Fortschr Neurol Psychiat 2009, 77:152-159.
31. Luntz BK, Widom CS: Antisocial personality disorder in abused and neglected children grown up. Am J Psychiatry 1994, 151:670-674.
32. Thomas C, Hyppönen E, Power C: Obesity and type 2 diabetes risk in midadult life: the role of childhood adversity. Pediatrics 2008, 121:e1240-1249.
33. Williamson DF, Thompson TJ, Anda RF, Dietz WH, Felitti V: Body weight and obesity in adults and self-reported abuse in childhood. Int J Obes Relat Metab Disord 2002, 26:1075-1082.
34. Rich-Edwards JW, Spiegelman D, Lividoti Hibert EN, Jun HJ, Todd TJ, Kawachi I, Wright RJ: Abuse in childhood and adolescence as a predictor of type 2 diabetes in adult women. Am J Prev Med 2010, 39:529-536.
35. Kendall-Tackett KA, Marshall R: Victimization and diabetes: an exploratory study. Child Abuse Negl 1999, 23:593-596.
36. Riley EH, Wright RJ, Jun HJ, Hibert EN, Rich-Edwards JW: Hypertension in adult survivors of child abuse: observations from the Nurses' health study II. J Epidemiol Community Health 2010, 64:413-418.
37. Stein DJ, Scott K, Haro Abad JM, Aguilar-Gaxiola S, Alonso J, Angermeyer M, Demytteneare K, de Girolamo G, Iwata N, Posada-Villa J, Kovess V, Lara C, Ormel J, Kessler RC, Von Korff M: Early childhood adversity and later hypertension: data from the World Mental Health Survey. Ann Clin Psychiatry 2010, 22:19-28.
38. Dong M, Giles WH, Felitti VJ, Dube SR, Williams JE, Chapman DP, Anda RF: Insights into causal pathways for ischemic heart disease: adverse childhood experiences study. Circulation 2004, 110:1761-1766.

39. Roy A, Janal MN, Roy M: Childhood trauma and prevalence of cardiovascular disease in patients with type 1 diabetes. Psychosom Med 2010, 72:833-838.
40. Fuller-Thomson E, Brennenstuhl S, Frank J: The association between childhood physical abuse and heart disease in adulthood: findings from a representative community sample. Child Abuse Negl 2010, 34:689-698.
41. Goodwin RD, Stein MB: Association between childhood trauma and physical disorders among adults in the United States. Psychol Med 2004, 34:509-520. German Institute of Medical Documentation and Information, DIMDI:
42. Internationale statistische Klassifikation der Krankheiten und verwandter Gesundheitsprobleme, 10. Revision, German Modification (ICD-10-GM), Version 2011.
43. Schmid M, Fegert JM, Petermann F: Traumaentwicklungsstörung: Pro und Contra. Kindheit und Entwicklung 2010, 19:47-63.
44. Knudsen EI, Heckman JJ, Cameron JL, Shonkoff JP: Economic, neurobiological, and behavioral perspectives on building America's future workforce. Proc Natl Acad Sci 2006, 103:10155-10162.
45. Anda RF, Felitti VJ, Bremner D, Walker JD, Whitfield C, Perry BD, Dube SR, Giles WH: he enduring effects of abuse and related adverse experiences in childhood. A convergence of evidence of neurobiology and epidemiology. Eur Arch Psychiatry Clin Neurosci 2006, 256:174-186.
46. Van der Kolk BA, Pynoos RS, Cicchetti D, Cloitre M, D'Andrea W, Ford JD, Lieberman AF, Putnam FW, Saxe G, Spinazzola J, Stolbach BC, Teicher M: Proposal to include a developmental trauma disorder diagnosis for children and adolescents in DSM-V.
47. Perkonigg A, Wittchen H-U, et al.: Prevalence and comorbidity of traumatic events and posttraumatic stress disorder in adolescents and young adults. In Posttraumatic stress disorder: a lifespan developmental perspective. 1st edition. Edited by Maercker A, Schützwohl M. Seattle, Toronto, Bern, Göttingen: Hogrefe & Huber; 1999:113-133.
48. Caspi A, McClay J, Moffitt TE, Mill J, Martin J, Craig IW, Taylor A, Poulton R: Role of genotype in the cycle of violence in maltreated children. Science 2002, 297:851-854.
49. Häfner S, Franz M, Lieberz K, Schepank H: Psychosoziale Risiko- und Schutzfaktoren für psychische Störungen: Stand der Forschung. Teil 2 Psychosoziale Schutzfaktoren. Psychotherapeut 2001, 46:403-408.
50. Werner EE: Vulnerable but invincible: High risk children from birth to adulthood. Eur Child Adolesc Psychiatry 1996, 5:47-51.
51. Meier-Gräwe U, Wagenknecht I: Expertise Kosten und Nutzen Früher Hilfen. Köln: Nationales Zentrum Frühe Hilfen; 2011.
52. Miller TR, Cohen MA, Wiersema B: Victim costs and consequences: a New look. Washington, DC: U.S: Department of Justice, National Institute of Justice; 1996.
53. Taylor P, Moore P, Pezzullo L, Tucci J, Goddard C, De Bortoli L: The cost of child abuse in Australia. Melbourne: Australian Childhood Foundation and Child Abuse Prevention Research Australia; 2008.
54. Wang C-T, Holton J: Total estimated cost of child abuse and neglect in the united states. Economic impact study. Chicago, Illinois: Prevent Child Abuse America; 2007.

55. Bowlus A, McKenna K, Day T, Wright D: The Economic Costs and Consequences of Child Abuse in Canada. Ottawa: Law Commission of Canada; 2003.
56. Caldwell RA: The costs of child abuse vs. Child abuse prevention: Michigan's experience. Lansing: Michigan Children's Trust Fund; 1992.
57. Noor I, Caldwell RA: The costs of child abuse vs. Child abuse prevention: a multiyear follow-up in Michigan. Lansing: Michigan Children's Trust Fund; 2005.
58. Nobuyasu S: Costs and Benefit Simulation Analysis of Catastrophic Maltreatment. In The cost of child maltreatment: Who pays? We all do. 1st edition. Edited by Franey K, Geffner R, Falconer R. San Diego: Family Violence and Sexual Assault Institute; 2001:199-210.
59. Statistisches Bundesamt – German Federal Statistical Office: Bevölkerung nach Altersgruppen, Familienstand und Religionszugehörigkeit. 2008.
60. The World Bank: PPP conversion factor, GDP (LCU per international $).
61. Zinsenberechnen.de: Inflationsrechner.http://www.zinsen-berechnen.de/inflationsrechner.php
62. Australian Bureau of Statistics: Australian Historical Population Statistics. 1. Population Size and Growth (cat. no. 3105.0.65.001). http://www.abs.gov.au/AUSSTATS/abs@.nsf/DetailsPage/3105.0.65.0012008?OpenDocument
63. Statistics Canada: Estimated population of Canada, 1605 to present. http://www.statcan.gc.ca/pub/98-187-x/4151287-eng.htm#table 3
64. Population Estimates Program, Population Division, U.S. Census Bureau: Resident population estimates of the united states by Age and Sex, selected years from 1990 to 2000. http://www.census.gov/popest/data/national/totals/1990s/tables/nat-agesex.txt
65. National Data Archive on Child Abuse and Neglect: Study of National Incidence and Prevalence of Child Abuse and Neglect. Ithaca: NIS-2; 1987.
66. Beske F, Drabinski T, Golbach U: Leistungskatalog des Gesundheitswesens im internationalen Vergleich. Eine Analyse von 14 Ländern. In Institut für Gesundheits-System-Forschung. Edited by Fritz B. Kiel: Schmidt & Klaunig; 2005. [Fritz Beske Institut für Gesundheits-System-Forschung (Series editor) Schriftenreihe / Institut für Gesundheits-System-Forschung Kiel, vol 104.]
67. Statistisches Bundesamt – German Federal Statistical Office: Bruttoinlandsprodukt für Deutschland. 2008. https://www.destatis.de/DE/PresseService/Presse/Pressekonferenzen/2009/BIP2008/Pressebroschuere_BIP2008.pdf?__blob=publicationFile
68. Tress W: Das Rätsel der seelischen Gesundheit. Traumatische Kindheit und früher Schutz gegen psychogene Störungen. Göttingen: Vandenhoeck & Ruprecht; 1986.
69. Tagay S, Gunzelmann T, Brähler E: Posttraumatische Belastungsstörungen alter Menschen. Psychotherapie 2009, 14:234-342.
70. De Bellis MD, Thomas LA: Biologic findings of post-traumatic stress disorder and child maltreatment. Curr Psychiatry Rep 2003, 5:108-117.
71. Sachs-Ericsson N, Blazer D, Plant EA, Arnow B: Childhood sexual and physical abuse and the 1-year prevalence of medical problems in the national comorbidity survey. Health Psychol 2005, 24:32-40.
72. Fergusson DM, Lynskey MT, Horwood LJ: Childhood sexual abuse and psychiatric disorder in young adulthood: I. Prevalence of sexual abuse and factors associated with sexual abuse. J Am Acad Child Adolesc Psychiatry 1996, 34:1355-1364.

73. Schulte-Markwort M, Bindt C: Psychotherapie im Kindes- und Jugendalter. Psychotherapeut. 2006, 51:72-79.
74. Fegert JM: Kinderschutz aus kinder- und jugendpsychiatrischer und psychotherapeutischer Sicht. Zeitschrift für Kindschaftsrecht und Jugendhilfe 2008, 4:136-139.
75. Fegert JM, Schnoor K, Kleidt S, Kindler H, Ziegenhain U: Lernen aus problematischen Kinderschutzverläufen - Machbarkeitsexpertise zur Verbesserung des Kinderschutzes durch systematische Fehleranalyse. In Bundesministerium für Familie, Senioren, Frauen und Jugend. Berlin: 2008; 2008. http://www.bmfsfj.de/RedaktionBMFSFJ/Broschuerenstelle/Pdf-Anlagen/Lernen-aus-problematischen-Kinderschutzverl_C3_A4ufen,property=pdf,bereich=bmfsfj,sprache=de,rwb=true.pdf
76. Krüger A, Brüggemann A, Holst P, Schulte-Markwort M: Psychisch traumatisierte Kinder: Vernetzung unabdingbar. Dtsch Arztebl 2006, 103:A2230-A2231.
77. Fegert JM, Ziegenhain U, Goldbeck L: Traumatisierte Kinder und Jugendliche in Deutschland. Analysen und Empfehlungen zu Versorgung und Betreuung. Weinheim, München: Juventa; 2010. Fegert JM, Ziegenhain U, Goldbeck L (Series editors): Studien und Praxishilfen zum Kinderschutz
78. Kraft S, Schepker R, Goldbeck L, Fegert JM: Behandlung der posttraumatischen Belastungsstörung bei Kindern und Jugendlichen: Eine Übersicht empirischer Wirksamkeitsstudien. Nervenheilkunde 2006, 25:709-716.
79. Cierpka M, Streeck-Fischer A: Kinder- und Jugendlichenpsychotherapie in Deutschland. Psychotherapeut 2006, 51:71.
80. Fegert JM: Sexueller Missbrauch an Kindern und Jugendlichen. Bundesgesundheitsblatt Gesundheitsforschung Gesundheitsschutz 2007, 50:78-89.
81. Fegert JM, Resch F: Editorial. Z Kinder Jugendpsychiatr Psychother 2009, 37:91-92.
82. Corso PS, Lutzker JR: The need for economic analysis in research on child maltreatment. Child Abuse Negl 2006, 30:727-738.

CHAPTER 3

Associations Between Trauma History and Juvenile Sexual Offending

LAURA E. W. LEENARTS, LARKIN S. MCREYNOLDS, ROBERT R. J. M. VERMEIREN, THEO A. H. DORELEIJERS, AND GAIL A. WASSERMAN

3.1 INTRODUCTION

Over the past two decades, researchers and clinicians have become increasingly interested in understanding the sexually delinquent behavior of juveniles [1]. Investigations have documented the high rates of histories of interpersonal trauma in juvenile sex offenders [2,3], as well as their high prevalence of mental health problems [4]. Exposure to interpersonal traumatic events is consistently associated with multiple mental health problems for justice system youths, regardless of the presence/absence of a history of sexual offending [5-9].

The higher rates of exposure to interpersonal traumatic events (e.g., sexual and physical abuse) among juvenile sexual offenders compared to juvenile non-sexual offenders [2,3], requires the need to take a closer look at the prevalence of mental health problems in juvenile sexual offenders.

Previous studies comparing juvenile sexual offenders with juvenile nonsexual offenders have shown inconsistent results, or have revealed few differences in rates of mental health problems between those with and without sex offending histories [10-12]. For example, rates of both conduct problems [12,13] and substance use disorders [14] have been found to be lower among juvenile sexual offenders than among juvenile nonsexual offenders. On the other hand, although many sexually abused individuals do not proceed to become offenders themselves [15]; research is consistent regarding both the high prevalence of sexual victimization among sex offenders and the links between these experiences and sexual offending behavior [2].

To an extent, inconsistent results when comparing juvenile sexual and nonsexual offenders may be a consequence of methodological differences among studies (e.g., different types of samples, measurements) and their design limitations, including small sample sizes and the use of nonstandardized instruments [11].

We sought to investigate the contributions of demographic characteristics, mental health problems and interpersonal trauma history to juvenile sexual offending, and the degree to which juvenile sexual offenders might differ from juvenile nonsexual interpersonal offenders. Such distinctions would be of clinical relevance in developing offender-specific treatment programs [16]. To address methodological limitations of earlier work, we relied on a large sample of youths from juvenile justice agencies across the United States of America (USA), whose mental health status was assessed on a well-researched computer-assisted self-interview [Voice Diagnostic Interview Schedule for Children: V-DISC].

3.2 METHOD

3.2.1 CONTEXT

This investigation relied on a large set (N=9819) of standardized psychiatric assessments resulting from nationwide collaborations with juvenile justice agencies (57 sites in 18 states) in the USA [8,17]. The collaborating agencies represent settings at three levels of increasingly restrictive justice system contact, including system intake sites (e.g., probation or family court intake), detention centers, and postadjudicatory correctional facilities.

3.1.2 PARTICIPANTS

Altogether 3803 (39%) juveniles were assessed at system intake, 1055 (11%) at detention intake, and 4961 (51%) at intake into postadjudicatory correctional facilities. For 6798 (69%) participants, local staff provided information on most serious current offense, utilizing an agreed-on rank ordering of offense seriousness, with sexual offenses designated a priori as the most serious, followed by nonsexual interpersonal offenses, and then by property offenses and substancerelated offenses. Youth with multiple current offenses were coded to the most serious offense. Note that by design, no juveniles considered nonsexual interpersonal offenders were also designated as sexual offenders. For 3021 (31%) participants, full information on all current offenses was available. We confined analysis to those with current interpersonal offenses (n=2920), comparing those whose current offense was indicated as a sexual offense (e.g., rape) versus a nonsexual interpersonal offense (e.g., aggravated assault). For 387 (4%), the most serious current offense was a sexual offense, representing offenders from 42 sites in 17 states; for 2533 (26%) across all settings, the most serious current offense was a nonsexual interpersonal offense. Because sites self-selected themselves for participation, the rate of sexual offenders in this sample is not an estimate of their prevalence among juvenile justice youth overall. Mean age of those with a current interpersonal offense was 15.5 (SD=1.6); about a quarter of these were female. The majority were African American (40%) or Caucasian (38%).

3.2.3 PROCEDURE

Sites used standardized data collection protocols, assessing the youth shortly after admission via universal or systematic random sampling, measuring a core set of disorders. Sites provided assessment results and deidentified demographic and offense information according to a protocol approved by their Institutional Review Boards.

3.2.4 MEASURES

Demographic (gender, age, race/ethnicity) and offense (nature of current offense, number of prior offenses, and age at first offense) characteristics were extracted by local staff from justice records. Following the rank ordering of offense seriousness noted earlier, we designated interpersonal offenders as those whose current offense was a sexual or nonsexual interpersonal offence. Nonsexual interpersonal offenses included assault, robbery, arson, homicide, and all weapons charges. Youths self-assessed their mental health status on the V-DISC (developed by National Institute for Mental Health and Columbia University New York, USA). The V-DISC measures 20 disorders in four clusters: substance use, disruptive behavior, anxiety, and affective disorder, based on past-month symptoms according to the DSM-IV, and utilizes an audio computer-assisted self-interview format; the DISC has been widely used in juvenile justice settings [18,19]. The V-DISC's posttraumatic stress disorder (PTSD) module inquires about eight types of traumatic exposure: being in a bad accident or natural disaster, seeing someone get badly hurt, seeing a dead body, being attacked or beaten badly, thinking that you or others would get badly hurt or die, experiencing forced sex or being threatened by a weapon. Of these eight types, following procedures described earlier [8], we considered reports of being attacked or beaten badly, or being threatened by a weapon as reflecting nonsexual trauma victimization. Those who reported exposure to forced sex were considered to be victims of sexual trauma; and those who reported nonsexual trauma and/or sexual trauma were considered as victims of any interpersonal trauma.

3.2.5 STATISTICAL ANALYSIS

First, we compared demographic, offense, and diagnostic characteristics of juvenile sexual offenders and nonsexual interpersonal offenders via t-test and chi-square analyses.

Next, via logistic regression, we examined the relationship between type of traumatic exposure and sex offender status (being juvenile sex offender versus being nonsexual interpersonal offender), adjusting for other significant demographic and diagnostic contributors. From the pool of potential covariates, gender, race/ethnicity, substance use disorder and lifetime history of a suicide attempt were retained in the final equation based on their significant ($p<.02$) associations with sex offender status in initial bivariate analyses. As we were interested in the contribution of types of interpersonal traumatic exposure to juvenile sex offender status, we constructed three models. The first considered demographic and diagnostic features and reported exposure to any type of interpersonal trauma compared to exposure to non-interpersonal trauma (e.g., being in a bad accident or natural disaster, seeing a dead body). The second model substituted reported exposure to nonsexual trauma for exposure to any interpersonal trauma, and the final model substituted exposure to sexual trauma.

3.3 RESULTS

Table 1 presents demographic, offense and diagnostic characteristics, as well as report of traumatic exposure for juvenile interpersonal offenders, and for sexual and nonsexual interpersonal offenders separately. Compared to juvenile nonsexual interpersonal offenders, sexual offenders were significantly less likely to be female, only 11 of 387 sexual offenders [$\chi^2(1)=114.28$, $p<.001$]; to be African American [$\chi^2(3)=94.22$, $p<.001$], or to meet criteria for a substance use disorder [$\chi^2(1)=8.57$, $p<.01$]. Juvenile sexual offenders were significantly more likely to report either a lifetime history of a suicide attempt [$\chi^2(1)=10.80$, $p<.01$], or exposure to sexual trauma [$\chi^2(1)=80.45$, $p<.001$]. There were no other significant differences between juvenile sexual offenders and nonsexual interpersonal offenders in age, race/ ethnicity, offense characteristics, or history of exposure to nonsexual trauma or to any interpersonal trauma.

Of the 1367 interpersonal offenders (290 weapon-related, 150 sexual offense, and 927 nonsexual interpersonal offense) for whom complete offense data was available, only 16 (1%) sexual offenders (of 42 sites) had also been charged with nonsexual interpersonal offenses.

Table 2 presents multivariate results predicting sexual offending status, adjusting for demographic and diagnostic characteristics. The first model, considering exposure to either type of interpersonal trauma, significantly

TABLE 1. Characteristics of Interpersonal Offenders, and Sexual and Nonsexual Interpersonal Offenders.

	Interpersonal offenders (n = 2920)	Sexual offenders (n = 387)	Nonsexual interpersonal offenders (n = 2533)
	n (%)	n (%)	n (%)
Female***	720 (24.7)	11 (2.8)	709 (28.0)
Age (years, M, SD)	15.5 (SD 1.6)	15.6 (SD 1.7)	15.4 (SD 1.6)
Race/ethnicity			
African American***	1162 (39.8)	80 (20.7)	1082 (42.7)
Hispanic	480 (16.4)	59 (15.2)	421 (16.6)
Caucasian	1111 (38.0)	229 (59.2)	1780 (71.9)
Other	167 (5.7)	19 (4.9)	743 (31.1)
Age at first offense (years, M, SD)	13.4 (2.0)	13.5 (2.1)	395 (16.0)
Repeat offender	2049 (72.0)	269 (73.3)	1387 (70.2)
Substance use disorder**	830 (30.1)	87 (23.6)	1304 (52.6)
Lifetime suicide at-tempt**	482 (16.9)	87 (22.7)	395 (16.0)
Traumatic exposure			
Any interpersonal trauma	1624 (70.7)	237 (73.8)	1387 (70.2)
Nonsexual trauma	1502 (52.5)	198 (52.0)	1304 (52.6)
Sexual trauma***	422 (14.8)	114 (29.9)	308 (12.4)

Note. Some entries are based on a slightly reduced n because of missing data.
M : Mean; SD: Standard Deviation
**p<.01, ***p<.001.

predicted sexual offending status [$\chi^2(7)=223.21$, $p<.001$, $R^2=.17$]. Females were less than a tenth (OR=.08, p<.001) as likely as males to be sexual offenders. Compared to African-Americans; Hispanics, Caucasians and other races were more likely to be sexual offenders [Hispanics were approximately 50% more likely (OR=1.54, p<.05), Caucasians were more than three times as likely (OR=3.27, p<.001), and the other races were twice as likely (OR=2.00, p<.05)]. Compared to juvenile nonsexual interpersonal offenders, sexual offenders were only half as likely to report a substance use disorder (OR=.54, p<.001) but were almost twice as likely

TABLE 2. Contributors to Sexual Offending.

	Model 1 (n = 2205) R^2 = .17		Model 2 (n = 2754) R^2 = .17		Model 3 (n = 2754) R^2 = .23	
	OR	95% CI	OR	95% CI	OR	95% CI
Female	.08***	[.04, .15]	.06***	[.03, .12]	.04***	[.02, .08]
Race/ethnicity (ref = African American)						
Hispanic	1.54*	[1.00, 2.36]	1.93**	[1.33, 2.82]	1.95**	[1.33, 2.86]
Caucasian	3.27***	[2.39, 4.47]	3.37***	[2.53, 4.48]	2.96***	[2.21, 3.96]
Other	2.00*	[1.11, 3.61]	2.10*	[1.19, 3.69]	2.11*	[1.19, 3.75]
Substance use disorder	.54***	[.40, .72]	.60***	[.45, .79]	.63**	[.48, .83]
Lifetime suicide attempt	1.75***	[1.29, 2.39]	1.87***	[1.39, 2.52]	1.31	[.96, 1.80]
Traumatic exposure						
Any interpersonal trauma	1.07	[.80, 1.43]	-	-	-	-
Nonsexual trauma	-	-	.86	[.67, 1.09]	-	-
Sexual trauma	-	-	-	-	5.02***	[3.67, 6.87]

Note. OR: Odds ratio; CI:Confidence interval; R^2:Nagelkerke R Square.
*p<.05, **p<.01, ***p<.001.

to report a lifetime history of a suicide attempt (OR=1.75, $p<.001$); exposure to any interpersonal trauma was unrelated to sexual offending.

Considering nonsexual trauma, the second model significantly predicted sexual offending status [$\chi^2(7)=267.00$, $p<.001$, $R^2=.17$], with contributions of demographic and diagnostic characteristics essentially unchanged, and explaining the same proportion of the variance as found for Model 1. Exposure to nonsexual trauma was unrelated to sexual offending.

The third model, considering exposure to sexual trauma, significantly predicted sexual offending status [$\chi^2(7)=364.01$, $p<.001$, $R^2=.23$], explaining 6% more of the variance than did either Model 1 or 2. The contribution of demographic and diagnostic characteristics remained essentially unchanged, except that history of a lifetime suicide attempt no longer contributed significantly to sexual offending status. Compared to juvenile nonsexual interpersonal offenders, sexual offenders were five times as likely to report a history of sexual trauma (OR=5.02, $p<.001$). When we substituted exposure to both nonsexual and sexual trauma [a total of 300 youths (10% of interpersonal offenders)], associations for demographic and diagnostic features were consistent with those found earlier, with a contribution of both types of trauma in between that found for Models 2 and 3 (OR=3.77, $p<.001$) (data not shown).

3.4 DISCUSSION

This exploratory study aimed to define the degree to which juvenile sexual offenders differed from nonsexual interpersonal offenders as well as the contribution of demographic characteristics, mental health problems and interpersonal trauma history to sexual offending. Compared to juvenile nonsexual interpersonal offenders, sexual offenders were significantly less likely to be female, to be African American, or to meet criteria for a substance use disorder; and were significantly more likely to report a lifetime history of a suicide attempt. These findings are in line with previous reports comparing juvenile sexual and nonsexual offenders [12,14,20,21]. The results concerning the sexual victimization of juvenile sexual offenders are also consistent with earlier findings [2,22,23] that highlight the role of sexual victimization in explaining sexually abusive behavior. However, it should be noted that for those sexual offenders without sexual trauma histories (70.1%), other factors most likely explain their sexually abusive behavior.

Collectively, the findings suggest that juvenile sexual offenders differ in key aspects from juvenile nonsexual interpersonal offenders. On the other hand, however, consistent with [24], we found sexual offenders were comparable to other offenders in their repeat offender status.

Unexpectedly, there were no differences between the two groups in their age at first offense; van Wijk et al. [24] found violent sexual offenders to be younger at first arrest than other violent offenders. Group differences in that study were significant but small, and discrepant results may have been a consequence of differences in the definitions of juvenile sexual and nonsexual offenders across investigations. In the earlier study [24] a juvenile was considered a violent sexual offender when he had committed a violent sex offense first before a possibly violent offense later on, for the group of violent offenders it was the other way around. In the current study we utilized a rank ordering of offense seriousness; with sexual offenses the most serious, followed by nonsexual interpersonal offenses; and juveniles with multiple current offenses were coded to the most serious offense. Also, the finding that only 1% of the sexual offenders had also been charged with nonsexual interpersonal offenses was remarkable. Whereas it is found that the majority of juvenile sexual offenders also frequently engage in nonsexual interpersonal offenses and antisocial behavior [25]. Such behavior could be explained by the fact that sexual offending is often accompanied by aggressive behavior, for example in case of rape. However, it is also found that most juvenile sexual offenders previously committed a nonsexual assault [25]. It should be noted that this 1%, compared to the other sexual offenders, revealed similar demographic, offense, or diagnostic characteristics. Unfortunately, given the low n of this group (16), comparisons lacked statistical power to test for significant differences.

A set of demographic and diagnostic characteristics contributed significantly to sexual offending, as did a reported history of sexual trauma. The finding that a history of a lifetime suicide attempt no longer contributed significantly to sexual offending status when we considered exposure to sexual trauma may reflect a power problem, as this concerned only 87 (3%) observations.

A number of shortcomings of the current study should be mentioned. The current study did not take into account heterogeneity among sexual offenders. Some prior studies have attempted to classify subgroups of juvenile sexual offenders (in e.g., those who victimize children versus those who victimize peers; those who commit sexual and nonsexual offenses versus those who commit only sexual offenses) and to describe differences between subgroups [26-28]. Subgroup analysis, however, has often led to inconsistent findings, with respect to sexual recidivism, social skills, and engagement in nonsexual offending [28]. Therefore, efforts will be needed to validate any such classification of subgroups of juvenile sexual offenders. Perhaps further study which takes into account relevant subgroups will more precisely delineate issues for youth who sexually offend and will have implications for the development of offender-specific interventions and risk prediction.

Another limitation is that the diagnostic measures and history of traumatic exposure were obtained via self-report. There is an ongoing debate about the use of self-report studies in juvenile justice populations, as youths' memory may limit the information that can be captured [29]. However, self-report is preferred over the use of official records to collect the prevalence of maltreatment in detained youth; as official records seriously underestimate the prevalence of maltreatment, especially in males [30]. In addition, self-report may actually be more accurate for internalizing disorders [31]. Furthermore, interpersonal trauma history was inquired about at intake, so that any victimization that occurred during incarceration (for those participants in secure care) would have been missed. Finally, although sub samples were not selected to be nationally or regionally representative, models accounted for clustering of individuals within setting, allowing adjustment for such jurisdictional differences.

Despite these limitations, the current study suggests ways in which future research might address issues of relevance for clinical practice. Consistent with other research, our results indicate that females are less likely than males to commit a sexual offense and that sexual victimization is related to sexual perpetration [2,24]. Although an extensive body of literature has demonstrated that girls in the juvenile justice system have higher rates of past sexual abuse than their male counterparts [32], there is less information about how the long-term negative consequences of sexual victimization (e.g., mental health problems, disruptive behavior, delinquency) differ across gender. Mechanisms related to these negative consequences should be studied and explored. Furthermore, as it has been demonstrated that juvenile sexual offenders may persist in their sexual offending behaviors if not treated [33], evidence-based interventions are required. However, as clinical trials evaluating specific interventions for juvenile sexual offenders are scarce [34,35], further research is desirable to pinpoint effective interventions for these youth.

REFERENCES

1. Barbaree HE, Marshall WL, Hudson SM (1993) The juvenile sex offender. New York, NY: Guilford Press.
2. Burton DL (2008) An exploratory evaluation of the contribution of personality and childhood sexual victimization to the development of sexually abusive behavior. Sex Abuse 20: 102-115.
3. Seto MC, LalumiÃ¨re ML (2010) What is so special about male adolescent sexual offending? A review and test of explanations through meta-analysis. Psychol Bull 136: 526-575.
4. Van Wijk AP, Blokland AA, Duits N, Vermeiren R, Harkink J (2007) Relating psychiatric disorders, offender and offence characteristics in a sample of adolescent sex offenders and non-sex offenders. Crim Behav Ment Health 17: 15-30.
5. Abram KM, Teplin LA, Charles DR, Longworth SL, McClelland GM, et al. (2004) Posttraumatic stress disorder and trauma in youth in juvenile detention. Arch Gen Psychiatry 61: 403-410.
6. Kerig PK, Ward RM, Vanderzee KL, Arnzen Moeddel M (2009) Posttraumatic stress as a mediator of the relationship between trauma and mental health problems among juvenile delinquents. J Youth Adolesc 38: 1214-1225.
7. Ruchkin VV, Schwab-Stone M, Koposov R, Vermeiren R, Steiner H (2002) Violence exposure, posttraumatic stress, and personality in juvenile delinquents. J Am Acad Child Adolesc Psychiatry 41: 322-329.
8. Wasserman GA, McReynolds LS (2011) Contributors to traumatic exposure and posttraumatic stress disorder in juvenile justice youths. J Trauma Stress 24: 422-429.
9. Wood J, Foy DW, Layne C, Pynoos R, James CB (2002) An examination of the relationships between violence exposure, posttraumatic stress symptomatology, and delinquent activity: An 'ecopathological' model of delinquent behavior among incarcerated adolescents. Journal of Aggression, Maltreatment and Trauma 6: 127-147.

10. Jacobs WL, Kennedy WA, Meyer JB (1997) Juvenile delinquents: A betweengroup comparison study of sexual and nonsexual offenders. Sexual Abuse: Journal of Research and Treatment 9: 201-217.
11. van Wijk A, Loeber R, Vermeiren R, Pardini D, Bullens R, et al. (2005) Violent juvenile sex offenders compared with violent juvenile nonsex offenders: explorative findings from the Pittsburgh Youth Study. Sex Abuse 17: 333-352.
12. van Wijk A, Vermeiren R, Loeber R, 't Hart-Kerkhoffs L, Doreleijers T, et al. (2006) Juvenile sex offenders compared to non-sex offenders: a review of the literature 1995-2005. Trauma Violence Abuse 7: 227-243.
13. Butler SM, Seto MC (2002) Distinguishing two types of adolescent sex offenders. J Am Acad Child Adolesc Psychiatry 41: 83-90.
14. Van Wijk AP, Vreugdenhil C, Bullens RAR (2004) Are juvenile sex offenders different from non-sexoffenders? Proces 5: 205-208.
15. Glasser M, Kolvin I, Campbell D, Glasser A, Leitch I, et al. (2001) Cycle of child sexual abuse: links between being a victim and becoming a perpetrator. Br J Psychiatry 179: 482-494.
16. Mulder E, Vermunt J, Brand E, Bullens R, van Marle H (2012) Recidivism in subgroups of serious juvenile offenders: different profiles, different risks? Crim Behav Ment Health 22: 122-135.
17. Wasserman GA, McReynolds LS, Schwalbe CS, Keating JM, Jones SA (2010) Psychiatric disorder, comorbidity, and suicidal behavior in juvenile justice youth. Criminal Justice and Behavior 37: 1361-1376.
18. Teplin LA, Abram KM, McClelland GM, Dulcan MK, Mericle AA (2002) Psychiatric disorders in youth in juvenile detention. Arch Gen Psychiatry 59: 1133-1143.
19. Wasserman GA, McReynolds LS, Ko SJ, Katz LM, Carpenter JR (2005) Gender differences in psychiatric disorders at juvenile probation intake. Am J Public Health 95: 131-137.
20. Heaton P, Davis RE, HappÃ© FG (2008) Research note: exceptional absolute pitch perception for spoken words in an able adult with autism. Neuropsychologia 46: 2095-2098.
21. Rantakallio P, Myhrman A, Koiranen M (1995) Juvenile offenders, with special reference to sex differences. Soc Psychiatry Psychiatr Epidemiol 30: 113-120.
22. Burton DL, Miller DL, Shill CT (2002) A social learning theory comparison of the sexual victimization of adolescent sexual offenders and nonsexual offending male delinquents. Child Abuse Negl 26: 893-907.
23. Veneziano C, Veneziano L, LeGrand S, Richards L (2004) Neuropsychological executive functions of adolescent sex offenders and nonsex offenders. Percept Mot Skills 98: 661-674.
24. van Wijk AP, Mali BR, Bullens RA, Vermeiren RR (2007) Criminal profiles of violent juvenile sex and violent juvenile non sex offenders: an explorative longitudinal study. J Interpers Violence 22: 1340-1355.
25. Righthand S, Welch C (2001) Juveniles who have sexually offended: A review of the professional literature (office of juvenile justice and delinquency prevention report). Washington, DC: Department of Justice.
26. Chu CM, Thomas SD (2010) Adolescent sexual offenders: the relationship between typology and recidivism. Sex Abuse 22: 218-233.

27. 't Hart-Kerkhoffs LA, Vermeiren RR, Jansen LM, Doreleijers TA (2011) Juvenile group sex offenders: a comparison of group leaders and followers. J Interpers Violence 26: 3-20.
28. Kemper TS, Kistner JA (2010) An evaluation of classification criteria for juvenile sex offenders. Sex Abuse 22: 172-190.
29. Snyder H, Sickmund M (2006) Juvenile offenders and victims: 2006 national report. Washington, DC: Office of Juvenile Justice and Delinquency Prevention.
30. Swahn MH, Whitaker DJ, Pippen CB, Leeb RT, Teplin LA, et al. (2006) Concordance between self-reported maltreatment and court records of abuse or neglect among high-risk youths. Am J Public Health 96: 1849-1853.
31. Martin JL, Ford CB, Dyer-Friedman J, Tang J, Huffman LC (2004) Patterns of agreement between parent and child ratings of emotional and behavioral problems in an outpatient clinical setting: when children endorse more problems. J Dev Behav Pediatr 25: 150-155.
32. Goodkind S, Ng I, Sarri RC (2006) The impact of sexual abuse in the lives of young women involved or at risk of involvement with the juvenile justice system. Violence Against Women 12: 456-477.
33. Efta-Breitbach J, Freeman KA (2004) Treatment of juveniles who sexually offend: an overview. J Child Sex Abus 13: 125-138.
34. Reitzel LR, Carbonell JL (2006) The effectiveness of sexual offender treatment for juveniles as measured by recidivism: a meta-analysis. Sex Abuse 18: 401- 421.
35. Walker DF, McGovern SK, Poey EL, Otis KE (2004) Treatment effectiveness for male adolescent sexual offenders: a meta-analysis and review. J Child Sex Abus 13: 281-293.

CHAPTER 4

Children's Exposure to Violence and the Intersection Between Delinquency and Victimization

CARLOS A. CUEVAS, DAVID FINKELHOR, ANNE SHATTUCK, HEATHER TURNER, AND SHERRY HAMBY

The association between delinquency and victimization is a common focus in juvenile justice research. Some observers have found that victimization and delinquency largely overlap, with most victims engaging in delinquency and most delinquents being victimized at some point in their lives (Lauritsen, Laub, and Sampson, 1992; Lauritsen, Sampson, and Laub, 1991; Singer, 1986). The literature in the bullying and peer victimization field paints a different picture. It points to three distinct groups of children: in addition to the children who are both victims and offenders (often referred to as bully-victims or, as in this bulletin, delinquent-victims), a second group are primarily victims and a third group are primarily offenders (Dodge et al., 1990; Olweus, 1978, 2000). One may explain the contrast in this way: many studies have relied simply on measures of association between delinquency and victimization (e.g., correlation or

Juvenile Justice Bulletin, October 2013, www.ojb.usdoj.gov. Government document from U.S. Department of Justice, Office of Justice Programs, Office of Juvenile Justice and Delinquency Prevention.

regression analyses) (see, e.g., Chang, Chen, and Brownson, 2003; Jensen and Brownfield, 1986; Sullivan, Farrell, and Kliewer, 2006). When researchers look beyond the association between delinquency and victimization (even when that association is strong), they are likely to find groups of children who are primarily victims or primarily offenders. Research has not fully explored how large these groups are and how their characteristics and experiences differ.

4.1 DEFINING DELINQUENTS, VICTIMS, AND DELINQUENT-VICTIMS IN THE NATSCEV STUDY GROUP

The National Survey of Children's Exposure to Violence (NatSCEV) is a national study that is both large and comprehensive in its assessment of victimization and delinquency (see "History of the National Survey of Children's Exposure to Violence"). Thus, it provides a look at how victimization and delinquency converge or diverge among youth of different ages.

Using the interview data from NatSCEV (see "Methodology" on page 7) (Finkelhor, Turner, Ormrod, and Hamby, 2009), the research team categorized adolescents ages 10 to 17 into one of four groups: those youth who were primarily delinquents and not victims (primarily delinquents), those who were primarily victims and not delinquents (primarily victims), those who were both delinquents and victims (delinquent-victims), and those who were neither victims nor delinquents. The criteria for defining these groups are based on work done in an earlier study (Cuevas et al., 2007) and take into account that many children have minor victimizations and that they engage in different kinds of delinquency, including violent delinquency, property delinquency, and forms of mild delinquency, such as skipping school or getting drunk.

In the interest of clarity, the researchers defined the subgroups in terms of key characteristics that the literature on victimization and delinquency suggests (Dodge et al., 1990; Jennings, Piquero, and Reingle, 2012; Malinosky-Rummell and Hansen, 1993; McGrath, Nilsen, and Kerley, 2011; Olweus, 1978, 2000; Windle and Mason, 2004). Table 1 illustrates the typology groups and defining criteria.

HISTORY OF THE NATIONAL SURVEY OF CHILDREN'S EXPOSURE TO VIOLENCE

Under the leadership of then-Deputy Attorney General Eric Holder in June 1999, the Office of Juvenile Justice and Delinquency Prevention (OJJDP) created the Safe Start initiative to prevent and reduce the impact of children's exposure to violence. As a part of this initiative and with a growing need to document the full extent of children's exposure to violence, OJJDP launched the National Survey of Children's Exposure to Violence (NatSCEV) with the support of the Centers for Disease Control and Prevention.

NatSCEV is the first national incidence and prevalence study to comprehensively examine the extent and nature of children's exposure to violence across all ages, settings, and timeframes. Conducted between January and May 2008, it measured the past-year and lifetime exposure to violence for children age 17 and younger across several major categories: conventional crime, child maltreatment, victimization by peers and siblings, sexual victimization, witnessing and indirect victimization (including exposure to community violence and family violence), school violence and threats, and Internet victimization. This survey marks the first attempt to measure children's exposure to violence in the home, school, and community across all age groups from 1 month to age 17, and the first attempt to measure the cumulative exposure to violence over the child's lifetime. The survey asked children and their adult caregivers about not only the incidents of violence that children suffered and witnessed themselves but also other related crime and threat exposures, such as theft or burglary from a child's household, being in a school that was the target of a credible bomb threat, and being in a war zone or an area where ethnic violence occurred.

OJJDP directed the development of the study, and the Crimes against Children Research Center at the University of New Hampshire designed and conducted the research. It provides data on the full extent of violence in the daily lives of children. NatSCEV documents the incidence and prevalence of children's exposure to a broad array of violent experiences across a wide developmental spectrum. The research team asked followup questions about specific events, including where the exposure to violence occurred, whether injury resulted, how often the child was exposed to a specific type of violence, and the child's relationship to the perpetrator and (when the child witnessed violence) the victim. In addition, the survey documents differences in exposure to violence across gender, race, socioeconomicstatus, family structure, region, urban/rural residence, and developmental stage of the child; specifies how different forms of violent victimization "cluster" or co-occur; identifies individual-, family-, and community-level predictors of violence exposure among children; examines associations between levels/types of exposure to violence and children's mental and emotional health; and assesses the extent to which children disclose incidents of violence to various individuals and the nature and source of assistance or treatment provided (if any).

4.1.1 DEFINITION OF VICTIMIZED VERSUS NONVICTIMIZED YOUTH

From previous analyses (Finkelhor, Hamby et al., 2005; Finkelhor, Ormrod et al., 2005a; Hamby et al., 2004), the researchers determined that one of the best measures of victimization intensity is the number of types of victimization per respondent based on the screening categories that the Juvenile Victimization Questionnaire (JVQ) uses (see "Methodology" on page 7). Although simply adding up the number of different types of victimization (including parental abuse, sex offenses, property offenses, and peer victimizations) does not take into account repeated victimizations of the same type, analyses have suggested that factoring in repeated victimizations and other measures of victimization severity does not produce substantively different results in identifying highly victimized youth (Finkelhor, Hamby et al., 2005; Finkelhor, Ormrod, and Turner, 2007).

For the purposes of this study, the researchers defined victimized youth as those who suffered three or more victimizations in the past year. They chose this number because the mean number of types of victimization in the past year per respondent in the NatSCEV study was 2.68 and because the JVQ and NatSCEV include many common kinds of victimizations, such as being hit by a sibling or having property stolen. Consequently, the researchers categorized non-/lowvictimized youth as those who suffered two victimizations or fewer in the past year.

4.1.2 DEFINITION OF DELINQUENT VERSUS NONDELINQUENT YOUTH

Based on the literature on delinquency (e.g., Snyder and Sickmund, 2006; Windle and Mason, 2004), the researchers considered it important to distinguish among types of delinquent behavior. The researchers clearly delineated the study's delinquency measures into the following types: those that involved violent behavior (assaults and carrying weapons), those that involved property delinquency (breaking something, stealing from a store), those that involved drug and alcohol use (drinking, smoking marijuana), and those that involved minor delinquency (truancy, cheating on tests). Violent behavior and property delinquency are categorized as separate types, and for the most part delinquency involving substance use or minor forms of rule violating is categorized as mild delinquency (see table 1).

As with victimized youth, some categories of delinquent youth are defined as those who committed more delinquent acts than the past-year mean (i.e., two or more types of delinquent acts within the past year). Given the inclusion of relatively minor and perhaps normative delinquent acts in the Frequency of Delinquency Behavior (Loeber and Dishion, 1983) (see "Methodology" on page 7), the researchers decided that defining those who committed fewer than the mean number of delinquent acts in the past year as nondelinquent would adequately identify youth with no or only minor delinquency.

4.1.3 CATEGORIES OF DELINQUENT-VICTIMS

The researchers first defined three groups of youth who fell into the delinquentvictim overlap category (see table 1). They defined "Violent Delinquent-Victims," consistent with descriptions from other studies of victimization and delinquency (Haynie et al., 2001; Olweus, 1978, 2000; Schwartz, Proctor, and Chien, 2001), as youth who in the past year engaged in violent, interpersonal acts or carried weapons and who experienced three or more violent victimizations in the past year. As suggested in the trauma response literature (Briere et al., 1997; Finkelhor, 1990; Kilpatrick et al., 2003; Wilsnack et al., 2004; Windle and Mason, 2004), the research team termed the second defined group as "Delinquent Sex/Maltreatment Victims," who had experienced sexual victimization or a form of child maltreatment and had engaged in two or more delinquent acts in the past year. They defined the third group, "Property Delinquent-Victims," as delinquent and highly victimized youth whose delinquencies were related solely to property crime and who had three or more victimizations of any type in the past year.

4.1.4 CATEGORIES OF PRIMARILY DELINQUENT YOUTH

In contrast to these three groups of delinquent-victims, the study also categorized some youth as primarily delinquent. These were youth who had rates of victimization below the mean of three in the past year, but who had engaged in violent (youth categorized as "Assaulters") or property delinquency (youth categorized as "Property Delinquents"), which were the most serious and least frequent delinquencies (see table 1).

4.1.5 CATEGORIES OF YOUTH WHO ARE PRIMARILY VICTIMS

The researchers defined two groups who were primarily victims but not delinquents. These were the "Mild Delinquency Victims," who had greater than mean levels of victimization (three or more victimizations within the past year) but no property or violent delinquency, and "Nondelinquent Sex/Maltreatment Victims," who had experienced a sexual victimization or a form of child maltreatment but had committed fewer than two delinquent acts in the past year (see table 1). This last group was distinguished as a separate category because the victimization literature suggests special seriousness for youth who experience even one incident of sexual victimization or child maltreatment, which are also acts that lead to the involvement of child protective services or police referrals (Briere et al., 1997; Egeland et al., 2002; Finkelhor, 1990; Kilpatrick et al., 2003; Wilsnack et al., 2004; Windle and Mason, 2004; Wood et al., 2002).

The grouping criteria illustrate, to some degree, the intricacy of establishing these categories given the complexity of victimization and delinquent behavior. As such, the categorizing approach examines both the number of types of behavior (above or below the mean for victimization and delinquency) and the type of delinquency or victimization (e.g., violent, property, sexual, or maltreatment). As a result, some youth may fit into more than one of the established categories. To keep the groups mutually exclusive, the researchers established a hierarchy for categorizing individuals who fell into more than one typology group (e.g., a youth who committed a violent act or carried a weapon within the previous year and had been sexually victimized in addition to undergoing three or more violent victimizations, and who therefore would fall into both the violent delinquent-victim and delinquent sex/maltreatment victim typology groups). The hierarchy is as follows, from the most severe to the least severe combination of delinquency and victimization: violent delinquent-victims, delinquent sex/ maltreatment victims, assaulters, nondelinquent sex/maltreatment victims, property delinquent-victims, property delinquents, mild delinquency victims, and mild delinquency non-/low-victimized youth (note that assaulters and nondelinquent sex/maltreatment victims, although they are categorized as primarily delinquent and primarily victims, respectively, are regarded as higher in the hierarchy than property delinquent-victims). This ordering was presented in the original typology using the Developmental Victimization Survey (DVS) data (Cuevas et al., 2007), which established this order according to which group of individuals was most similar based on their demographic characteristics.

TABLE 1. Delinquency and Victimization Criteria for Typology Groups

	Name	Delinquency Criteria	Victimization Criteria
Delinquent-victims	Violent Delinquent-Victims	Any interpersonal violence	≥3 violent
	Delinquent Sex/ Maltreatment Victims	≥2 delinquencies	Any sexual victimizations or child maltreatment
	Property Delinquent-Victims	Property delinquency, no interpersonal violence	≥3 victimizations
Primarily delin-quent	Assaulters	Any interpersonal violence or weapon carrying	<3 violent victimizations
	Property Delinquents	Property delinquency, no interpersonal violence	<3 victimizations
Primarily victims	Nondelinquent Sex/ Maltreatment Victims	<2 delinquencies	Any sexual victimizations or child maltreatment
	Mild Delinquency Victims	No violent and no property delinquency	≥3 victimizations
Low delinquency/ victimization	Mild Delinquency Non-/ Low-Victimized Youth	No violent and no property delinquency	<3 victimizations

For consistency, the ordering remained the same for the purposes of this analysis based on the NatSCEV data.

4.2 FINDINGS BY GENDER AND TYPOLOGY GROUP FOR DELINQUENTS, VICTIMS, AND DELINQUENT-VICTIMS

4.2.1 VICTIMIZATION AND DELINQUENCY PATTERNS AMONG BOYS

Among boys overall, the primarily delinquent group comprised 20.8 percent of the total sample (see "Methodology" on page 7 for sample size). Boys who were primarily victims with little or no delinquency comprised

17.9 percent of the total sample, and the group who were both victimized and delinquent comprised 18.1 percent (figure 1). Substantial percentages of all three groups were evident throughout the developmental course for boys ages 10 to 17 (figure 2). However, the proportion of boys in the primarily victim group differed between ages 12 and 13 (declining from 27.8 percent to 15.5 percent). At ages 13 and 14, the proportion of boys in the delinquent-victim group increased from 14.7 percent to 28.2 percent and was elevated through age 17.

The boys in the delinquent-victim group had considerably more victimization than the boys who were primarily victims, disclosing 6.3 and 4.5 different kinds of victimization in the past year, respectively (table 2). This delinquent-victim group had a greater percentage of victims than the primarily victim group in every category of victimization except for bullying victimization. These boys had particularly greater percentages of sexual victimization (which includes sexual harassment) (40 percent for delinquent-victim boys versus 13 percent for primarily victim boys), witnessing family violence (26 percent for delinquent-victim boys versus 12 percent for primarily victim boys), and Internet victimization (14 percent for delinquentvictim boys versus 1 percent for primarily victim boys). The primarily victim group of boys had a greater percentage of victims than the delinquent-victim group in only one victimization category— bullying victimization (58 percent versus 40 percent).

The boys in the delinquent-victim group were also more delinquent than the primarily delinquent group (3.9 and 2.7 delinquent activities in the past year, respectively) (see table 2), which may be in part a function of the definitional criteria that set a higher threshold of delinquent activities for delinquent-victim boys than for primarily delinquent boys. The elevation of their drugs/minor delinquency score was particularly large (1.4 for delinquent-victims versus 0.8 for the primarily delinquent group).

4.2.2 VICTIMIZATION AND DELINQUENCY PATTERNS AMONG GIRLS

Girls had different patterns in both typology groups and age of changes in victimization and delinquency. Except for the group of girls who were

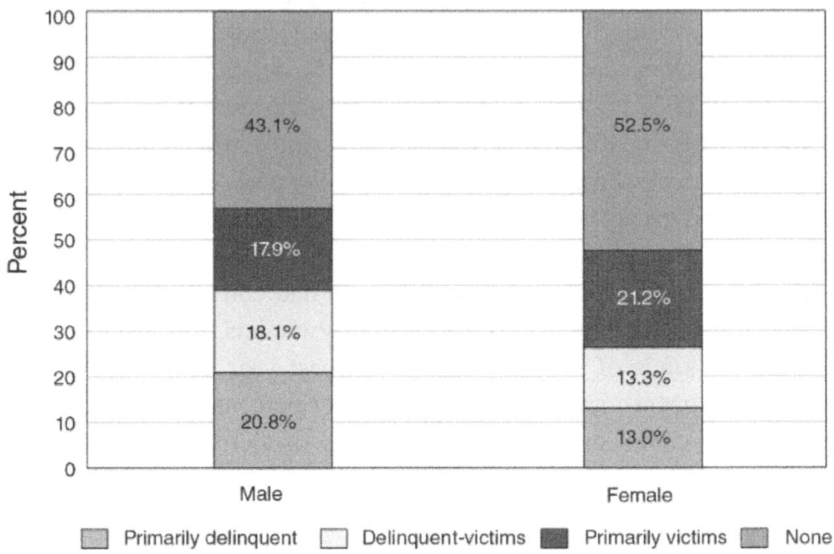

Figure 1. Victimization-Delinquency Co-occurrence by Gender, Ages 10 to 17.

neither victims nor delinquents (52.5 percent), the largest group of girls was the primarily victim group (21.2 percent). The primarily delinquent group (13 percent) and delinquentvictim group (13.3 percent) were smaller than the comparable groups among boys, reflecting that girls tend to engage in less delinquency than boys. A rise in both delinquency and victimization for girls appeared particularly notable between ages 11 and 12 (figure 3); as girls got older, the victimization component remained stable and then rose, while the delinquency component rose and then fell.

The patterns of victimization and delinquency for girls are generally similar to those for boys in terms of both the number and types of victimizations and delinquent acts. The delinquent-victim girls were more victimized than the primarily victim girls, disclosing 6.4 and 4.2 different victimizations in the past year, respectively (table 2). (This is not a function of the definitional criteria that set a higher threshold of victimizations for delinquent-victim girls than for primarily victim girls.) The

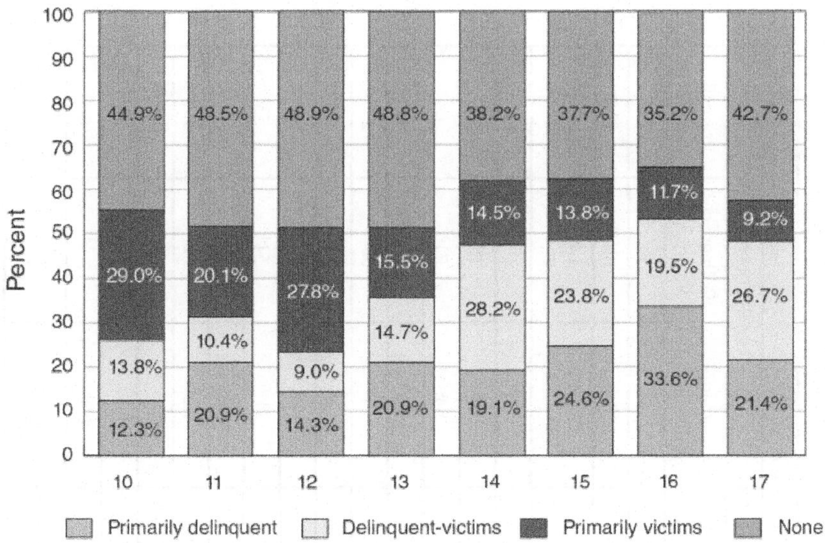

Figure 2. Victimization-Delinquency Co-occurrence by Males Ages 10 to 17.

delinquent-victim girls had greater percentages of victimization in every category of victimization except bullying victimization. Their victimization rates were particularly higher for sexual victimization, for which the rate among delinquent-victim girls (58 percent) was more than twice that among the primarily victim girls (27 percent); and Internet victimization, for which the rate among delinquent-victim girls was more than four times higher than among the primarily victim girls (33 percent versus 7 percent) and much higher than the equivalent rate among delinquent-victim boys (14 percent).

Delinquent-victim girls were also more delinquent than the primarily delinquent girls (3.3 and 2.0 delinquent activities in the past year, respectively). As with the boys, their drugs/minor delinquency scores were particularly elevated (1.7 for delinquent-victim girls versus 0.6 for primarily delinquent girls).

TABLE 2. Characteristics by Delinquent/Victim Group and Gender.

NatSCEV 10- to 17-year-olds N = 2,090 (unweighted)	Delinquent/Victim Group					
	Males (n = 1,039)			Males (n = 1,039)		
	Primarily Delinquent (a)	Delinquent-Victims (b)	Primarily Victims (c)	Primarily Delinquent (d)	Delinquent-Victims (e)	Primarily Victims (f)
Total n (unweighted)	222	198	167	140	155	214
Age	13.9[c]	14.2[c]	12.7[a,b]	13.9	14.4[f]	13.3[e]
Total number of victimization screeners	2.0[b,c]	6.3[a,c]	4.5[a,c]	2.7[e,f]	6.4[d,f]	4.2[d,e]
Victimization type (% yes)						
Witness family violence	15[b]	26[a,c]	1[2b]	18[e]	36[d,f]	19[e]
Exposure to community violence	49[b,c]	70[a]	63[a]	54[e]	71[d]	63
Assault	57[b,c]	91[a,c]	80[a,b]	62[e]	90[d,f]	68[e]
Sexual victimization	0[b,c]	40[a,c]	13[a,b]	7[e,f]	58[d,f]	27[d,e]
Property victimization	24[b,c]	56[a,c]	43[a,b]	38[e]	63[d,f]	45[e]
Maltreatment	1[b,c]	45[a,c]	25[a,b]	4[e,f]	59[d,f]	33[d,e]
Bullying	16[b,c]	40[a,c]	58[a,b]	34[e,f]	51[d]	53[d]
Internet victimization	5[b]	14[a,c]	1[b]	12[e]	33[d,f]	7[e]
Past-year adversity score (mean)	1.1[b]	1.9[a,c]	1.1[b]	1.6[e]	2.2[d,f]	1.6[e]
Total delinquency score (mean)	2.7[b,c]	3.9[a,c]	0.3[a,b]	2.0[e,f]	3.3[d,f]	0.3[d,e]
Violent delinquency (mean)	1.3[b,c]	1.5[a,c]	0.0[a,b]	1.0[e,f]	0.8[d,f]	0.0[d,e]
Property delinquency (mean)	0.6[b,c]	0.9[a,c]	0.0[a,b]	0.4[e,f]	0.8[d,f]	0.0[d,e]
Drugs/minor delinquency score (mean)	0.8[b,c]	1.4[a,c]	0.3[a,b]	0.6[e,f]	1.7[d,f]	0.2[d,e]

TABLE 2. CONTINUED.

Mental health symptoms (mean)						
Anger	9.8b	11.3^{a,c}	9.3^{b}	10.8^{e,f}	12.4^{d,f}	9.7^{d,e}
Depression	11.5^{b}	12.3^{a}	11.7	13.2^{e}	15.3^{d,f}	12.6^{e}
Anxiety	6.4^{b}	7.2^{a}	6.9	7.5^{e,f}	8.3^{d,f}	6.6^{d,e}
Parenting characteristics (mean scale scores)						
Warmth	38.0	37.9	38.5	38.5	37.9	38.1
Inconsistency/harshness	11.2	11.3	10.6	10.4^{e}	11.8^{d,f}	10.8^{e}
Supervision/monitoring	4.9	5.0	4.8	4.7	5.0	4.8
Social support score	27.1^{b}	25.7^{a,c}	27.5^{b}	27.6^{e}	24.7^{d,f}	27.1^{e}

Notes: Estimates are weighted. Sample sizes are unweighted. Superscript letters indicate that a value is significantly different from the value in the column labeled with the same letter in parentheses. Comparisons were made using one-way analysis of variance and post-hoc Bonferroni tests.

Past-year adversity score: total number of adverse events, out of 15 possible, that the youth experienced in the past year. Examples of items: natural disaster, a parent going to prison, and homelessness.

Total delinquency score: total number of delinquency types, out of 15 possible, that the youth committed in the past year. Violent, property, and drugs/minor delinquency scores are subsets of total delinquency. Violent delinquency items: destruction or damage of property, physical assault against a peer or adult, carrying a weapon, and injuring someone enough to require medical care. Property delinquency items: theft at school, theft at home, theft from a store, graffiti, and avoiding paying for things such as movies or bus rides. Drugs/minor delinquency items: cheating on tests at school, skipping school, tobacco use, marijuana use, and other drug use.

Scores for mental health symptoms, parenting characteristics, and social support are adjusted for age.

Mental health symptoms were measured using the anger, depression, and anxiety subscales of a shortened version of the Trauma Symptom Checklist for Children (Briere, 1996).

Parenting characteristics are sum scores of items rated on four-point scales asking how often parents engage in certain parenting behaviors. Higher scores indicate more frequent behavior associated with each characteristic. Warmth scale: 10 items such as encouraged a child to talk about his/her troubles, gave comfort and understanding when a child was upset, and hugged a child to express affection. Inconsistent/harsh parenting: five items such as lost control of temper when child misbehaved and punishments given to child depend on parent's mood. Supervision/monitoring scale: four items such as child is home without adult supervision overnight and child goes out with friends whom parent does not know.

Social support score is a sum score of eight items rated on a four-point scale asking about the child's perception of support available from family and friends, with higher scores indicating higher levels of perceived support. Examples of items: "I can talk about my problems with my family" and "I can count on my friends when things go wrong."

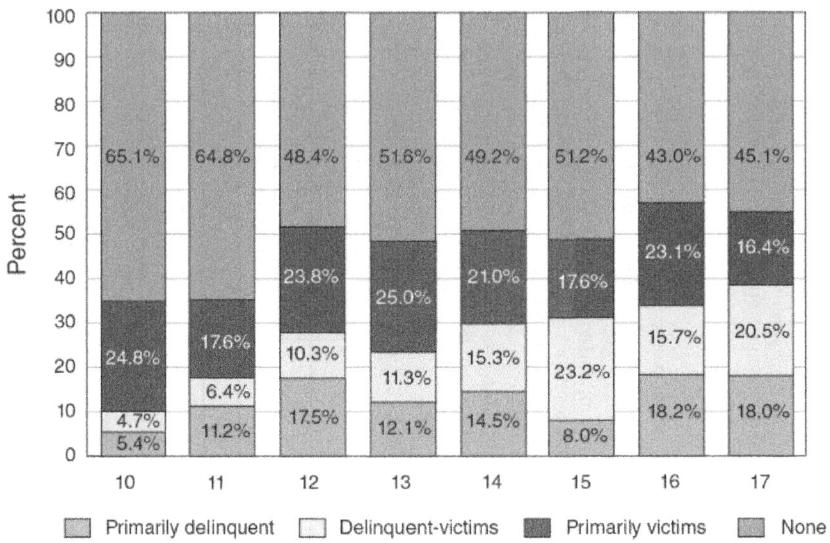

Figure 3. Victimization-Delinquency Co-occurrence by Females Ages 10 to 17.

4.2.3 FINDINGS REGARDING OTHER DIMENSIONS OF ADVERSITY

As table 2 shows, the groups differ on some additional dimensions as well. Among both boys and girls, delinquentvictims tended to experience more life adversities and mental health symptoms than other groups. They also received less social support. Delinquent-victim girls experienced higher rates of inconsistent/harsh parenting. There were few significant differences among the primarily delinquent, primarily victim, and delinquent-victim groups on features such as socioeconomic status, ethnicity, family structure, disability status, school performance, or physical features.

4.3 IMPLICATIONS FOR ADOLESCENT DEVELOPMENT AND FOR INTERVENTION BY PRACTITIONERS

4.3.1 AGE ONSET OF INCREASING RISK FOR VICTIMIZATION AND DELINQUENCY

Delinquency and victimization are widespread among youth ages 10 to 17, and they are statistically associated. However, in addition to those who experience both, it is possible to identify large groups within this age range who are victimized but not delinquent as well as those who are delinquent but experienced few types of victimization.

The relative sizes of these various groups appear to change as children age; they also differ by gender. The delinquentvictim group among boys is larger overall and increases substantially between ages 13 and 14. This may reflect an increase in delinquent activities around the time they enter high school among those who had previously been primarily victims. The high school environment may expose them to older delinquent role models and present them with conditions of more independence and less supervision than middle school.

For girls, the pattern change appears to occur earlier (between ages 11 and 12) and is associated with an increase in both victimization and delinquency, but particularly victimization. This is likely related to the onset of pubertal changes in girls and shows up in the data as a particularly marked increase in sexual harassment.

4.3.2 INCREASED RISK OF BOTH DELINQUENCY AND VICTIMIZATION FOR DELINQUENT-VICTIMS

For both genders, the data reveal worrying facts about the group who are both victimized and delinquent. This group manifests higher levels of both victimization and delinquency than either the primarily victim or primarily delinquent group. This group also has more additional adversities, lower levels of social support, and higher rates of mental health symptoms (see table 2). This is consistent with observations from the bullying literature that the so-called "bully-victims" are often the most distressed children (Cuevas et al., 2007; Haynie et al., 2001; Olweus, 1978, 2000; Schwartz, Proctor, and Chien, 2001). Improving strategies for identifying and helping this group of children is an obvious priority.

4.3.3 TIMING OF INTERVENTIONS TO REDUCE VICTIMIZATION AND DELINQUENCY

The current study is not longitudinal, and so it is limited in the inferences that can be made about how to identify children who are on track to become distressed delinquent-victims. This group does not appear to be discernible on the basis of demographic, family, or school variables collected in this study. The age comparisons suggest that victims who have additional adversities and higher levels of victimization and mental health symptoms may also be those at greatest risk of moving into delinquent activities. Targeting prevention at highly victimized youth with mental health symptoms may be important.

The study points clearly to the importance of early intervention. For girls, a large jump in victimization and delinquency occurs between ages 11 and 12; for boys, the delinquent-victim group increases between ages 13 and 14. This strongly suggests that delinquency and victimization prevention efforts need to be marshaled around or before the fifth grade, and they need to include components that minimize sexual aggression and harassment.

The transition to high school may also be a crucial juncture, especially for boys. Further study may better determine how children at this juncture both are targeted as victims and initiate multiple delinquent activities. Better early-warning systems may identify students who need special guidance and education from early in their high school careers.

METHODOLOGY

The National Survey of Children's Exposure to Violence (NatSCEV) was designed to obtain past-year and lifetime prevalence estimates of a wide range of childhood victimizations and was conducted between January and May 2008. NatSCEV documented the experiences of a nationally representative sample of 4,549 children ages 1 month to 17 years living in the contiguous United States. This study focuses on the 2,090 children (1,039 male and 1,051 female) who were 10 to 17 years old at the time of the survey. These children were surveyed on both their victimization experiences and their participation in 15 different kinds of delinquent behavior.

SAMPLING TECHNIQUES

The interviews with parents and youth were conducted over the phone. Sample households were drawn from a nationwide sampling frame of residential telephone numbers through random-digit dialing. To ensure that the study included an adequate number of minority and low-income respondents for more accurate subgroup analyses, the researchers oversampled telephone exchanges that had high concentrations of African American, Hispanic, or low-income households. Sample weights were applied to adjust for differential probability of selection due to (1) study design, (2) demographic variations in nonresponse, and (3) variations in eligibility within households. Additional information on sampling methods and procedures has been provided elsewhere (Finkelhor, Turner, Ormrod, and Hamby, 2009; Finkelhor, Turner, Ormrod, Hamby, and Kracke, 2009).

Interviewers first spoke with an adult caregiver in each household to obtain family demographic information. They then randomly selected the child with the most recent birthday to be interviewed. Interviewers spoke directly with children ages 10 to 17. For children younger than age 10, they interviewed the caregiver who "is most familiar with the child's daily routine and experiences."

SOURCES AND ANALYSIS OF INFORMATION REGARDING VICTIMIZATION

Researchers obtained reports of victimization using the Juvenile Victimization Questionnaire (JVQ), an inventory of childhood victimization (Finkelhor, Hamby et al., 2005; Finkelhor, Ormrod et al., 2005a; Hamby et al., 2004). The JVQ obtains reports on 48 forms of youth victimization covering 5 general areas of interest: conventional crime, maltreatment, victimization by peers and siblings, sexual victimization, and witnessing and exposure to violence (Finkelhor, Ormrod et al., 2005b).

Followup questions for each victimization item gathered additional information about each event, including perpetrator characteristics, weapon use (use of a knife, gun, or other object that could cause physical harm), injury, whether the event occurred in the past year, and whether it was known to school officials or police. The analysis for this bulletin examined victimizations that occurred in the past year. The researchers constructed 8 aggregate types of victimization from 32 of the JVQ's 48 victimization screeners: physical assault, sexual victimization, maltreatment, property victimization, witnessing family violence, exposure to community violence, bullying, and Internet victimization.

SOURCES AND ANALYSIS OF INFORMATION REGARDING DELINQUENCY

Researchers used the Frequency of Delinquency Behavior (FDB) that Loeber and Dishion (1983) originally developed to measure self-reported delinquency. For this study, the researchers adapted the FDB scale from its most recently published format (Dahlberg, Toal, and Behrens, 1998; Loeber and Stouthamer-Loeber, 1987).* The adapted form asked participants only whether they had committed the listed delinquency in the past year rather than how often they had committed each delinquent behavior. Researchers asked all NatSCEV participants between the ages of 5 and 17 about a total of 15 delinquency items. This study focuses on the 2,090 respondents aged 10 to 17.

REFERENCES

1. Briere, J. 1996. Trauma Symptoms Checklist for Children (TSCC): Professional Manual. Odessa, FL: Psychological Assessment Resources.
2. Briere, J., Woo, R., McRae, B., Foltz, J., and Sitzman, R. 1997. Lifetime victimization history, demographics, and clinical status in female psychiatric emergency room patients. Journal of Nervous and Mental Disease 185:95–101.
3. Chang, J.J., Chen, J.J., and Brownson, R.C. 2003. The role of repeat victimization in adolescent delinquent behaviors and recidivism. Journal of Adolescent Health 32(4):272–280.
4. Cuevas, C., Finkelhor, D., Turner, H.A., and Ormrod, R.K. 2007. Juvenile delinquency and victimization: A theoretical typology. Journal of Interpersonal Violence 22:1581–1602.
5. Dahlberg, L.L., Toal, S.B., and Behrens, C.B. 1998. Measuring Violence-Related Attitudes, Beliefs, and Behaviors Among Youth: A Compendium of Assessment Tools. Atlanta, GA: Centers for Disease Control and Prevention, National Center for Injury Prevention and Control.
6. Dodge, K.A., Coie, J.D., Pettit, G.S., and Price, J.M. 1990. Peer status and aggression in boys' groups: Developmental and contextual analyses. Child Development 61(5):1289–1309.
7. Egeland, B., Yates, T., Appleyard, K., and van Dulmen, M. 2002. The long-term consequences of maltreatment in the early years: A developmental pathway model to antisocial behavior. Children's Services: Social Policy, Research, and Practice 5:249–260.
8. Finkelhor, D. 1990. Early and long-term effects of child sexual abuse: An update. Professional Psychology Research and Practice 21:325–330.
9. Finkelhor, D., Hamby, S.L., Ormrod, R.K., and Turner, H.A. 2005. The JVQ: Reliability, validity, and national norms. Child Abuse & Neglect 29(4):383–412.
10. Finkelhor, D., Ormrod, R.K., and Turner, H.A. 2007. Poly-victimization: A neglected component in child victimization trauma. Child Abuse & Neglect 31:7–26.
11. Finkelhor, D., Ormrod, R.K., Turner, H.A., and Hamby, S.L. 2005a. Measuring polyvictimization using the JVQ. Child Abuse & Neglect 29(11):1297–1312.
12. Finkelhor, D., Ormrod, R.K., Turner, H.A., and Hamby, S.L. 2005b. The victimization of children and youth: A comprehensive, national survey. Child Maltreatment 10(1):5–25.
13. Finkelhor, D., Turner, H., Ormrod, R., and Hamby, S.L. 2009. Violence, abuse, and crime exposure in a national sample of children and youth. Pediatrics 124(5):1–13.
14. Finkelhor, D., Turner, H., Ormrod, R., Hamby, S., and Kracke, K. 2009. Children's Exposure to Violence: A Comprehensive National Survey. Bulletin. Washington, DC: U.S. Department of Justice, Office of Justice Programs, Office of Juvenile Justice and Delinquency Prevention.
15. Hamby, S.L., Finkelhor, D., Ormrod, R.K., and Turner, H.A. 2004. The Juvenile Victimization Questionnaire (JVQ): Administration and Scoring Manual. Durham, NH: Crimes against Children Research Center.

16. Haynie, D.L., Nansel, T., Eitel, P., Crump, A.D., Saylor, K., Yu, K., and Simons-Morton, B. 2001. Bullies, victims, and bully/victims: Distinct groups of at-risk youth. The Journal of Early Adolescence 21:29–49.
17. Jennings, W.G., Piquero, A.R., and Reingle, J.M. 2012. On the overlap between victimization and offending: A review of the literature. Aggression and Violent Behavior 17:16–26.
18. Jensen, G.F., and Brownfield, D. 1986. Gender, lifestyles, and victimization: Beyond routine activity, Violence and Victims 1(2):85–99.
19. Kilpatrick, D.G., Ruggiero, K.J., Acierno, R., Saunders, B.E., Resnick, H.S., and Best, C.L. 2003. Violence and risk of PTSD, major depression, substance abuse/dependence, and comorbidity: Results from the national survey of adolescents. Journal of Consulting and Clinical Psychology 71:692–700.
20. Lauritsen, J.L., Laub, J.H., and Sampson, R.J. 1992. Conventional and delinquent activities: Implications for the prevention of violent victimization among adolescents. Violence and Victims 7(2):91–108.
21. Lauritsen, J.L., Sampson, R.J., and Laub, J.H. 1991. The link between offending and victimization among adolescents. Criminology 29:265–292.
22. Loeber, R., and Dishion, T.J. 1983. Early predictors of male delinquency: A review. Psychological Bulletin 94:68–94.
23. Loeber, R., and Stouthamer-Loeber, M. 1987. The prediction of delinquency. In Handbook of Juvenile Delinquency, edited by H.C. Quay. New York, NY: Wiley, pp. 325–382.
24. Malinosky-Rummell, R., and Hansen, D.J. 1993. Long-term consequences of childhood physical abuse. Psychological Bulletin 114:68–79.
25. McGrath, S.A., Nilsen, A.A., and Kerley, K.R. 2011. Sexual victimization in childhood and the propensity for juvenile delinquency and adult criminal behavior: A systematic review. Aggression and Violent Behavior 16:485–492.
26. Olweus, D. 1978. Aggression in the Schools: Bullies and Whipping Boys. Oxford, England: Hemisphere.
27. Olweus, D. 2000. Bullying. In Encyclopedia of Psychology, vol. 1, edited by A.E. Kazdin. Washington, DC: American Psychological Association, pp. 487–489.
28. Schwartz, D., Proctor, L.J., and Chien, D.H. 2001. The aggressive victim of bullying: Emotional and behavioral dysregulation as a pathway to victimization by peers. In Peer Harassment in School: The Plight of the Vulnerable and Victimized, edited by J. Juvonen and S. Graham. New York, NY: Guilford Press, pp. 147–174.
29. Singer, S.I. 1986. Victims of serious violence and their criminal behavior: Subcultural theory and beyond. Victims and Violence 1:61–70.
30. Snyder, H.N., and Sickmund, M. 2006. Juvenile Offenders and Victims: 2006 National Report. Washington, DC: U.S. Department of Justice, Office of Justice Programs, Office of Juvenile Justice and Delinquency Prevention.
31. Sullivan, T.N., Farrell, A.D., and Kliewer, W. 2006. Peer victimization in early adolescence: Association between physical and relational victimization and drug use, aggression, and delinquent behaviors among urban middle school students. Development and Psychopathology 18(1):119–137.
32. Wilsnack, S.C., Wilsnack, R.W., Kristjanson, A.F., Vogeltanz-Holm, N.D., and Harris, T.R. 2004. Child sexual abuse and alcohol use among women: Setting the stage

for risky sexual behavior. In From Child Sexual Abuse to Adult Sexual Risk: Trauma, Revictimization, and Intervention, edited by L.J. Koenig, L.S. Doll, A. O'Leary, and W. Pequegnat. Washington, DC: American Psychological Association, pp. 181–200.

33. Windle, M., and Mason, W.A. 2004. General and specific predictors of behavioral and emotional problems among adolescents. Journal of Emotional and Behavioral Disorders 12:49–61.
34. Wood, J., Foy, D.W., Goguen, C.A., Pynoos, R., and James, C.B. 2002. Violence exposure and PTSD among delinquent girls. Journal of Aggression, Maltreatment, and Trauma 6:109–126.

CHAPTER 5

Early Trauma and Increased Risk for Physical Aggression During Adulthood: The Moderating Role of MAOA Genotype

GIOVANNI FRAZZETTO, GIORGIO DI LORENZO, VALERIA CAROLA, LUCA PROIETTI, EWA SOKOLOWSKA, ALBERTO SIRACUSANO, CORNELIUS GROSS, AND ALFONSO TROISI

5.1 INTRODUCTION

Expressions of violent behavior such as aggression are influenced by a complex and dynamic interplay of biological, psychological and social variables. Individual differences in aggressive behavior are at least partly heritable and presumably result from the interaction between genetic and environmental factors [1]. Gene-environment interactions (G×E) refer to genetic differences in susceptibility to particular environmental risk factors. It is well documented that early life environmental risk factors have detrimental effects on the long-term mental health of individuals and increasing evidence suggests that genotype can moderate the capacity of early environmental pathogens to alter risk for mental disorders [2]. In the development of adult antisocial and violent behavior, the environmental factors considered influential include in utero exposure to pathogens and birth complications [3], childhood abuse or neglect [4], [5], and family relationships, home environment, and other social variables [6].

The clearest genetic link to aggressive behavior exists for the monoamine oxidase A (MAOA) gene which plays a key role in the catabolism of monoamines, including dopamine (DA), norepinephrine (NE), and serotonin (5-HT) [7]. MAOA knockout (KO) mice display elevated levels of DA, NE and 5-HT and male KO mice exhibit increased aggressive behavior [8]. Forebrain-restricted transgenic expression of MAOA in MAOA KO mice results in lower levels of DA, NE and 5-HT and in a reversal of the aggressive phenotype, suggesting that lack of enzyme activity in the forebrain of MAOA KO mice underlies their behavioral phenotype [9]. In humans, a missense mutation was found in the MAOA gene (Xp11.23-11.4) in a Dutch kindred whose members exhibited a pattern of impulsively violent behavior for generations [10]. Since MAOA is an X-linked gene [11], hemizygous males from this family effectively represent functional gene knockouts. However, this mutation is extremely rare and has not been found in any other pedigree. More recently, a common variable number tandem repeat (VNTR) polymorphism lying 1.2 kb upstream of the transcription initiation site of MAOA has been shown to affect transcriptional activity of the gene in transfected cells. The 3.5-and 4-repeat forms show high MAOA mRNA expression and high enzyme activity, while the 2-, 3-and 5-repeat forms show low MAOA mRNA expression and low enzyme activity [12], [13].

Recently, a large longitudinal study of children followed for 26 years since birth showed that MAOA VNTR genotype moderates the association between childhood maltreatment and violent and antisocial behavior [14]. Although several studies have replicated this G×E effect [15]–[17], other studies have failed to replicate the original findings reported by Caspi and co-workers [18]–[20]. Explanations for these conflicting findings are manifold, including the use of different measures of the behavioral phenotype and of environmental risk factors. In this work, we studied a mixed population of psychiatric outpatients and healthy volunteers to test the hypothesis that the MAOA VNTR polymorphism moderates the association between early traumatic life events experienced during the first fifteen years of life and the display of physical aggression during adulthood. We found that the risk for displaying physical aggression during adulthood was significantly increased by the combination of low MAOA activity and exposure to early trauma.

5.2 RESULTS

5.2.1 DISTRIBUTION OF ALLELE FREQUENCIES AND POPULATION SUBGROUPS

Because MAOA is an X-linked gene, male subjects were straightforwardly assigned to one of two genotype groups: 1) subjects carrying one low activity allele (2-, 3-or 5-repeat form), and 2) subjects carrying one high activity allele (3.5-or 4-repeat form). Females were assigned to three genotype groups: 1) homozygous subjects carrying two low activity alleles, 2) homozygous subjects carrying two high activity alleles, and 3) heterozygous subjects carrying one low and one high activity allele. Expression studies have demonstrated that in female skin fibroblasts the MAOA gene undergoes X-inactivation and shows mono-allelic expression [21]. Although the extent of X-inactivation in human brain is not known, these findings suggest that heterozygous low-high females are mosaic for different MAOA alleles and are likely to have intermediate enzymatic activity. A functional discrimination analysis showed that in our sample the three female genotypes were indistinguishable by physical aggression scores of the Aggression Questionnaire (Wilk's $\lambda = 0.99$; $F_{2,170} = 0.74$, $P = 0.47$; AQ-PA, see Materials and Methods [22]) and thus, for the purposes of our analysis, we grouped heterozygous female participants together with low-low homozygous females following the convention of a previous study [23]. The low and high enzyme activity groups accounted respectively for 43% and 57% of the total male participants (N = 82) and 54% and 46% of the total female participants (N = 153). Genotype frequencies within the sample did not significantly deviate from those reported for other Caucasian populations ($\chi^2 = 2.51$, df = 4, $P = 0.64$) [12], [14].

Participants were divided into two groups according to self-reported exposure to early traumatic life events: 1) those reporting none, and 2) those reporting one or more traumatic events. Thirty-four percent of the participants experienced at least one traumatic life event between 0 and 15 years of age, with some participants reporting the occurrence of multiple traumatic events (Table 1).

Before assessing the effect of ETLE exposure and MAOA genotype on risk for increased physical aggression, we first tested whether subgroups in our sample differed significantly for the distribution of psychiatric diagnosis, ETLE exposure, and MAOA genotype. Such deviations might confound the interpretation of subsequent findings and reveal the existence of gene-by-environment correlation effects. Men and women did not differ in the distribution of psychiatric diagnosis ($\chi^2 = 0.92$, df = 1, P = 0.34) and exposure to ETLE ($\chi^2 = 0.03$, df = 1, P = 0.87). Compared to healthy controls, exposure to ETLE between 0 and 15 years of age was more frequent among psychiatric patients ($\chi^2 = 3.67$, df = 1, P = 0.05). Importantly, the ETLE groups did not differ significantly in MAOA genotype distribution, arguing against the possibility that genotype influenced exposure to traumatic events ($\chi^2 = 0.21$, df = 1, P = 0.64). Finally, the distribution of MAOA genotype did not differ between the healthy and psychiatric patient groups ($\chi^2 = 0.35$, df = 1, P = 0.56).

Scores on the AQ-PA scale in our sample ranged from 9 to 41 (median: 14.0). The percentage of psychiatric patients included in the subgroup of participants who scored in the top 25% of the score distribution (AQ-PA $\geq$ 19) was higher than that included in the subgroup of participants who scored in the bottom 25% (AQ-PA$\leq$11) (50 vs. 28%, $\chi^2 = 6.41$, df = 1, P<0.01).

5.2.2 EFFECTS OF GENDER, EARLY TRAUMATIC LIFE EVENTS, AND MAOA GENOTYPE ON PHYSICAL AGGRESSION

Effects of gender, ETLE, and MAOA genotype were assessed using an ANOVA model with the AQ-PA score as the dependent variable. Statistical analysis revealed significant main effects of gender ($F_{1,227} = 36.77$, P<0.0001) and ETLE ($F_{1,227} = 27.50$, P<0.0001), but no main effect of MAOA genotype ($F_{1,227} = 0.10$, P = 0.75). As expected, physical aggression scores were higher among males and participants reporting exposure to early traumatic life events. The importance of MAOA genotype

TABLE 1. Number of participants and relative percentage who reported early traumatic life events (ETLE) during the first 15 years of their lives*.

Early Traumatic Life Events	
Death of mother	2 (0.84%)
Long absence of the mother due to illness (>100 days)	9 (3.79%)
Absence of the mother due to adoption	1 (0.42%)
Absence of the mother due to upbringing in a foster home	1 (0.42%)
Long absence of the mother due to upbringing by other family kin or unrelated persons	6 (2.53%)
Long absence of the mother due to divorce or separation of parents	0
Death of the father	11 (4.64%)
Long absence of the father due to illness (>100 days)	4 (1.68%)
Absence of the father due to adoption	1 (0.42%)
Absence of the father due to upbringing in a foster home	0
Long absence of the mother due to upbringing by other family kin or unrelated persons	3 (1.26%)
Long absence of the father due to war service or war imprisonment	0
Long absence due to imprisonment	1 (0.42%)
Long absence of the father due to separation or divorce of parents	8 (3.37%)
Separation from parents due to illness of the proband (>100 days)	1 (0.42%)
Severe physical handicap of the subject during childhood	3 (1.26%)
Severe physical handicap of sibling	11 (4.64%)
Parents' marital problems	62 (26.16%)
Alcohol addiction of one or both parents	22 (9.28%)
Severe psychiatric illness of mother or father (other than alcohol dependence)	13 (5.48%)
Violence in the family	32 (13.50%)
Sexual molestation or abuse	8 (3.37%)

* The sum of percentages is greater than 100 because some participantsreported more than one ETLE.

in modulating the impact of early trauma on adult physical aggression emerged when interaction effects were examined. We found significant MAOA×ETLE ($F_{1,227}$ = 8.20, P = 0.005) and gender×MAOA×ETLE ($F_{1,227}$ = 7.04, P = 0.009) interaction effects. The cumulative variance in the physical aggression score explained by the ANOVA effects involving

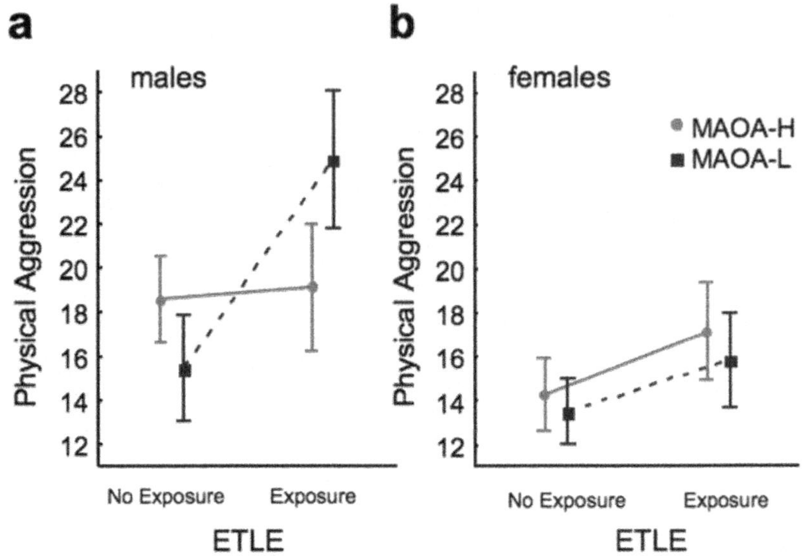

Figure 1. MAOA genotype moderates the association between early traumatic life events and physical aggression. Interactions between gender, MAOA genotype, and early traumatic life events (ETLE) predicted AQ-PA physical aggression scores in (a) males and (b) females. In the male group, carriers of the low, but not the high MAOA activity allele reporting exposure to early traumatic life events showed significantly greater physical aggression scores.

the MAOA allele was 6.6%. Physical aggression scores were higher in men who had experienced early traumatic life events and who carried low MAOA activity alleles (Table 2 and Figure 1).

We repeated the ANOVA in the subgroup of healthy volunteers (N = 145) to exclude that the G×E interactions we found were due to the inclusion of psychiatric patients in our sample and were not generalizable to the population at large. The results for the subgroup of healthy volunteers were identical to those for the entire sample. We found significant main effects of gender ($F_{1,137} = 37.53$, $P<0.0001$) and ETLE ($F_{1,137} = 10.34$, $P = 0.002$), no main effect of MAOA genotype ($F_{1,137} = 0.86$, $P = 0.35$), and

TABLE 2. Descriptive statistics and ANOVA results for physical aggression in the entire sample. η_p^2: partial eta squared.

Gender	ETLE	MAO-A Activity	Mean	N
Females	No Exposure	High	13.65	43
		Low	13.33	58
		Total	13.47	101
	Exposure	High	16.37	27
		Low	16.40	25
		Total	16.38	52
	Total	High	14.70	70
		Low	14.25	83
		Total	14.46	153
Males	No Exposure	High	19.06	33
		Low	15.09	22
		Total	17.47	55
	Exposure	High	20.36	14
		Low	25.69	13
		Total	22.93	27
	Total	High	19.45	47
		Low	19.03	35
		Total	19.27	82
Total	No Exposure	High	16.00	76
		Low	13.81	80
		Total	14.88	156
	Exposure	High	17.73	41
		Low	19.58	38
		Total	18.62	79
	Total	High	16.61	117
		Low	15.67	118
		Total	16.14	235

Effects: Gender: $F_{1,227} = 36.77$, $p<0.0001$, $\eta_p^2 = 0.14$; ETLE: $F_{1,227} = 27.51$, $p<0.0001$, $\eta_p^2 = 0.11$; MAO-A: $F_{1,227} = 0.10$, $p = 0.75$, $\eta_p^2 = 0.00$; Gender Ч ETLE: $F_{1,227} = 3.28$, $p = 0.07$, $\eta_p^2 = 0.01$; Gender Ч MAO-A: $F_{1,227} = 0.24$, $p = 0.62$, $\eta_p^2 = 0.00$; ETLE Ч MAO-A: $F_{1,227} = 8.20$, $p = 0.005$, $\eta_p^2 = 0.04$, Gender Ч ETLE Ч MAO-A: $F_{1,227} = 7.04$, $p = 0.009$, $\eta_p^2 = 0.03$.

significant interaction effects for MAOA×ETLE ($F_{1,137}$ = 10.13, P = 0.002) and for gender×MAOA×ETLE ($F_{1,137}$ = 6.66, P = 0.01). The cumulative variance in the physical aggression score explained by the ANOVA effects involving the MAOA allele was 12.1% (Table 3).

5.3 DISCUSSION

We studied a mixed population of psychiatric outpatients and healthy volunteers in order to examine the gene-environment interaction effect of MAOA genotype and early trauma on the increased risk for self-reported levels of physical aggression during adulthood. We found that levels of physical aggression were significantly higher in men who had experienced traumatic events during the first 15 years of life and who carried the low expression allele (MAOA-L). When we repeated the analysis in the subsample of healthy volunteers, the results did not change. Our results are consistent with the majority of previous reports [14]–[17], [24] and point toward the MAOA genotype as a genetic factor that moderates the impact of early traumatic life events on the developmental pathway leading to later-life aggression.

Based on the findings of several independent studies, the relationship between the MAOA polymorphism and aggression appears to be fairly consistent. Yet, the intervening neural and psychological mechanisms are still unclear. One promising line of research has investigated the possibility that individuals with the low expression allele might be more sensitive to negative social experiences, which might ultimately result in defensively aggressive behavior. A recent fMRI study showed that the MAOA genotype at risk for impulsivity and violent behavior is associated with reduced gray matter volumes in limbic regions such as the amygdala, dorsal anterior cingulated cortex (dACC), and subgenual ACC and greater amygdala and subgenual ACC responsivity to negative emotional faces [25]. Consistent with the social hypersensitivity hypothesis, Eisenberger et al. (2007) have found that, compared to individuals with the high expression allele, healthy men and women with the MAOA-L reported higher trait aggression, higher interpersonal sensitivity and showed greater dorsal anterior cingulated cortex activity (associated with rejection-related distress)

TABLE 3. Descriptive statistics and ANOVA results for physical aggression in the sub-sample of healthy volunteers. η_p^2: partial eta squared.

Gender	ETLE	MAO-A Activity	Mean	N
Females	No Exposure	High	12.46	26
		Low	12.69	36
		Total	12.60	62
	Exposure	High	13.86	14
		Low	15.13	15
		Total	14.52	29
	Total	High	12.95	40
		Low	13.41	51
		Total	13.21	91
Males	No Exposure	High	19.09	22
		Low	14.95	19
		Total	17.17	41
	Exposure	High	17.75	8
		Low	23.60	5
		Total	20.00	13
	Total	High	18.73	30
		Low	16.75	24
		Total	17.85	54
Total	No Exposure	High	15.50	48
		Low	13.47	55
		Total	14.42	103
	Exposure	High	15.27	22
		Low	17.25	20
		Total	16.21	42
	Total	High	15.43	70
		Low	14.48	75
		Total	14.94	145

Effects: Gender: $F_{1,227} = 37.53$, $p<0.0001$, $\eta_p^2 = 0.22$; ETLE: $F_{1,227} = 10.33$, $p = 0.002$, $\eta_p^2 = 0.07$; MAO-A: $F_{1,227} = 0.86$, $p = 0.36$, $\eta_p^2 = 0.01$; Gender Ч ETLE: $F_{1,227} = 1.01$, $p = 0.32$, $\eta_p^2 = 0.01$; Gender Ч MAO-A: $F_{1,227} = 0.00$, $p = 0.96$, $\eta_p^2 = 0.00$; ETLE Ч MAO-A: $F_{1,227} = 10.13$, $p = 0.002$, $\eta_p^2 = 0.07$, Gender Ч ETLE Ч MAO-A: $F_{1,227} = 6.66$, $p = 0.01$, $\eta_p^2 = 0.05$.

in response to social exclusion [26]. If replicated by future studies, these preliminary findings suggest that the MAOA-L would confer a vulnerability to negative social experiences, including early trauma, and a specific proclivity toward reactive aggression, i.e. that type of aggression triggered by exaggerated levels of negative emotion, such as anger and anxiety.

Although recent research has demonstrated that the allele×environment strategy is promising for detecting individual vulnerability to environmental risk, reported associations between gene variants and complex behaviors are in general weak. This is likely to reflect the fact that a number of several alleles contribute in various small ways to the interplay between environmental risk factors and development of complex behaviors. In the case of G×E interactions involving MAOA alleles and predicting antisocial behavior and/or conduct disorder, effect sizes reported to date are small on average. In this regard, the present study is no exception. The cumulative variance in the physical aggression score explained by the ANOVA effects involving the MAOA allele was 6.6% in the entire sample and 12.1% in the sub-sample of healthy volunteers. However, the significant G×E interaction effects found in the present study are remarkable considering its relatively small sample (N = 235) and require a methodological comment.

The questionnaire we used to measure the occurrence of early traumatic life events explored a variety of adverse experiences other than physical and sexual abuse. There is a large body of evidence in the clinical literature demonstrating that childhood attachment-related trauma [27], [28], such as prolonged separation from parents or chronic conflict within the family (which were the most frequently reported events among the participants of our study), and lack of parental warmth [29] can increase the risk for aggressive behavior during adolescence and adulthood. The exclusive or limited focus on physical abuse and maltreatment might in part explain the failure of some previous studies to confirm the role of MAOA genotype in moderating the relationship between early stress and subsequent aggressive behavior [18]–[20].

Another important difference between the present study and previous ones is the measure used to assess the behavioral phenotype. As dependent variable, we used the physical aggression scale of the Aggression Questionnaire [22], a continuous measure that assesses individual propensity toward aggression and that can be administered to individuals in the normative range of aggressive behavior. In contrast, most previous studies have used relatively indirect measures of aggressive behavior, such as incarceration, criminal conviction, or a diagnosis of antisocial behavior or conduct disorder. The problem with these measures is that antisocial behavior or conduct disorder include a number of behaviors other than aggression and that they are dichotomous (presence or absence of the behavioral phenotype), which may lead to a corresponding loss of discriminatory power. Our findings suggest that the use of psychometric tools assessing behavioral aspects of aggression ranging from normative levels to pathological extremes may increase the likelihood of detecting interactions of MAOA genotype with early traumatic events.

This study has several limitations, the first of which is the small sample size. Studies relating genetic polymorphisms to behavioral or self-report assessments typically use much larger samples. Thus, the present results should be interpreted with caution until these findings have been replicated in larger samples. However, the within-study replication in psychiatric patients and healthy volunteers justifies a fairly high level of confidence. Second, we used a retrospective measure to assess the occurrence of traumatic events during childhood. When the type of events assessed is not limited to objective trauma (e.g., death of mother) but also includes perceived situations (e.g., parental marital problems), retrospective data may be subject to faulty recall or systematic distortions, even though the construct validity of our measure of early trauma was supported by its strong association with later-life aggression, in accordance with most other studies related to this topic. Although prospective studies are clearly desirable in delineating the role of early environment in the development of later-life aggressive behavior, such investigations face daunting methodological difficulties. Until such methodological problems can be overcome, reliance will have to be placed on a variety of sources of information, including retrospective data, to study G×E. Third, we used a self-report measure of aggression, and the social desirability bias of some subjects might have affected their self-reporting of aggression. Subjects motivated by need for social approval may not report as much aggression as those to whom social approval is less important. Such a bias, however, probably reduced our ability to detect interaction effects and thus implies that the findings are conservative estimates of G×E. Fourth, we included women in our sample to assess the impact of gender on the MAOA-early trauma interaction. Few studies investigating MAOA-related aggression have included female subjects [25], [26]. Inclusion of women in such studies is complicated by the fact that somatic MAOA allele mosaicism, due to X-chromosome inactivation, makes classification of heterozygous females problematic. Previous research has shown that female heterozygotes show patterns of neural activity intermediate between MAOA-L and MAOA-H male hemizygotes and that female homozygotes show patterns of neural activity comparable to male hemizygotes [25]. Because, in our sample physical aggression scores were indistinguishable among the three female genotypes, we were not able to draw conclusions about the status of heterozygous female subjects.

In conclusion, despite its limitations, this study supports and extends the findings of previous reports showing that the MAOA polymorphism in combination with early experience modulates individual proclivity to later-life physical aggression. Its major methodological contribution is that the use of continuous self-report measures of aggression ranging from normative levels to pathological extremes and a wider focus in assessing early trauma may increase the likelihood of detecting interactions between the MAOA gene and childhood environment.

5.4 MATERIALS AND METHODS

5.4.1 POPULATION SAMPLE AND RECRUITMENT

The population sample of this study consisted of 90 outpatients (69% women; mean±SD age: 32.18±8.66 years) consecutively admitted to the day hospital of the psychiatric clinic at the University of Rome Tor Vergata and 145 healthy volunteers (63% women; mean±SD age: 29.59±6.73 years). All participants were of Caucasian origin. Diagnostic assessment was made by experienced clinical psychiatrists using the Structured Clinical Interview for DSM-IV Axis I Disorders (SCID-CV) [30] and the Schedule for Interviewing DSM-IV Personality Disorders-IV (SIDP-IV) [31]. Patients with medical or neurological disorders, mental retardation, or psychotic disorders were excluded from the sample. The diagnostic composition of the clinical group was as follows: anxiety disorders, 28%; major depressive disorder, 27%; eating disorders, 21%; cluster B personality disorders, 13%; bipolar disorder, 11%. All patients were interviewed when they had partially improved and reached the drug treatment dosage prescribed for maintenance therapy. Healthy volunteers were recruited among students in the medical school, paramedic staff members, and conscripts of the Italian army. Inclusion in the control group required the absence of current or past psychiatric disorders, as confirmed by diagnostic interview.

All data were obtained under informed consent and using procedures and protocols approved by the University of Rome Tor Vergata Intramural Ethics Committee and the EMBL Bioethics Internal Advisory Committee (BIAC).

5.4.2 DNA EXTRACTION AND GENOTYPING

For all participants DNA was obtained from buccal samples [32] and DNA was extracted using standard procedures. PCR was carried out using the following conditions: initial 5-min denaturing step at 95.0 C, followed by 35 cycles at 94.0 C for 1 min, 53.8 C for 1 min and 72.0 C for 1 min 30 s, and a final extension phase at 72.0 C for 10 min. Primer sequences were those described by Sabol et al. (1998): MAO-F (5′-ACAGCCTGACCGTGGAGAAG-3′) and MAO-R (5′-GAACGGACGCTCCATTCGGA-3′). Reactions were performed in 25 μl total volume with 50 ng genomic DNA, 1.5 mM $MgCl_2$, 10 pmoles of each primer, 0.33 mM dNTPs, and 1.5 U of native Taq (Promega, Madison, WI). PCR products were assayed on a 3% agarose gel. The primers used yielded 290, 320, 335, 350 and 380 bp fragments corresponding to the 2-, 3-, 3.5-, 4-and 5-repeat alleles, respectively [12].

5.4.3 ASSESSMENT OF PHYSICAL AGGRESSION

On the same day when DNA was collected, each subject completed the Aggression Questionnaire (AQ) [22]. AQ is a 29-item scale divided into four subscales: physical aggression (9 items), verbal aggression (5 items), anger (7 items), and hostility (8 items). Each statement was assessed by a five-point Likert scale (from 1 = never or hardly ever applies to me, to 5 = very often applies to me). Two items were reverse scored. In addition to the scores on each subscale, a total score was also calculated. AQ measures aggressive attitudes that are consistent across an extended time frame and characterological in nature, and is therefore considered a trait measure of aggression [33]. AQ is related to other self-report measures of aggression as well as behavioral indicators of aggression. The AQ subscales have high levels of internal consistency and moderate to high levels of test-retest reliability [34]. In the present study, data analysis was based on the physical aggression (AQ-PA) subscale. Statements rating AQ-PA included: "I have become so mad that I have broken things", "Once in a while I can't control the urge to strike another person", "Given enough provocation, I may hit another person" and "If somebody hits me, I hit back".

5.4.4 ASSESSMENT OF EARLY TRAUMATIC LIFE EVENTS

The occurrence of traumatic life events during childhood was assessed using a questionnaire developed by Bandelow et al. [35] to measure exposure to a variety of adverse early experiences including: separation from father/mother due to death or long absence (>100 days) associated with illness, adoption, or separation or divorce of parents; occurrence of severe handicap in the subject or subject's siblings; severe parental marital problems; parental mental illness, alcoholism, or violence in the family (including physical abuse of the subject); and sexual abuse of the subject. Prevalence of early traumatic life events (ETLE) occurring between 0 and 15 years of age was recorded (Table 1).

5.4.5 STATISTICAL ANALYSIS

Functional discrimination analysis was used to detect differences in levels of physical aggression among genotype groups of female participants.

Chi-square tests were used to test differences between categorical variables. Main and interaction effects of gender, ETLE, and MAOA genotype on the physical aggression score were calculated by using three-way analysis of variance (ANOVA). All statistical analyses were carried out with the help of Statistica (StatSoft, Tulsa, OK) and SPSS (SPSS, Chicago, IL) software.

REFERENCES

1. Lesch KP,Merschdorf U (2000) Impulsivity, aggression, and serotonin: a molecular psychobiological perspective. Behav Sci Law 18: 581–604.
2. Moffitt T,Caspi A (2005) Strategy for Investigating Interactions Between Measured Genes and Measured Environments. Arch Gen Psychiatry 62: 473–481.
3. Raine A,Brennan P,Mednick SA (1997) Interaction between birth complications and early maternal rejection in predisposing individuals to adult violence: specificity to serious, early-onset violence. Am J Psychiatry 154: 1265–1271.
4. Luntz BK,Widom CS (1994) Antisocial personality disorder in abused and neglected children grown up. Am J Psychiatry 151: 670–674.
5. Johnson JG,Cohen P,Brown J,Smailes EM,Bernstein DP (1999) Childhood maltreatment increases risk for personality disorders during early adulthood. Arch Gen Psychiatry 56: 600–606.
6. Raine A,Brennan P,Mednick B,Mednick SA (1996) High rates of violence, crime, academic problems, and behavioral problems in males with both early neuromotor deficits and unstable family environments. Arch Gen Psychiatry 53: 544–549.
7. Shih JC,Chen K,Ridd MU (1999) Monoamine oxidase: From genes to behavior. Annu Rev Neurosci 22: 197–212.
8. Cases O,Seif I,Grimsby J,Gaspar P,Chen K,et al. (1995) Aggressive behavior and altered amounts of brain serotonin and norepinephrine in mice lacking MAOA. Science 268: 1763–1766.
9. Chen K,Cases O,Rebrin I,Wu W,Gallaher TK,et al. (2006) Forebrain specific expression of monoamine oxidase A reduces neurotransmitter levels, restores the brain structure and rescues aggressive behavior in monoamine oxidase A deficient mice. J Biol Chem 282: 115–123.
10. Brunner HG,Nelen M,Breakefield XO,Ropers HH,van Oost BA (1993) Abnormal behavior associated with a point mutation in the structural gene for monoamine oxidase A. Science 262: 578–580.
11. Levy ER,Powell JF,Buckle VJ,Hsu YP,Breakefield XO,et al. (1989) Localisation of human monamine oxidase-A gene to Xp11.23-11.4 by in situ hypbridisation: implications for Norrie disease. Genomics 5: 368–370.
12. Sabol S,Hu S,Hamer D (1998) A functional polymorphism in the monamine oxidase A gene promoter. Hum Genet 103: 273–279.

13. Deckert J,Catalano M,Syagailo YV,Bosi M,Okladnova O,et al. (1999) Excess of high activity monoamine oxidase A gene promoter alleles in female patients with panic disorder. Hum Mol Genet 8: 621–624.
14. Caspi A,McClay J,Moffitt TE,Mill J,Martin J,et al. (2002) Role of genotype in the cycle of violence in maltreated children. Science 297: 851–854.
15. Nilsson KW,Sjoeberg RL,Damberg M,Leppert J,Oerhvik J,et al. (2005) Role of Monoamine Oxidase A Genotype and Psychosocial Factors in Male Adolescent Criminal Activity. Biol Psychiatry 59: 121–127.
16. Foley D,Eaves LJ,Wornley B,Silberg JL,Maes HH,et al. (2004) Childhood adversity, monoamine oxidase A genotype, and risk for conduct disorder. Arch Gen Psychiatry 61: 738–744.
17. Kim-Cohen J,Caspi A,Taylor A,Williams B,Newcombe R,et al. (2006) MAOA, maltreatment and gene-environment interaction predicting children's mental health: new evidence and a meta-analysis. Mol Psychiatry 11: 903–913.
18. Haberstick BC,Lessem JM,Hopfer CJ,Smolen A,Ehringer MA,et al. (2005) Monoamine oxidase A (MAOA) and antisocial behaviors in the presence of childhood and adolescent maltreatment. Am J Med Genet B Neuropsychiatr Genet 135: 59–64.
19. Young SE,Smolen A,Hewitt JK,Haberstick BC,Stalings MC,et al. (2006) Interaction between MAO-A genotype and maltreatment in the risk for conduct disorder: failure to confirm in adolescent patients. Am J Psychiatry 163: 1019–1025.
20. Huizinga D,Haberstick BC,Smolen A,Menard S,Young SE,et al. (2006) Childhood maltreatment, subsequent antisocial behavior, and the role of monoamine oxidase A genotype. Biol Psychiatry 60: 677–683.
21. Nordquist N,Oreland L (2006) Monoallelic expression of MAOA in skin fibroblasts. Biochem Biophys Res Commun 348: 763–767.
22. Buss AH,Perry M (1992) The aggression questionnaire. J Pers Soc Psychol 63: 452–459.
23. Fan J,Fossella J,Sommer T,Wu Y,Posner MI (2003) Mapping the genetic variation of executive attention onto brain activity. Proc Natl Acad Sci U S A 100: 7406–7411.
24. Reif A,Roesler M,Freitag CM,Schneider M,Eujen A,et al. (2007) Nature and nurture predispose to violent behavior: serotonergic genes and adverse childhood environment. Neuropsychopharmacology In Press.
25. Meyer-Lindenberg A,Buckholtz JW,Kolachana B,Hariri A,Pezawas L,Blasi G,et al. (2006) Neural mechanisms of genetic risk for impulsivity and violence in humans. Proc Natl Acad Sci USA 103: 6269–6274.
26. Eisenberger N,Way BM,Taylor SE,Welch WT,Lieberman MD (2007) Understanding Genetic Risk for Aggression: Clues from the Brain's Response to Social Exclusion. Biol Psychiatry 61: 1100–1108.
27. Renn P (2002) The link between childhood trauma and later violent offending: the application of attachment theory in a probation setting. Attach Hum Dev 4: 294–317.
28. Troisi A,D'Argenio A (2004) The relationship between anger and depression in a clinical sample of young men: the role of insecure attachment. J Affect Disorders 79: 269–272.
29. Feinberg M,Button TM,Neiderhiser JM,Reiss D,Hetherington M (2007) Parenting and Adolescent Antisocial Behavior and Depression. Arch Gen Psychiatry 64: 457–465.

30. First MB,spitzer RL,Gibbon M,et al. (1997) Structured Clinical Interview for DSM-IV Axis I Disorders-Clinician Version. Washington DC: American Psychiatric Association.
31. Pfohl B,Blum N,Zimmerman M (1995) Structured Interview for DSM-IV Personality Disorders SIDP-IV. Iowa City, , Iowa: Department of Psychiatry, University of Iowa.
32. Freeman B,Smith N,Curtis C,Huckett L,Mill J,et al. (2003) DNA from buccal swabs recruited by mail: evaluation of storage effects on long term stability and suitability for multiplex polymerase chain reaction genotyping Behav Genet 33: 67–72.
33. Suris A,Lind L,Emmet G,Bormann PD,Kashner M,et al. (2004) Measures of Aggressive Behavior: Overview of clinical and research instruments. Aggress Violent Beh 9: 165–227.
34. Harris JA (1997) A further evaluation of the Aggression Questionnaire: issues of validity and reliability. Behav Res Ther 35: 1047–1053.
35. Bandelow B,Spaeth C,Tichauer GA,Broocks A,Hajak G,et al. (2002) Early traumatic life events, parental attitudes, family history and birth risk factors in patients with panic disorder. Compr Psychiat 43: 269–278.

PART II

EFFECTS OF EARLY TRAUMA ON HEALTH BEHAVIORS AND MENTAL HEALTH

CHAPTER 6

Lessons Learned from Child Sexual Abuse Research: Prevalence, Outcomes, and Preventive Strategies (continued)

DELPHINE COLLIN-VÉZINA, ISABELLE DAIGNEAULT, AND MARTINE HÉBERT

6.1 MENTAL HEALTH OUTCOMES: WHAT ARE THE EFFECTS OF CSA?

Several models have been developed in an attempt to explain the adverse negative impact of CSA [36]. Among the most established conceptual frameworks on the impact of CSA is the Four-Factor Traumagenics Model [37]. This model suggests that CSA alters a child's cognitive and emotional orientation to the world and causes trauma by distorting their self-concept and affective capacities. This model underscores the issues of trust and intimacy that are particularly pronounced among victims of CSA. The unique nature of CSA as a form of maltreatment is highlighted by the four trauma-causing factors that victims may experience, which are traumatic sexualization, betrayal, powerlessness, and stigmatization. Traumatic sexualization refers to the sexuality of the victims that is shaped and distorted by the sexual abuse. Betrayal is the loss of trust in the perpetrator who shattered the relationship and in other adults who are perceived as not having protected the child from being abused in the first place, or having not supported her upon disclosure. Powerlessness is experienced through power issues at play in CSA, where victims are unable to alter the situation despite feeling the threat of harm and the violation of their personal space. Stigmatization is the incorporation of perceptions, reinforced by the perpetrator's manipulative discourse or by dominant social negative attitudes towards victims, of being bad or deserving and responsible for the abuse.

Several reviews and meta-analyses published in the 90s and early years of 2000 suggested that a wide range of psychological and behavioral disturbances were associated with the experience of CSA, which led experts in the field to conclude that CSA was a substantial risk factor in the development of a host of negative consequences in both childhood, adolescence and adulthood [38-41]. More recently, systematic reviews have confirmed that, given the vast array of etiological factors that interact in predicting mental health outcomes, CSA is considered a significant, though general and nonspecific, risk factor for psychopathology in children and adolescents [42-44].

Among the wealth of psychopathologies that have been studied among CSA victims, post-traumatic stress and dissociation symptoms have received great attention. Overall, victims have been shown to present significantly more of these symptoms than non-abused children, or than victims of other forms of trauma. In one of our studies that compared 67 sexually abused school-aged girls with a matched group, CSA was found to significantly increase the odds of presenting with a clinical level of dissociation and PTSD symptoms, respectively, by eightfold and fourfold [45]. These results have echoed previous research conducted among cohorts of sexually abused school-aged children and teenagers where about a third to a half of all victims showed clinical levels of post-traumatic stress symptoms [46-50]. Only a few studies have been conducted with younger cohorts of children, yet high levels of dissociation were documented among sexually abused preschoolers [51,52]. In that vein, results from one of our recent inquiries revealed higher frequencies of dissociative symptoms among a group of 76 sexually abused children aged 4 to 6 than children of the comparison group [53]. These symptoms were found to persist over a period of a year following disclosure [54]. In contrast to children who have experienced other forms of trauma, it was also found that CSA victims are more likely to present post-traumatic stress symptoms [55]. Using a prospective method in which sexually abused children were followed over 36 months, Maikovich, Koenen, and Jaffe [25] demonstrated that boys were as likely as girls to exhibit post-traumatic stress symptoms.

Aside from post-traumatic stress and dissociation symptoms, a significant number of other mental health and behavioral disturbances have been linked to CSA. High levels of mood disorders, such as major depressive episodes, are found in cohorts of children and teenagers who have been sexually abused [56,57]. Sexually abused children are more likely than their non-abused counterparts to present behavior problems, such as inappropriate sexualized behaviors [58]. In the teenage years, they are found to more often exhibit conduct problems [59] and engage in at-risk sexual behaviors [60,61]. Victims are more prone to abusing substances, to engaging in self-harm behaviors, and to attempting or committing suicide [62-65]. Adolescents sexually abused in childhood are five times more likely to report non-clinical psychotic experiences such as delusions and hallucinations than their non-abused counterparts [66].

The mental health outcomes of CSA victims are likely to continue into adulthood as the link of CSA to lifetime psychopathology has been demonstrated [67-72]. Even more worrisome is the fact that CSA victims are more at risk than non-CSA youth to experience violence in their early romantic relationships [73,74] and that they are 2–5 times more at risk of being sexually revictimized in adulthood than women not sexually abused in childhood [75-77]. In adulthood, CSA survivors are more likely to experience difficulties in their psychosexual functioning [78,79]. A 23-year longitudinal study of the impact of intrafamilial sexual abuse on female development confirmed the deleterious impact of CSA across stages of life, including all of the mental health issues mentioned above, but also hypothalamic–pituitary–adrenal attenuation in victims, as well as asymmetrical stress responses, high rates of obesity, and healthcare utilization [80]. The impact of CSA as a predictor of major illnesses is garnering increasing attention, including gastrointestinal disorders, gynecologic or reproductive health problems, pain, cardiopulmonary symptoms, and diabetes [81-83]. In all cases, early assessment and intervention to offset the exacerbation and continuation of negative outcomes is highlighted, according to several studies [84], as symptoms can develop at a later age [3] or may not be apparent at first [85].

Indeed, despite overwhelming evidence of deleterious outcomes of CSA, it is commonly agreed that the impact of CSA is highly variable and that a significant portion of victims do not exhibit clinical levels of symptoms [86]. Some authors have suggested that about a third of victims may not manifest any clinical symptoms at the time the abuse is disclosed [87]. This can be explained, in part, by the extremely diverse characteristics of CSA which lead to a wide range of potential outcomes [86]. Other common reasons thought to account for asymptomatic survivors of sexual abuse include: (1) insufficient severity of abuse, (2) the fact that symptoms may not be detected by practitioners, (3) development of avoidant coping styles that mask victims' distress, (4) or that asymptomatic survivors may be more resilient than the survivors who show symptoms [88]. Related to this latter explanation, among an array of variables potentially influencing the resilience capacities of CSA victims, children who receive support from their non-offending parents [89] and those who have not experienced prior abuse [90] seem to fare better in spite of the sexual abuse adversity. Among other personal and relational factors that promote resilience in victims are: less reliance on avoidant coping strategies to deal with the traumatic event [91-93], higher emotional self-control [94], interpersonal trust and feelings of empowerment [85], less personal attributions of blame and of stigmatization [95,96], and high family functioning and secure attachment relationships [97,98]. This scholarship points to the importance of using a broad ecological framework when researching and intervening on the factors that promote resilience in victims of CSA [88].

Three promising lines of research have recently emerged that shed new light on the relationships between CSA and psychopathology. First, results from the growing field of polyvictimization, which is the study of the impact of multiple types of victimization (from peers, family, crime, community violence, physical assaults, and sexual assaults), call for a de-compartmentalization of violence research by pointing out that cumulative experiences of victimizations are more detrimental to the child's well-being than are any single experiences, including those of a sexual nature [99]. This suggests that measuring the impact of all forms of victimization alongside CSA is warranted in order to fully capture the influence of violence and abuse on the development of children and youth mental health outcomes. Second, recognizing the great diversity of symptom presentations in sexually abused cohorts, several scholars have attempted to identify the different profiles or sub-categories of victims. For example, Trickett and colleagues [100] found distinct profiles in their sample of girls sexually abused by family members, including victims of multiple perpetrators, characterized by significantly higher levels of dissociation, and victims of father-daughter incest who presented higher levels of disturbances across domains, including internalized (e.g. depression) and externalized (e.g. delinquency) behaviors. Hébert and colleagues [101] further contributed to this scholarship by identifying four different profiles among a sample of sexually abused children: (1) the chronically abused children displaying anxiety symptoms, (2) the severely abused children presenting a host of both internalized and externalized problems, (3) the less severely abused children displaying fewer symptoms, (4) and the less severely impaired children despite severe experiences of CSA, which the authors referred to as the resilient group. As a whole, these studies call for a better tailoring of the services offered to sexually abused children, so that services can well match the mental health needs of victims [102]. Third, drawing from epigenetics [103], cutting-edge inquiries are developing in CSA research on the interaction of CSA with other environmental factors and with genetic factors to predict mental health and behavioral outcomes, for example, violent behavior [104], or suicidal gesture [105]. These inquiries confirm the relevance of studying the psychobiology of child maltreatment [106] as a promising route to better our understanding of the unique contribution of CSA to mental health disturbances, relative to other factors, as well as of the complex nature of the interactions at play. This knowledge could eventually benefit the elaboration of effective intervention programs.

REFERENCES

36. Freeman KA, Morris TL: A review of conceptual models explaining the effects of child sexual abuse. Aggress Violent Beh 2001, 6:357–373.
37. Finkelhor D, Browne A: The traumatic impact of child sexual abuse: A Conceptualization. J Orthopsychiat 1985, 55:530–541.
38. Jumper SA: A meta-analysis of the relationship of child sexual abuse to adult psychological adjustment. Child Abuse Negl 1995, 19:715–728.

39. Neumann DA: Houskamp, BM, Pollock, VE, Briere, J: The long-term sequelae of childhood sexual abuse in women: A meta-analytic review. Child Maltreat 1996, 1:6–16.
40. Paolucci EO, Genuis ML, Violato C: A meta-analysis of the published research on the effects of child sexual abuse. J Psychol 2001, 135:17–36.
41. Tyler KA: Social and emotional outcomes of childhood sexual abuse: A review of recent research. Aggress Violent Beh 2002, 7:567–589.
42. Hillberg T, Hamilton-Giachritsis C, Dixon L: Review of meta-analyses on the association between child sexual abuse and adult mental health difficulties: A systematic approach. Trauma Violence Abuse 2011, 12:38–49.
43. Managlio R: Child sexual abuse in the etiology of anxiety disorders: A systematic review of reviews. Trauma Violence Abuse 2013, 14:96–112.
44 McMahon SD, Grant KE, Compas BE, Thurm AE, Ey S: Stress and psychopathology in children and adolescents: Is there evidence of specificity. J Child Psychol Psychiatry 2003, 44:107–133.
45. Collin-Vézina D, Hébert M: Comparing dissociation and PTSD in sexually abused school-aged girls. Journal of Nervous Mental Disorders 2005, 193:47–52.
46. Ackerman PT, Newton JEO, McPherson WB, Jones JG, Dykman RA: Prevalence of post-traumatic stress disorder and other psychiatric diagnoses in three groups of abused children (sexual, physical, and both). Child Abuse Negl 1998, 22:759–774.
47. Boney-McCoy S, Finkelhor D: Prior victimization: A risk factor for child sexual abuse and for PTSD-related symptomatology among sexually abused youth. Child Abuse Negl 1995, 19:1401–1421.
48. Tremblay C, Hébert M, Piche C: Type I and type II posttraumatic stress disorder in sexually abused children. J Child Sex Abus 2000, 9:65–90.
49. Wolfe DA, Sas L, Wekerle C: Factors associated with the development of post-traumatic stress disorder among child victims of sexual abuse. Child Abuse Negl 1994, 18:37–50.
50. Daigneault I, Tourigny M, Cyr M: Description of trauma and resilience in sexually abused adolescents: An integrated assessment. Journal of Trauma Practice 2004, 3:23–47.
51. Macfie J, Cicchetti D, Toth SL: The development of dissociation in maltreated preschool-aged children. Developmental Psychopathology 2001, 13:233–254.
52. Macfie J, Cicchetti D, Toth SL: Dissociation in maltreated versus nonmaltreated preschool-aged children. Child Abuse Negl 2001, 25:1253–1267.
53. Bernier MJ, Hébert M, Collin-Vézina D: Symptômes de dissociation chez les enfants d'âge préscolaire ayant dévoilé une agression sexuelle. J Int de Victimologie 2011, 26:318–332.
54. Bernier MJ, Hébert M, Collin-Vézina D: Dissociative symptoms over a year in a sample of sexually abused children. Journal of Trauma and Dissociation 2013, 14:455–472.
55. Berliner L: Child sexual abuse: Definitions, prevalence, and consequences. In The APSAC Handbook on Child Maltreatment. Thousand Oaks (CA): SAGE Publications; 2011:215–232.
56. Pollio E, Deblinger E, Runyon M: Mental health treatment for the effects of child sexual abuse. In The APSAC Handbook on Child Maltreatment. Thousand Oaks (CA): SAGE Publications; 2011:267–288.

57. Sadowski H, Trowell J, Kolvin I, Weeramanthri T, Berelowitz M, Gilbert LH: Sexually abused girls: Patterns of psychopathology and exploration of risk factors. Eur Child Adolesc Psychiatry 2003, 12:221–230.
58. Friedrich WN, Davies W, Fehrer E, Wright J: Sexual behavior problems in preteen children: Developmental, ecological, and behavioral correlates. Ann NY Acad Sci 2004, 989:95–104.
59. Danielson CK, Macdonald A, Amstadter AB, Hanson R, de Arellano MA, Saunders BE, Kilpatrick DG: Risky behaviors and depression in conjunction with—or in the absence of—lifetime history of PTSD among sexually abused adolescents. Child Maltreat 2010, 15:101–107.
60. Houck CD, Nugent NR, Lescano CM, Peters A, Brown LK: Sexual abuse and sexual risk behavior: Beyond the impact of psychiatric problems. J Pediatr Psychol 2010, 35:473–483.
61. Lalor K, McElvaney R: Child sexual abuse, links to later sexual exploitation/ high-risk sexual behavior, and prevention/treatment programs. Trauma Violence Abuse 2010, 11:159–177.
62. Brezo J, Paris J, Tremblay R, Vitaro F, Hébert M, Turecki G: Identifying correlates of suicide attempts in suicidal ideators: A population-based study. Psychological Medicine: A Journal of Research in Psychiatry and the Allied Sciences 2007, 31:1551–1562.
63. Kilpatrick DG, Acierno R, Saunders B, Resnick HS, Best CL, Schnurr PP: Risk factors for adolescent substance abuse and dependence: Data from a national sample. J Consult Clin Psychol 2000, 68:19–30.
64. Wright J, Friedrich WN, Cinq-Mars C, Cyr M, McDuff P: Self-destructive and delinquent behaviors of adolescent female victims of child sexual abuse: Rates and covariates in clinical and nonclinical samples. Violence Vict 2004, 19:627–643.
65. Shin SH, Edwards EM, Heeren T: Child abuse and neglect: Relations to adolescent binge drinking in the National Longitudinal Study of Adolescent Health (AddHealth) Study. Addiction Behaviors 2010, 34:277–280.
66. Lataster T, van Os J, Drukker M, Henquet C, Feron F, Gunther N, MyinGermeys I: Childhood victimisation and developmental expression of non-clinical delusional ideation and hallucinatory experiences: victimisation and non-clinical psychotic experiences. Soc Psychiatry Psychiatr Epidemiol 2006, 41:423–428.
67. Cutajar MC, Mullen PE, Ogloff JRP, Thomas SD, Wells DL, Spataro J: Psychopathology in a large cohort of sexually abused children followed up to 43 years. Child Abuse Negl 2010, 34:813–822.
68. Fergusson DM, Boden JM, Horwood LJ: Exposure to childhood sexual and physical abuse and adjustment in early adulthood. Child Abuse Negl 2008, 32:607–619.
69. Kendler KS, Bulik CM, Silberg J, Hettema JM, Myers J, Prescott CA: Childhood sexual abuse and adult psychiatric and substance abuse disorders in women: An epidemiological and co-twin control analysis. Archive of General Psychiatry 2000, 57:953–959.
70. MacMillan HL, Fleming JE, Streiner DL, Lin E, Boyle MH, Jamieson E, Duki EK, Walsh CA, Wong MY, Beardslee WR: Childhood abuse and lifetime psychopathology in a community sample. Am J Psychiatry 2001, 158:1878–1883.
71. Spataro J, Mullen PE, Burgess PM, Wells DL, Moss SA: Impact of child sexual abuse on mental health: Prospective study in males and females. Br J Psychiatry 2004, 184:416–421.

72. Bebbington P, Jonas S, Kuipers E, King M, Cooper C, Brugha T, Meltzer H, McManus S, Jenkins R: Childhood sexual abuse and psychosis: Data from a cross-sectional national psychiatric survey in England. Br J Psychiatry 2011, 199:29–37.
73. Vezina J, Hébert M: Risk factors for victimization in romantic relationships of young women: a review of empirical studies and implications for prevention. Trauma Violence Abuse 2007, 8:33–66.
74. Hébert M, Lavoie F, Vitaro F, McDuff P, Tremblay RE: Association of child sexual abuse and dating victimization with mental health disorder in a sample of female adolescents. J Trauma Stress 2008, 21:181–189.
75. Classen CC, Palesh OG, Aggarwal R: Sexual revictimization: A review of the empirical literature. Trauma Violence Abuse 2005, 6:103–129.
76. Noll JG, Horowitz LA, Bonanno GA, Trickett PK, Putnam FW: Revictimization and self-harm in females who experienced childhood sexual abuse. J Interpers Violence 2003, 18:1452–1471.
77. Daigneault I, Hébert M, McDuff P: Men's and women's childhood sexual abuse and victimization in adult partner relationships: A study of risk factors. Child Abuse Negl 2009, 33:638–647.
78. Meston C, Rellini A, Heiman J: Women's history of sexual abuse, their sexuality, and sexual self-schemas. J Consult Clin Psychol 2006, 74:229–236.
79. Easton SD, Coohey C, O'Leary P, Zhang Y, Hua L: The effect of childhood sexual abuse on psychosexual functioning during adulthood. J Fam Violence 2011, 26:47–50.
80. Trickett PK, Noll JG, Putnam FW: The impact of sexual abuse on female development: Lessons from a multigenerational longitudinal research study. Dev Psychopathol 2011, 23:453–476.
81. Irish L, Kobayashi I, Delahanty DL: Long-term physical health consequences of childhood sexual abuse: a meta-analytic review. J Pediatr Psychol 2010, 35:50–461.
82. Lacelle C, Hébert M, Lavoie F, Vitaro F, Tremblay RE: Sexual health in women reporting a history of child sexual abuse. Child Abuse Negl 2012, 36:247–259.
83. Rich-Edwards JW, Spiegelman D: Lividoti Hibert EN, Jun HJ, Todd TJ, Kawachi I, Wright RJ: Abuse in childhood and adolescence as a predictor of type 2 diabetes in adult women. Am J Prev Med 2010, 39:529–536.
84. Briere J, Elliott DM: Immediate and long-term impacts of child sexual abuse. Future Child 1994, 4:54–69.
85. Daigneault I, Hébert M, Tourigny M: Personal and interpersonal characteristics related to resilient developmental pathways of sexually abused adolescents. Child Adolesc Psychiatr Clin N Am 2007, 16:415–434.
86. Saywitz KJ, Mannarino AP, Berliner L, Cohen JA: Treatment for sexually abused children and adolescents. Am Psychol 2000, 55:1040–1049. Kendall-Tackett K, Meyer-Williams L, Finkelhor D: Impact of sexual abuse on children: A review and synthesis of recent empirical studies. Psychol Bull 1993, 113:164–180.
88. Williams J, Nelson-Gardell D: Predicting resilience in sexually abused adolescents. Child Abuse Negl 2012, 36:53–63.
89. Elliott AN, Carnes CN: Reactions of nonoffending parents to the sexual abuse of their child: a review of the literature. Child Maltreat 2001, 6:314–341.
90. Hébert M, Collin-Vézina D, Daigneault I, Parent N, Tremblay C: Factors linked to outcomes in sexually abused girls: a regression tree analysis. Compr Psychiatry 2006, 47:443–455.

91. Bal S, Van Oost P, De Bourdeaudhuij I, Crombez G: Avoidant coping as a mediator between self-reported sexual abuse and stress-related symptoms in adolescents. Child Abuse Negl 2003, 27:883–897.
92. Banyard VL: Explaining the link between sexual abuse and psychological distress: Identifying mediating processes. Child Abuse Negl 2003, 27:869–875.
93. Tremblay C, Hébert M, Piché C: Coping strategies and social support as mediators of consequences in child sexual abuse victims. Child Abuse Negl 1999, 23:929–945.
94 Kassis W, Artz S, Scambor C, Scambor E, Moldenhauer S: Finding the way out: A non-dichotomous understanding of violence and depression resilience of adolescents who are exposed to family violence. Child Abuse Negl 2012, 37:181–199.
95. Daigneault I, Hébert M, Tourigny M: Attributions and coping in sexually abused adolescents referred for group treatment. J Child Sex Abus 2006, 15:35–59.
96. Feiring C, Miller-Johnson S, Cleland CM: Potential pathways from stigmatization and internalizing symptoms to delinquency in sexually abused youth. Child Maltreat 2007, 12:220–232.
97. Bal S, De Bourdeaudhuij I, Crombez G, Van Oost P: Differences in trauma symptoms and family functioning in intra- and extrafamilial sexually abused adolescents. J Interpers Violence 2004, 19:108–123.
98. Beaudoin G, Hébert M, Bernier A: Contribution of attachment security to the prediction of internalizing and externalizing behavior problems in preschoolers victims of sexual abuse. Revue Européenne de Psychologie Appliquée 2013, 63:147–157.
99. Finkelhor D, Ormrod RK, Turner HA: Poly-victimization: A neglected component in child victimization. Child Abuse Negl 2007, 31:7–26.
100. Trickett PK, Noll JG, Reiffman A, Putnam FW: Variants of intrafamilial sexual abuse experience: Implications for short- and long-term development. Dev Psychopathol 2001, 13:1001–1019.
101. Hébert M, Parent N, Daignault I, Tourigny M: Typological analysis of behavioral profiles of sexually abused children. Child Maltreat 2006, 11:203–216.
102. McCrae JS, Chapman MV, Christ SL: Profile of children investigated for sexual abuse: Association with psychopathology symptoms and services. Am J Orthopsychiatry 2006, 76:468–481.
103. McGowan PO, Szyf M: The epigenetics of social adversity in early life: Implications for mental health outcomes. Neurobiol Dis 2010, 30:66–72.
104. Beaver KM: The interaction between genetic risk and childhood sexual abuse in the prediction of adolescent violent behavior. Sexual Abuse: A Journal or Research and Treatment 2008, 20:426–443.
105. Roy A, Hodgkinson CA, DeLuca V, Goldman D, Enoch MA: Two HPA axis genes, CRHBP and FKBP5, interact with childhood trauma to increase the risk for suicidal behavior. J Psychiatr Res 2012, 46:72–79.
106. De Bellis MD, Putnam FW: The psychobiology of childhood maltreatment.Child Adolesc Psychiatr Clin N Am 1994, 3:663–677.

This article is continued on page 315.

CHAPTER 7

Interpersonal Trauma Exposure and Cognitive Development in Children to Age 8 Years: A Longitudinal Study

MICHELLE BOSQUET ENLOW, BYRON EGELAND, EMILY A. BLOOD, ROBERT O. WRIGHT, AND ROSALIND J. WRIGHT

7.1 INTRODUCTION

Childhood exposure to traumatic events has significant effects on long-term cognitive development, as evidenced by negative associations with intelligence quotient (IQ) scores, language development and academic achievement. [1, 3] The impact of timing of exposure is not well understood, though current knowledge regarding brain development suggests that the type, magnitude and persistence of effects depends on when in development exposure occurs. [1, 4] In early development, particularly from birth to age 2 years, the brain undergoes rapid growth and reorganisation, a process heavily influenced by environmental factors. [5, 6] Structural and functional reorganisation that occurs during this sensitive period may become permanent, influencing subsequent development, even after environmental conditions change. Therefore, early childhood trauma may have considerable and enduring effects on cognitive development, though empirical evidence in this area is needed. [1]

The goal of the current study was to examine the impact of a specific type of early trauma exposure, interpersonal trauma (IPT) involving the primary caregiver, on child cognitive outcomes. IPT, including maltreatment and interparental violence, is a particularly potent stressor for young children, given the critical role of the attachment relationship in shaping the developing nervous system. [7] Furthermore, maltreatment and interparental violence are often chronic events.1 Though previous research has associated such exposures with impairments in cognitive domains (eg, IQ, executive functioning, reading and math abilities) [1–3 8–10] and brain structure (eg, reduced volumes of the cerebral cortex, hippocampus and corpus callosum) and functioning (eg, event-related potential and electroencephalography abnormalities), [1, 4, 6] the immediate and long-term effects of such exposures specifically in the first years of life have not been well researched.

The current study addresses this gap by examining the impact of IP-Texposure from birth to age 5 on longitudinal assessments of cognitive functioning in a prospective birth cohort sample. Analyses distinguished between exposures from 0 to 24 months and from 24 to 64 months and controlled for several potential confounders, including socio-demographic factors, maternal IQ, birth complications, birth weight and quality of cognitive stimulation in the home.

7.2 METHODS

7.2.1 PARTICIPANTS

Participants (N=206) were from the Minnesota Longitudinal Study of Parents and Children, a prospective examination of adaptation in low-income families. [11] English-speaking pregnant women were recruited during the third trimester from the Minneapolis Department of Public Health Clinic and the Hennepin County General Hospital between 1975 and 1977. Mothers were eligible if the pregnancy was their first (primiparous) and if they qualified for public assistance for prenatal care and delivery (ie, their income was below the official poverty line); 267 women consented and were enrolled. An additional 147 mothers were approached but declined to participate (mother's partner refused to allow participation, too busy) or were unable to participate (planned to move, delivered prior to prenatal assessment, infant adopted out, infant died at delivery, mother did not speak English fluently enough to complete study measures). There were no significant differences between families who did and did not consent to study participation on maternal age, education, occupation or clinic staff assessment of family risk. All procedures were approved by the Institutional Review Board of the University of Minnesota. Mothers provided written informed consent. Participant attrition from 267 to 206 occurred largely during the first 2 years of the study. There were no differences between enrolled families who did and did not complete the current study activities on maternal marital status, education level, age or socioeconomic status (SES) at the child's birth or child race/ethnicity, gender or birth weight. Table 1 summarises participant demographic characteristics.

7.2.2 PROCEDURES AND MEASURES

7.2.2.1 INTERPERSONAL TRAUMA EXPOSURE

Interpersonal trauma exposure (IPT) events included experiencing child maltreatment and witnessing partner violence against the mother. Two dichotomous (yes/no) scores were derived based on timing of IPT exposure: exposed in infancy (0–24 months) and exposed in preschool (24–64 months). All IPT assessments were made blind to the cognitive results.

7.2.2.1.1 CHILD MALTREATMENT

Child maltreatment was identified prospectively based on the following: home observations at 7–10 days, 3, 6 and 9 months and twice at 12 months; laboratory observations at 9, 12 (two visits), 18, 24 and 42 months; maternal interviews throughout assessment periods; and reviews of medical records and child protection records at 24 and 64 months. Children were classified

TABLE 1. Characteristics of mother and child participants at child's birth (N=206).

Variable	%	Mean	SD	Range
Maternal age		20.67 years	3.78 years	12–34 years
Maternal education				
Less than high school	37			
High school graduate	40			
Some college education or greater	23			
Maternal marital status				
Single/separated/ divorced/widowed	65			
Married	35			
Child gender, male	56			
Birth complications, any	30			
Child birth weight		3262 g	545 g	1580–4400 g
Child race/ethnicity				
White, non-Hispanic	65.5			
Multiracial	17			
Black	12			
Native American	4			
Asian	0.5			
Hispanic	1			

as maltreated between 0 and 24 months if there was evidence of any of the following: (a) physical abuse, defined as parental acts resulting in physical damage (eg, bruises, cuts, burns); (b) psychological maltreatment, defined as verbal abuse (eg, constant harassment or berating, chronically finding fault, harsh criticism) or psychological unavailability (eg, interacting only as necessary, emotional unresponsiveness) or (c) neglect, defined as incompetent and irresponsible management of the child's day-to-day care, inadequate nutritional or health care, or dangerous home environment due to insufficient supervision. Between 24 and 64 months, sexual abuse was added as a maltreatment category and was defined as genital contact between the child and a person ≥5 years older than the child (all perpetrators were adolescents or adults). [12] Psychological unavailability but not verbal abuse was rated as a form of psychological maltreatment due to conceptual and methodological difficultiesi in assessing verbal abuse during this time period. [12] Project staff conferenced and classified each child into the above categories, reaching near perfect agreement regarding classification. Validation for the identification of maltreatment cases has been previously reported. [12, 13]

7.2.2.1.2 EXPOSURE TO MATERNAL PARTNER VIOLENCE

Child exposure to partner violence against the mother was based on maternal interviews and questionnaires and interviewer observations of the families at 12, 18, 24, 30, 42, 48, 54 and 64 months. [14] Inter-rater reliability was calculated at each time point on the basis of 50 ratings completed by two developmental psychology graduate students (rs=0.930.99). Children exposed to severe maternal partner violence were classified as IPT-exposed, given prior research showing a similar magnitude of IQ effects among children exposed to high levels of domestic violence as among maltreated children. [10]

7.2.2.2 POTENTIAL CONFOUNDERS

7.2.2.2.1 SOCIO-DEMOGRAPHICS

Factors previously associated with cognitive development [15, 16] were considered as potential confounders: child gender, child race/ethnicity and SES, assessed during pregnancy and when the child was 42 and 96 months old. SES was based on the mean standardised scores from at least two of three sources: the revised Duncan Socioeconomic Index household score, [17, 18] maternal education and household income. Greater scores indicate higher SES.

7.2.2.2.2 BIRTH-RELATED FACTORS

A variable reflecting the presence or absence of birth complications was based on data extracted from labour and delivery records. Presence of any of the following problems was coded as positive for a birth complication:

maternal heart massage required; Rh-/fetal blood incompatibility; fetal tachycardia, bradycardia, asphyxia or hypoxia; intrauterine growth restriction; elevated bilirubin; infant respiratory distress, hypoglycemia, pulmonary flow murmur, infection or severe abnormal scalp formation; Potter's syndrome (atypical physical appearance due to decreased amniotic fluid); Holt-Oram Syndrome (abnormalities of the upper limbs and heart); wet lung syndrome (excessive fluid retained in the lungs) and gestational age <37 weeks or >42 weeks. Birth weight was also extracted from medical records.

7.2.2.2.3 MATERNAL IQ

Maternal IQ was estimated by summing scores on the Comprehension, Similarities and Block Design subscales of the Wechsler Adult Intelligence Scale, [19, 20] ascertained when the child was 48 months of age. The measure is a reasonable estimate of maternal IQ throughout the child's life, given the stability of IQ in adulthood [21] and the high reliability, validity and stability of the Wechsler Adult Intelligence Scale. [22]

7.2.2.2.4 QUALITY OF COGNITIVE STIMULATION

The Home Observation for Measurement of the Environment (HOME) was administered at 30 months to assess the support available to promote the child's social and cognitive development. The scale has demonstrated moderate stability across time, [23] and prior research has documented associations between child IQ and HOME subscales. [24] A cognitive stimulation scale (HOME) was created by summing standardised scores from the subscales focused on cognitive support, including organisation of the physical and temporal environment, provision of appropriate play materials and opportunity for variety and daily stimulation. Higher scores indicate greater stimulation.

7.2.2.3 COGNITIVE OUTCOMES

The cognitive battery conforms to recent suggestions for assessing cognitive trajectories in longitudinal studies of children. [25]

7.2.2.3.1 BAYLEY MENTAL DEVELOPMENT SCALE

At 24 months, children were administered the Bayley Scales of Infant Development [26], which provide standardised scores (M=100, SD=15) on scales of infant mental and motor development. For these analyses, the mental development scale (BMD) was used, which assesses the following: sensory/perceptual acuities, discriminations and responses; acquisition of object constancy; memory learning and problem solving; vocalisation and beginning of verbal communication; basis of abstract thinking; habituation; mental mapping; complex language; and mathematical concept formation.

7.2.2.3.2 WECHSLER PRESCHOOL AND PRIMARY SCALE OF INTELLIGENCE

At 64 months, children were administered a short form of the Wechsler Preschool and Primary Scale of Intelligence (WPPSI), [27] including the Vocabulary, Block Design and Animal House subtests. Prorated IQ scores (M=100, SD=15) were derived using Sattler's formula. [20] The short form has high reliability and validity and correlates highly with full-scale IQ scores. [20, 24]

7.2.2.3.3 WECHSLER INTELLIGENCE SCALE FOR CHILDREN—REVISED

At 96 months, children were administered a short form of the Wechsler Intelligence Scale for Children–Revised (WISC-R), [28] including the Vocabulary, Similarities and Block Design subtests. [20] Prorated IQ scores (M=100, SD=15) were derived using Sattler's formula. [20] The short form has high reliability and validity and correlates highly with full-scale IQ scores. [20, 24]`

7.2.2.4 DATA ANALYTIC PLAN

Differences among children never exposed to IPT, children exposed to IPT in infancy only, children exposed to IPT in preschool only and children exposed to IPT in both infancy and preschool on cognitive scores were examined separately at 24, 64 and 96 months via one-way analyses of variance followed by pairwise t tests if the overall F test was significant. Associations among the study variables were tested in bivariate correlational analyses. To test whether IPT exposure was associated with cognitive scores from 24 to 96 months, mixed effects models with a random intercept were implemented. These models accounted for repeated cognition measures within participants, took advantage of the longitudinal nature of the data, increased statistical power (when compared with analysing separately at each time point) and enhanced possible inferences regarding associations between IPT exposure and cognitive functioning over time. Longitudinal models were possible given that all the cognitive measures are standardised to have the same mean (M=100) and SD (SD=15). An indicator variable was included in the model that allowed IPT in preschool to affect cognitive outcomes only at 64 and 96 months. This ensured that IPT in preschool could not affect 24-month cognitive outcomes.

In the first step of the model, a three-way interaction term among IPT in infancy, IPT in preschool and time of cognitive testing (ie, 24, 64 or 96 months) and all possible two-way interaction and main effect terms were included. The three-way interaction term tested whether the effect of IPT in infancy on cognitive scores differed over time depending on the presence or absence of IPT exposure in preschool (IPT in infancy 3 time 3 IPT in preschool). Once found non-significant, the three-way interaction was removed and the remaining two-way interactions were tested. The two-way interactions tested (a) whether the effect of IPT in one time period (infancy or preschool) on cognitive scores differed by whether IPT in the other time period (preschool or infancy) was experienced (IPT in infancy 3 IPT in preschool), (b) whether the effect of IPT in infancy on cognitive scores changed over time (IPT in infancy 3 time) and (c) whether the effect of IPT in preschool on cognitive scores changed over time (IPT in preschool 3 time). Any non-significant two-way interaction terms were removed from the model. In the final step, covariates were added to test the effects of IPT exposure independent of other known risk factors, including child gender, race, SES, maternal IQ, birth weight, birth complications and cognitive stimulation in the home. SES was included as a time-varying covariate in the model, with SES during pregnancy used for predicting

24-month cognitive scores, SES at 42 months for predicting 64-month cognitive scores and SES at 96 months for predicting 96-month cognitive scores. In addition, a main effect term for time was included to test whether there were differences in mean cognitive scores over time. For all analyses, a p value <0.05 was considered statistically significant.

A set of multiple regression analyses were also run using comparable models to predict cognitive scores separately at each age (24, 64 and 96 months). Results from these analyses produced similar conclusions and are available online (see supplementary file online).

7.2.2.4.1 DATA IMPUTATION

Participants were included in the analyses if they had data for at least one of the cognitive outcomes; 199 completed the BMD, 174 completed the WPPSI and 177 completed the WISC-R. Missing data in the predictor, covariate and outcome variables were imputed using the Markov Chain Monte Carlo method [29] of multiple imputation, implemented in SAS PROC MI, which produces unbiased results if the data are missing at random. Analyses were conducted on the multiple imputed data sets and then summarised for inference purposes according to the rules developed by Rubin, [30 31] implemented in SAS PROC MIANALYZE. One hundred and thirty-one participants had complete data for all variables, and 75 had missing data for at least one variable. Ten data sets were imputed, each with 206 observations. Results from the imputed data sets did not differ qualitatively from results from the complete case data set, and both sets produced similar conclusions. Results based on imputed data are presented.

7.3 RESULTS

By 64 months, 36.5% of the sample had experienced IPT, with 4.8% exposed in infancy only, 13.0% in preschool only and 18.7% in both infancy and preschool. Table 2 displays mean cognitive test scores by IPT exposure. Analyses of variance showed that IPT groups differed significantly on BMD scores at 24 months (p=0.0003), WPPSI scores at 64 months (p<0.0001) and WISC-R scores at 96 months (p=0.0006). Follow-up pairwise t tests revealed that children exposed to IPT in infancy only and children exposed in infancy + preschool had lower BMD and WPPSI scores than children exposed in preschool only and unexposed children. Children exposed to IPT in infancy + preschool had significantly lower WISC-R scores than unexposed children. The remaining pairwise comparisons were not significantly different. Table 3 presents the bivariate correlation coefficients among the study variables.

In the mixed effects models predicting cognitive scores from 24 to 96 months, none of the interaction terms were significant, signifying that (a) IPT exposure in infancy had a similar magnitude of effect on cognitive scores at 24, 64 and 96 months (non-significant IPT in infancy × time); (b) IPT exposure in preschool had a similar magnitude of effect on cognitive scores at 64 and 96 months (non-significant IPT in preschool × time); (c) the impact of IPT exposure in one time period (infancy or preschool) on cognitive scores did not vary by the presence/absence of IPTexposure in the other time period (non-significant IPT in infancy × IPT in preschool) and (d) the impact of IPT exposure in infancy on cognitive scores over time did not vary by the presence/absence of IPT exposure in preschool (non-significant IPT in infancy × time 3 IPT in preschool). Therefore, the interaction terms were removed from the final model, summarised in table 4. In this model, IPT exposure in infancy but not in preschool was significantly associated with cognitive outcomes. Specifically, those with IPT exposure in infancy had cognitive scores that were on average 7.25 points lower than those without exposure in infancy. Additionally, male gender, lower birth weight, lower maternal IQ, lower SES, and lesser cognitive stimulation in the home predicted lower cognitive scores. The time main effect term was not significant, indicating similar mean scores on the cognitive tests over time.

7.4 DISCUSSION

This is the first study to examine prospectively the impact of early IPT—specifically maltreatment or witnessing maternal partner violence—on cognitive functioning from infancy through the early school years with repeated assessments on the same children. The results suggest that IPT in early childhood, particularly during the first 2 years, has significant

TABLE 2. Cognitive scores by interpersonal trauma exposure.

	BMD, 24 months		WPPSI, 64 months		WISC-R, 96 months	
	Mean	95% CI	Mean	95% CI	Mean	95% CI
No exposure	103.73	100.44 to 107.02	108.34	105.90 to 110.77	107.08	104.22 to 109.94
Exposure infancy* only	86.62	74.71 to 98.52	90.89	81.00 to 100.78	95.91	78.27 to 113.55
Exposure pre-schooly only	102.12	94.73 to 109.50	104.66	99.00 to 110.32	101.11	94.76 to 107.47
Exposure infancy* + preschool**	90.25	85.50 to 94.99	95.44	90.79 to 100.09	93.89	87.94 to 99.83

*Infancy = 0–24 months.
**Preschool = 24–64 months.
BMD, Bayley Mental Development Scale; WISC-R, Wechsler Intelligence Scale for ChildrendRevised; WPPSI, Wechsler Preschool and Primary Scale of Intelligence.

and enduring effects on cognitive development, even after adjusting for gender, race/ethnicity, SES, maternal IQ, birth complications, birth weight and quality of cognitive stimulation in the home. These findings are consistent with other studies documenting vulnerability in the early years to fundamental changes in neural circuitry and brain structure related to social adversity and trauma. [1, 6] In contrast to many studies in this area, subjects were drawn from the community rather than mental health clinics or domestic violence shelters or via child protection records, thereby broadening the generalisability of the findings.

Several hypotheses have been proposed to account for the impact of trauma on childhood cognitive development. Certain forms of maltreatment may cause direct injury to the brain, such as physical abuse involving the head or neglect resulting in malnutrition. Other forms of IPT that do not involve frank neurological injury (eg, sexual abuse, witnessing domestic violence) have also been associated with adverse cognitive development, leading some to hypothesise that trauma affects cognitive outcomes through stress pathways. [1, 10] Extreme stress has been associated with enduring changes in the secretion and processing of numerous stress hormones and neurotransmitters. [1, 8] These responses may be associated with altered neural structure and functioning, particularly in the early years when the brain is undergoing its most rapid phase of growth, differentiation and synaptic organisation. [1] Because early brain organisation frames later neurological development, changes in early development may have lifelong consequences.

The significant association between IPT and child cognitive outcomes may also reflect the role of the parent-child relationship in promoting child cognitive development. Child maltreatment represents the most extreme form of poor caregiving, and maltreating parents demonstrate a host of characteristics predictive of various negative child outcomes. [3] Exposure to partner violence may also compromise mothers' caregiving abilities. [32] Poorer quality parent-child interactions, in turn, have been associated with depressed child cognitive development. [24, 33]

Trauma-induced psychological symptoms (eg, posttraumatic stress disorder [PTSD]) may contribute to cognitive deficits by impeding the ability to engage the environment effectively and learn new skills. [3] Some studies have found that neural/cognitive effects from trauma exposure are evident only among participants with PTSD, whereas others have documented effects regardless of psychiatric status. [6, 8, 9] Conversely, low IQ by age 5 has been identified as a risk factor for the development of PTSD. [34] Therefore, there are likely complex, multidirectional transactional associations over time among emotional/behavioural symptomatology, cognitive functioning and brain development that shape children's responses to IPT. Future studies may consider whether psychological disorders such as PTSD mediate or moderate the effects of early trauma exposure on cognitive development.

Of note, short forms of the WPPSI and WISC-R were used, a validated method in developmental research and the recommended approach for assessing child IQ in longitudinal studies. [25] However, trauma exposure may have different effects on the various domains of cognitive functioning, including domains not assessed with the short forms. Therefore, future research should consider use of more comprehensive neurocognitive batteries to examine whether subscales are differentially affected by early trauma exposure.

TABLE 3. Correlation coefficients among study variables.

Variable	1	2	3	4	5	6	7	8	9	10	11	12	13
1. IPT, 0–24 months	–												
2. IPT, 24–64 months	0.59***	–											
3. Child gender[a]	–0.10	–0.03	–										
4. Child race/ ethnicity[b]	0.14	0.09	–0.05	–									
5. SES, pre-natal	–0.20**	–0.17	–0.07	–0.15*	–								
6. SES, 42 months	–0.16*	–0.25**	–0.08	–0.04	0.67***	–							
7. SES, 96 months	–0.21**	–0.27**	0.03	–0.12	0.55***	0.69***	–						
8. Maternal IQ (WAIS)	–0.17*	–0.26**	–0.09	–0.15*	47***	0.54**	0.50***	–					
9. Birth complications	–0.07	–0.08	–0.05	0.00	0.14*	0.13	0.12	–0.03	–				
10. Child birth weight	–0.02	0.03	0.03	–0.03	–0.10	–0.06	–0.03	0.09	–0.24**	–			

TABLE 3. CONTINUED.

11. HOME, 30 months	–0.37***	–0.34***	0.03	–0.37***	0.24***	0.29***	0.39**	0.30***	0.05	–0.07	–		
12. BMD, 24 months	–0.31***	–0.19**	0.19**	–0.18**	0.19**	0.20**	0.28***	0.27***	–0.06	0.21**	0.35***	–	
13. WPPSI, 64 months	–0.38***	–0.26***	0.15*	–0.16*	0.35***	0.40***	0.38***	0.46***	0.05	0.16*	0.37***	0.55***	–
14. WISC-R, 96 months	–0.30***	–0.27***	0.04	–0.17*	0.27***	0.29***	0.41***	0.47***	0.02	0.20**	0.33***	0.52***	0.72***

*p<0.05, **p<0.01, ***p<0.001.
aMale children were coded '1'; female children were coded '2.'
bWhite, non-Hispanic children were coded '1'; racial/ethnic minority children were coded '2.'
BMD, Bayley Mental Development Scale; HOME, Home Observation for Measurement of the Environment composite summary scale; IPT, interpersonal trauma exposure; IQ, intelligence quotient; SES, socioeconomic status; WAIS, Wechsler Adult Intelligence Scale; WISC-R, Wechsler Intelligence Scale for ChildrendRevised; WPPSI, Wechsler Preschool and Primary Scale of Intelligence.

TABLE 4. Associations between IPT and child cognitive scores from 24 to 96 months: final mixed effects model.

Variable	Parameter estimate	SE	p Value
IPT exposure, 0–24 months	−7.25	2.30	0.002
IPT exposure, 24–64 months	−0.37	1.82	0.84
Time*	−0.04	0.04	0.31
Gender[a]	4.85	1.63	0.003
Race/ethnicity[b]	−0.39	1.81	0.83
SES[c]	0.17	0.07	0.02
Maternal IQ (WAIS)	0.52	0.12	<0.0001
Birth weight	0.01	0.002	0.0007
Birth complications	0.23	1.78	0.90
Cognitive stimulation in the home	1.27	0.43	0.003

* The time term tested whether there were differences in mean cognitive scores over time.
a Males are the reference group.
b White, non-Hispanic children are the reference group.
c SES during pregnancy was used for predicting 24-month cognitive scores, SES at 42 months for predicting 64-month cognitive scores and SES at 96 months for predicting 96-month cognitive scores.
IPT, interpersonal trauma exposure; IQ, intelligence quotient; SES, socioeconomic status;
WAIS, Wechsler Adult Intelligence Scale.

7.4.1 LIMITATIONS

A significant limitation of the current study is the relatively small sample size, particularly the small number of children exposed to IPT in infancy only. Because the large majority of children exposed to IPT in infancy were also exposed in the preschool period, the power to distinguish timing effects from chronicity effects was limited. Previous studies have demonstrated that longer exposure to maltreatment is associated with smaller intracranial volume and greater IQ suppression, though length of exposure is often confounded with age of onset. [6] That IPT exposure in infancy but not in the preschool period emerged as a significant predictor and that exposure in infancy had similar effects on cognitive scores across development and regardless of preschool exposure suggests that the first two years of life may be a period of particular vulnerability to negative, enduring effects of trauma exposure on cognitive development.

Changes to the maltreatment coding scheme after 24 months may have resulted in an underidentification of maltreatment cases during both time periods. Notably, among the identified cases of verbal abuse and sexual abuse, 79% and 64%, respectively, experienced at least one other form of maltreatment. Therefore, the majority of unidentified verbal and sexual abuse cases were likely identified as IPT-exposed for other forms of maltreatment. Given the frequency of overlap among different IPT exposures, examining cognition effects by exposure type was not possible.

Other factors not assessed within the current study may, in part, account for associations between IPT and child cognitive functioning, including maternal prenatal substance use (eg, alcohol, tobacco, narcotics) and child lead exposure. The current analyses adjusted for birth complications and low birth weight, pathways through which prenatal substance use may affect cognitive outcomes. [35, 36] Analyses also adjusted for SES, which is strongly associated with lead exposure. [37] Because participants were all low SES, the results may not generalise to higher SES populations.

7.5 CONCLUSIONS

Each year in the USA, there are approximately 750,000 validated cases of child maltreatment, [38] and 3–10 million children witness domestic violence. [39] Children under the age of 4 are most likely to be victimized/exposed, with infants from birth to 1 year especially vulnerable. [38] The current findings suggest that the first years of life is a period of heightened sensitivity to substantial and enduring cognitive effects from such exposures. Depressed cognitive functioning in early development has been shown to result in long-term damaging consequences, including poor academic performance throughout schooling and poor adjustment throughout life. [1, 40] These findings highlight the importance of identifying at-risk families and preventing IPT in early life to promote positive cognitive development throughout childhood.

REFERENCES

1. Pechtel P, Pizzagalli DA. Effects of early life stress on cognitive and affective function: an integrated review of human literature. Psychopharmacology (Berl) 2011;214:55–70.
2. Perez CM, Widom CM, Spatz C. Childhood victimization and long-term intellectual and academic outcomes. Child Abuse Negl 1994;18:617–33.
3. Veltman MWM, Browne KD. Three decades of child maltreatment research: implications for the school years. Trauma Violence Abuse 2001;2:215–39.
4. Andersen SL, Tomada A, Vincow ES, et al. Preliminary evidence for sensitive periods in the effect of childhood sexual abuse on regional brain development. J Neuropsychiatry Clin Neurosci 2008;20:292–301.
5. Huttenlocher PR, Dabholkar AS. Regional differences in synaptogenesis in human cerebral cortex. J Comp Neurol 1997;387:167–78.
6. De Bellis M, Keshavan MS, Clark DB, et al. Developmental traumatology. Part II: brain development. Biol Psychiatry 1999;45:1271–84.
7. Schore AN. The neurobiology of attachment and early personality organization. J Prenat Perinat Psychol Health 2002;16:249–63.
8. De Bellis M. Developmental traumatology: the psychobiological development of maltreated children and its implications for research, treatment, and policy. Dev Psychopathol 2001;13:539–64.
9. DePrince AP, Weinzierl KM, Combs MD. Executive function performance and trauma exposure in a community sample of children. Child Abuse Negl 2009;33:353–61.
10. Koenen KC, Moffitt TE, Caspi A, et al. Domestic violence is associated with environmental suppression of IQ in young children. Dev Psychopathol 2003;15:297e311.
11. Sroufe LA, Egeland B, Carlson EA, et al. The Development of the Person. New York, NY: Guilford, 2005.
12. Pianta R, Egeland B, Erickson MF. The antecedents of maltreatment: results of the mother-child interaction research project. In: Cicchetti D, Carlson V, eds. Child Maltreatment: Theory and Research on the Causes and Consequences of Child Abuse and Neglect. Cambridge, United Kingdom: Cambridge University Press, 1989:203–53.
13. Shaffer A, Huston L, Egeland B. Identification of child maltreatment using prospective and self-report methodologies: a comparison of maltreatment incidence and relation to later psychopathology. Child Abuse Negl 2008;32:682–92.
14. Dodds M. The Impact Of Exposure To Interparental Violence On Child Behavior Problems. Minneapolis, MN: Institute of Child Development, University of Minnesota, 1995. Unpublished doctoral dissertation.
15. Dickens WT, Flynn JR. Black Americans reduce the racial IQ gap: evidence from standardization samples. Psychol Sci 2006;17:913–20.
16. Gutman LM, Sameroff AJ, Cole R. Academic growth curve trajectories from 1st grade to 12th grade: effects of multiple social risk factors and preschool child factors. Dev Psychol 2003;39:777–90.
17. Duncan O. A socioeconomic index for all occupations. In: Reiss AJ Jr, ed. Occupations and Social Status. New York, NY: Free Press, 1961:109–38.

18. Stevens G, Featherman DL. A revised socioeconomic index of occupational status. Soc Sci Res 1981;10:364–95.
19. Wechsler D. Manual for the Wechsler Adult Intelligence Scale. San Antonio, TX: The Psychological Corporation, 1955.
20. Sattler JM. Assessment of Children. 3rd edn. San Diego, CA, 1992. Author.
21. Schuerger JM, Witt AC. The temporal stability of individually tested intelligence. J Clin Psychol 1989;45:294–302.
22. Parker KCH, Hanson RK, Hunsley J. MMPI, Rorschach, and WJS: a meta-analytic comparison of reliability, stability, and validity. Psychol Bul 1988;103:367–73.
23. Bradley RH. The use of the HOME inventory in longitudinal studies of child development. In: Bornstein MH, Krasnegor NA, eds. Stability and Continuity in Mental Development: Behavioral and Biological Perspectives. Hillsdale, NJ: Lawrence Erlbaum, 1989:191–215.
24. Pianta RC, Egeland B. Predictors of instability in children's mental test performance at 24, 48, and 96 months. Intelligence 1994;18:145–63.
25. White RF, Campbell R, Echeverria D, et al. Assessment of cognitive trajectories in longitudinal population-based studies of children. J Epidemiol Community Health 2009;63:i15–26.
26. Bayley N. Bayley Scales of Infant Development. New York, NY: Psychological Corporation, 1969.
27. Wechsler D. Manual for the Wechsler Preschool and Primary Scale of Intelligence. San Antonio, TX: The Psychological Corporation, 1967.
28. Wechsler D. Manual for the Wechsler Intelligence Scale for Children-Revised. San Antonio, TX: The Psychological Corporation, 1974.
29. Shafer JL. Analysis of Incomplete Multivariate Data. New York, NY: Chapman and Hall, 1997.
30. Rubin DB. Inference and missing data. Biometrika 1976;63:581–92.
31. Rubin DB. Multiple Imputation for Nonresponse in Surveys. New York, NY: John Wiley & Sons, 1987.
32. McIntosh JE. Thought in the face of violence: a child's need. Child Abuse Negl 2002;26:229–41.
33. Burchinal M, Vernon-Feagans L, Cox M; Key family life project investigators. Cumulative social risk, parenting, and infant development in rural low-income communities. Parent Sci Pract 2008;8:41–69.
34. Koenen KC, Moffitt TE, Poulton R, et al. Early childhood factors associated with the development of post-traumatic stress disorder: results from a longitudinal birth cohort. Psychol Med 2007;37:181–92.
35. Dombrowski SC, Kelly N, Martin RP. Low birth weight and cognitive outcomes: evidence for a gradient relationship in an urban, poor, African American birth cohort. Sch Psychol Q 2007;22:26–43.
36. Visscher WA, Feder M, Burns AM, et al. The impact of smoking and other substance use by urban women on the birthweight of their infants. Subst Use Misuse 2003;38:1063–93.
37. Bellinger DC. Lead neurotoxicity and socioeconomic status: conceptual and analytical issues. Neurotoxicology 2008;29:828–32.

38. U.S. Department of Health and Human Services. Administration on Children, Youth and families. Child maltreatment, 2009. http://www.acf.hhs.gov/programs/cb/ pubs/cm09/index.htm (accessed 6 Jun 2011).
39. American Psychological Association. Intimate Partner Abuse And Relationship Violence Working Group. Intimate Partner Abuse and Relationship Violence. http://www.apa.org/pi/women/programs/violence/partner-violence.pdf (accessed 25 Jan 2010).
40. Gottfredson LS. Why g matters: the complexity of everyday life. Intelligence 1997;24:79–132.

CHAPTER 8

Adverse Childhood Experiences: Retrospective Study to Determine Their Impact on Adult Health Behaviours and Health Outcomes in a UK Population

MARK A. BELLIS, HELEN LOWEY, NICOLA LECKENBY, KAREN HUGHES, AND DOMINIC HARRISON

8.1 INTRODUCTION

Studies are increasingly exposing relationships between childhood trauma and the emergence of health damaging behaviours and poor health and social outcomes in adulthood. [1– 3] The first large-scale adverse childhood experiences (ACE) study in the USA began to quantify the impacts of ACEs on health and behaviour throughout the life course. [4] This and subsequent studies have identified a set of ACEs including: growing up in a household with someone who is depressed, mentally ill, a substance abuser or has been incarcerated in the criminal justice system; exposure to child maltreatment or domestic violence and losing a parent through divorce, separation or death. [4,5] Exposure to such ACEs has been associated with poor health outcomes including substance use, mental ill-health, obesity, heart disease and cancer, as well as unemployment and continued involvement in violence. [4,6,7] Importantly, the impact of ACEs appears to be cumulative, with risks of poor outcomes increasing with the number of ACEs suffered. [4,8,9]

The relationships between ACEs and pressures on health and social systems [e.g. from non-communicable diseases (NCDs)] should be a critical element in informing health policy and strategic investment. [10,11] That ACEs appear linked to important outcomes for other public services (e.g. criminal justice, education) means an understanding of ACEs should inform work across government departments. However, such intelligence is rare outside the USA, even in high-income countries. [11] Thus, global public health efforts are focusing on developing and implementing standardized methodologies for measuring the impact of ACEs across populations. [11] As Europe increasingly embraces a social determinants approach to health, [12] understanding relationships between deprivation, ACEs and adult outcomes becomes paramount. [13 – 16]

We present findings from a general population ACE study in a relatively deprived and culturally diverse part of the UK. The study was designed to examine associations between ACEs and poor health and social outcomes over the life course. Controlling for demographics and deprivation, we explore the strength of ACEs as predictors of poor behaviour, health, criminal justice and educational outcomes, and discuss the implications for health policy.

8.2 METHODS

In collaboration with the National Health Service, a diverse geography covering a range of income levels and ethnic groups was identified. Its population is 150 000, relatively young (26% of residents aged 0–17 years compared with England 21%), [17] with higher than national residential ethnic minority levels (White British 74.6%, Indian 9.2%, Pakistani 8.9%, other ethnicities 7.3%) [18] and high levels of material deprivation and child poverty. [18,19]

8.2.1 QUESTIONNAIRE

The questionnaire used tested ACE categories and other survey tools. ACE questions were based on the Centers for Disease Control and Prevention short ACE tool11 (Table 1). Outcomes potentially associated with ACEs were identified from US studies (substance use, sexual behaviour, exercise, disease diagnoses, health service use, employment, obesity and violence involvement) [4,7,20,21] with additional variables relating to UK health policy (diet, mental wellbeing, life satisfaction, educational attainment, incarceration; Table 2). Alcohol consumption was measured using AUDIT-C questions, [22] including information on what constitutes a standard drink (UK = 10 ml pure alcohol). [23] Heavy drinking was defined as consuming ≥6 standard drinks/ occasion at least once a week. Mental wellbeing was measured using the Short Warwick-Edinburgh Mental Wellbeing Scale (SWEMWBS). [24,25] Low mental wellbeing was categorized as SWEMWBS score <23 based on a larger mental wellbeing survey undertaken in the same region. [25] This survey was also used to set the threshold for low life satisfaction as ≤5 on a 10-point Likert scale. Body mass index (BMI) was calculated based on participants' selfreported height and weight. Individuals were considered obese if their BMI was ≥30 and morbidly obese at ≥40. [26] To minimize self-diagnosis of health conditions, respondents were asked if (and when) they had ever been diagnosed by a doctor or nurse with each condition. Ethnicity was selfdefined based on standard UK Census categories. The questionnaire was developed for delivery by trained researchers through face-to-face interviews or self-completion under researcher supervision.

A pilot of 152 residents in the study area resulted in the questionnaire being shortened through changes to wording and removal of superfluous questions. The final tool contained 42 questions and took 10 min to complete. The questionnaire was available in English, Urdu, Gujarati, Hindi and Polish.

8.2.2 SAMPLE

The inclusion criteria were resident in the study area; aged 18–70 years and cognitively able to participate in a face-to-face interview. ACEs in the pilot ranged in prevalence from 2.6% for forced sex to 21.9% for being sworn at, insulted, and put down. Based on the pilot a sample of 1500 was identified for the survey and a random sampling methodology stratified by deprivation quintile was used to ensure an approximate match to the local population. Deprivation was based on index of multiple deprivation (IMD) 2010; a composite measure including 38 economic and social indicators. [27] The Postcode Address File [28] was used to identify houses in each national deprivation quintile and, to allow for non-compliance as indicated in the pilot, 3000 households were selected.

Letters were sent to sampled households prior to researchers visiting, providing study information and the opportunity to withdraw (via post, email or telephone); 120 (4.0%) households opted out at this stage. Households were given a second opportunity to opt out when researchers arrived. Those that did were replaced by a neighbouring household. At least three attempted visits were made to each sampled household. A total of 2162 sampled houses were occupied when visited; of these 511 (23.6%) opted out and 151 (7.0%) were ineligible. Sampling was completed once the 1500 target was reached. Compliance was 74.6% across eligible occupied households excluding the 120 opting out at the letter stage; 70.4% including them. Under the research team's instruction, a professional survey company delivered the questionnaire (August to October 2012). After explaining the voluntary and anonymous nature of the survey and its rationale, respondents could choose to complete the questionnaire through a face-to-face interview or self-complete.

As problematic substance users were likely to be underrepresented in door-to-door surveys, a specialist sample (n = 67) was surveyed at three substance use services in the same locality. This sample was self-selected; staff informed eligible clients of the study during routine appointments and invited them to attend survey sessions held by researchers at the services. Clients attending appointments on survey days were also invited to participate. This sample has been treated separately for analysis but is included to provide information on a group with potentially multiple ACEs likely to be missed in household surveys. [29]

Ethical approval for the household study was granted by Liverpool John Moores University Research Ethics Committee and for the substance user sample by the NHS Research Ethics Committee.

TABLE 1. Percentage of each adverse childhood experience (ACE) in total sample and in individuals with different ACE counts.

ACE definitions:	n	All	ACE count			Odds ratio	x^2_{trend} [a]	P
while you were growing up, before the age of 18 years			1 (n = 287)	2–3 (n = 234)	4+ (n = 185)	4+ to 1		
Did you live with anyone who								
Was depressed, mentally ill or suicidal?	1497	11.10	11.50	23.10	43.40	5.90	61.207	<0.001
Was a problem drinker or alcoholic?	1494	9.40	4.90	17.90	47.50	17.63	118.861	<0.001
Used illegal street drugs or who abused prescription medications?	1495	3.90	0.70	6.40	22.80	42.03	66.856	<0.001
Was sentenced to serve time in a prison or young offenders institution?	1492	4.00	0.30	6.40	24.90	94.62	78.292	<0.001
Were your parents ever separated or divorced?	1492	23.70	48.40	43.20	65.50	2.03	9.803	0.002
Did your parents or adults in your home ever								
Slap, hit, kick, punch or beat each other up?	1487	14.10	13.20	28.20	62.80	11.06	118.265	<0.001
Hit, beat, kick or physically hurt you in any way?[b]	1491	15.20	5.60	42.70	63.60	29.64	178.338	<0.001
Swear at you, insult you or put you down?	1486	20.10	14.60	54.30	77.20	19.74	182.769	<0.001
Did anyone at least 5 years older than you (including adults)								
Ever touch you sexually?	1485	4.30	0.30	5.10	30.60	126.03	103.047	<0.001
Try to make you touch them sexually?	1485	3.40	0.30	3.00	25.30	96.84	85.667	<0.001
Force you to have sex?	1485	2.10	0.00	1.70	15.90	NC	55.435	<0.001

NC, not calculable.

[a] x^2 for a trend measures increasing representation of each ACE in categories of higher ACE count.

[b] This excluded gentle smacking for punishment.

8.2.3 ANALYSIS

Analyses used PASW Statistics v18. Having any ACE was highly correlated with having any other ACE (all P<0.001). Therefore, in line with other studies, [4,20] an ACE count was used to classify respondents into, here, four ACE categories (0 ACEs, n = 794; 1 ACE, n = 287; 2–3 ACEs, n = 234; 4+ ACES, n = 185). Dependent variables of interest were dichotomized for the purpose of calculating adjusted odds ratios (AORs) for health and behavioural outcomes. Individuals were allocated an IMD based on the lower super output area (a nationally defined set of small geographies) containing their residential postcode and then categorized into national deprivation quintiles. [30] Bivariate analyses used x^2. Multinomial logistic regression (LR) was used to examine independent associations between ACE counts and demographic variables (age, sex, ethnicity, deprivation; Table 3). Binary LR was used to control for such associations when calculating independent relationships between outcome measures and ACE count. In each binary LR model (Tables 4 and 5) AORs [±95% confidence intervals (CIs)] represent changes in odds of each outcome with changing ACE count after correcting for demographics. [31] Where individuals did not answer all questions adjusted sample sizes are presented.

8.3 RESULTS

Across the population sample, 47.1% of individuals reported at least one ACE, with ACE count categories 1, 2–3 and 4+ representing 19.1, 15.6 and 12.3%, respectively. Being forced to have sex by an older individual had the lowest prevalence (Table 1). ACEs involving sexual abuse, living with someone incarcerated or abusing drugs were most strongly associated with higher numbers of ACEs. Compared with those with no ACEs, individuals with >1 ACE were more likely to be aged <60 years. White British respondents were more likely to report ACEs than individuals of Indian or Pakistani ethnicity. There were no significant relationships between deprivation quintile and having 1 or 2–3 ACEs, yet having 4+ ACEs was strongly associated with higher deprivation (quintiles 4 and 5; Table 3).

TABLE 2. Relationships between number of ACEs and behavioural, social and health outcomes.

Outcome	All		ACE count				x^2_{trend} [a]	P
	%	n	0 %	1 %	2-3 %	4+ %		
Sexual behaviour								
Had/caused unintentional pregnancy <18 years	9.0	1487	5.0	8.7	11.2	24.3	60.398	<0.001
Had sex <16 years	20.5	1388	13.4	22.6	27.7	37.9	61.056	<0.001
Mental health and wellbeing[a]								
Low mental wellbeing score	18.8	1500	14.2	16.0	25.2	34.6	45.190	<0.001
Low life satisfaction	12.8	1338	8.5	9.0	17.9	29.9	54.828	<0.001
Substance use								
Current daily smoker	31.1	1494	20.5	32.2	43.2	59.5	125.663	<0.001
Drink ≥6 drinks[b] per occasion ≥1/week	12.5	1487	7.5	11.3	16.9	30.3	69.937	<0.001
Ever used cannabis	17.6	1492	9.2	15.7	28.8	42.3	132.317	<0.001
Ever used heroin or crack cocaine	2.9	1482	1.1	1.8	2.2	13.4	51.404	<0.001
Violence and criminal justice								
Been hit by someone in last 12 months	6.0	1494	3.4	3.5	8.1	18.8	52.787	<0.001
Hit someone in last 12 months	5.7	1495	2.6	3.8	8.5	18.2	62.730	<0.001

TABLE 2. Continued.

Ever spent ≥1 night in police station/prison	5.2	1491	1.9	1.7	11.1	17.2	82.049	<0.001
Diet, weight and exercise								
≤1 portion of fruit or vegetables a day	15.3	1500	12.0	15.7	18.8	24.3	20.487	<0.001
Obese (BMI ≥ 30)	17.9	1497	16.3	17.4	21.5	21.1	4.210	0.040
Morbidly obese (BMI ≥ 40)	2.7	1500	2.1	2.4	2.1	5.9	5.012	0.025
≤2 30 min sessions of exercise/week	44.8	1500	47.1	41.8	45.3	38.9	3.503	0.061
Education and employment								
No qualifications (vocational, school, other)	31.5	1500	29.8	31.4	35.0	34.1	2.519	0.113
Currently unemployed/on long-term sickness	22.4	1474	16.5	20.2	31.6	39.5	55.684	<0.001
Health								
Ever broken a bone in your own body	42.3	1500	35.3	41.1	54.7	58.9	50.333	<0.001
Spent ≥ 1 night in hospital in last 12 months	12.0	1494	11.0	9.1	16.7	15.3	5.357	0.021
Spent ≥ 6 nights in hospital ever	30.7	1496	26.6	31.7	37.2	38.8	16.068	<0.001

TABLE 2. Continued.

Ever diagnosed with								
STI	2.1	1486	0.3	2.4	3.0	8.3	43.397	<0.001
Cancer	3.6	1487	2.9	5.3	4.3	2.8	0.269	0.604
Type II diabetes	7.4	1491	8.9	5.6	6.0	5.5	4.041	0.044
Cardiovascular conditions[c]	4.4	1496	4.3	3.8	6.0	3.8	0.090	0.765
Respiratory disease	5.4	1489	4.6	4.9	6.0	9.4	5.814	0.016
Digestive/liver disease	3.3	1496	2.3	2.1	7.3	4.4	8.301	0.004

STI, sexually transmitted infection; BMI, body mass index.
a Low mental wellbeing was categorized as a score of <23 on the Short Warwick-Edinburgh Mental Wellbeing Scale (SWEMWBS) and low life satisfaction as ≤5 on a Likert 10-point scale (see the section Methods).
b A drink is a standard UK unit of alcohol equivalent to 10 ml pure alcohol.
c Including coronary heart disease, myocardial infarction and stroke.

TABLE 3. Multinomial LR analysis of relationship between number of ACEs, deprivation and other demographics.

	Total sample		ACE count (reference category: 0 ACEs)								
	n	%	1			2–3			4+		
			AOR	95% CI	P	AOR	95% CI	P	AOR	95% CI	P
Age (years)											
<30 (ref)	357	23.9									
30–39	319	21.3	1.28	(0.86–1.91)	0.224	1.11	(0.71–1.75)	0.639	1.08	(0.67–1.75)	0.748
40–49	327	21.9	0.56	(0.37–0.86)	0.008	0.70	(0.44–1.09)	0.112	0.74	(0.46–1.18)	0.199
50–59	223	14.9	0.77	(0.49–1.22)	0.264	0.87	(0.53–1.41)	0.560	0.64	(0.37–1.11)	0.115
60+	270	18.0	0.56	(0.36–0.86)	0.009	0.56	(0.35–0.90)	0.017	0.31	(0.17–0.55)	<0.001
Ethnicity											
White British (ref)	1038	69.2									
Pakistani	204	13.6	0.44	(0.28–0.68)	<0.001	0.37	(0.23–0.60)	<0.001	0.17	(0.09–0.33)	<0.001
Indian	166	11.1	0.40	(0.24–0.65)	<0.001	0.39	(0.23–0.66)	<0.001	0.16	(0.07–0.34)	<0.001
Other	92	6.1	0.73	(0.41–1.32)	0.301	0.59	(0.30–1.16)	0.127	0.74	(0.39–1.41)	0.361

TABLE 3. Continued.

Deprivation quintile											
(Least deprived) 1 (ref)	82	5.5									
2	153	10.2	0.69	(0.33–1.43)	0.316	1.08	(0.47–2.47)	0.859	2.30	(0.80–6.62)	0.122
3	122	8.1	0.66	(1.18–0.57)	0.657	2.41	(0.32–2.07)	0.672	1.52	(0.46–4.98)	0.494
4	216	14.4	0.98	(0.50–1.92)	0.942	1.67	(0.77–3.63)	0.195	3.08	(1.10–8.64)	0.032
(Most deprived) 5	927	61.8	1.20	(0.67–2.17)	0.537	1.81	(0.90–3.63)	0.097	3.58	(1.38–9.29)	0.009
Gender											
Female (ref)	882	60.2									
Male	584	39.8	1.08	(0.81–1.44)	0.621	1.85	(1.36–2.51)	<0.001	1.15	(0.81–1.62)	0.436

AOR, adjusted odds ratio; 95% CI, 95% confidence intervals; ref, reference category.

For sexual behaviour, ACEs increased with prevalence of having (females)/causing (males) unintentional pregnancy age <18 years and having had sex <16 years (Table 2). Multivariate analysis, accounting for confounding effects, confirmed increases in both unintentional pregnancy and early sex in those with .1 ACE (reference group 0 ACEs; Table 4). Relationships between sex <16 years and having >1 ACE remained significant even when individuals whose ACEs included being forced to have sex were removed from analysis (2–3 ACEs, $P<0.05$; 4+ ACEs, $P<0.001$; reference group 0 ACEs).

For wellbeing, the prevalence of low life satisfaction increased from 8.5% in those with no ACEs to 29.9% in those with 4+ ACEs, with 34.6% of this ACE category also having low mental wellbeing (Table 2). Accounting for demographics, having one ACE (cv no ACEs) did not impact on life satisfaction or mental wellbeing but subsequent increases in ACEs were associated with reductions in both (Table 4).

All substance use measures increased in prevalence with increasing ACEs. The prevalence of heavy drinking increased 2-fold from 0 to 4+ ACEs (Table 2). Demographically adjusted comparisons identified no impact of one ACE on substance use, but increases in risk of heavy drinking, daily smoking and having ever used cannabis in those with >1 ACE. Odds of having used heroin or crack cocaine did not differ significantly from those with no ACEs until 4+ ACEs (Table 4).

Increasing ACEs were associated with higher prevalence of both having been hit and hitting someone else in the last 12 months (Table 2). Accounting for demographics, odds of having been hit were only significantly elevated in those with 4+ ACEs, while odds of having hit someone else were increased in those with >1 ACE (Table 4). Having spent ≥1 night in prison or a police station in the last 12 months did not increase with one ACE but were over four and eight times higher in those with 2–3 and 4+ ACEs, respectively (Table 4).

ACE counts were not associated with exercise frequency (Tables 2 and 4). However, low fruit and vegetable intake was significantly more likely in those with 4+ ACEs. While obesity (BMI ≥30) was associated with increased ACE count in bivariate analyses (Table 2), this relationship disappeared when demographic confounders were accounted for (Table 4).

TABLE 4. Relationships between number of ACEs and behavioural, social and health outcomes.

Outcome measure	n	P[a]	ACE count (reference category: 0 ACEs)						Demographic factors[c]			
			1		2–3		4+		Ethnicity	Age	Gender	IMD
			AOR (95% CI)	P[b]	AOR (95% CI)	P[b]	AOR (95% CI)	P[b]				
Sexual behaviour												
Had/caused unintentional pregnancy <18 years	1452	***	1.52 (0.88–2.62)	ns	2.19 (1.27–3.78)	**	4.46 (2.73– 7.30)	***	W***	ns	F***	D*
Had sex <16 years	1355	***	1.41 (0.96–2.09)	ns	1.76 (1.17–2.63)	**	2.49 (1.65–3.77)	***	W***	Y***	M**	D*
Mental health and wellbeing[a]												
Low mental wellbeing score	1464	***	1.20 (0.81–1.75)	ns	2.03 (1.41–2.92)	***	3.48 (2.40–5.04)	***	ns	Y***	ns	ns
Low life satisfaction	1305	***	1.04 (0.62–1.75)	ns	2.20 (1.39–3.47)	***	4.65 (2.99–7.25)	***	ns	***	ns	D***
Substance use												
Current daily smoker	1460	***	1.36 (0.98–1.90)	ns	2.08 (1.48–2.93)	***	3.96 (2.74–5.73)	***	W***	Y***	M***	D***
Drink ≥ 6 drinks[b] per occasion ≥ 1/week	1451	***	1.22 (0.75–1.98)	ns	1.74 (1.09–2.79)	*	3.72 (2.37–5.85)	***	W*	Y***	M***	ns
Ever used cannabis	1457	***	1.39 (0.90–2.15)	ns	3.00 (1.97–4.57)	***	5.48 (3.58–8.38)	***	W***	Y***	M***	ns
Ever used heroin or crack cocaine	1447	***	1.27 (0.41–3.94)	ns	1.26 (0.41–3.89)	ns	9.69 (4.24–22.10)	***	W*	ns	M***	ns
Violence and criminal justice												
Been hit by someone in last 12 months	1458	***	0.79 (0.37–1.72)	ns	1.70 (0.89–3.25)	ns	5.18 (2.87–9.36)	***	ns	Y***	M***	ns
Hit someone in last 12 months	1459	***	1.39 (0.65–2.98)	ns	2.95 (1.54–5.67)	**	7.92 (4.34–14.45)	***	ns	Y***	M***	ns

TABLE 4. Continued.

Ever spent ≥1 night in police station/ prison	1455	***	0.75 (0.26– 2.14)	ns	4.28 (2.14–8.55)	***	8.83 (4.42–17.62)	***	W*	Y*	M***	ns
Diet, weight and exercise												
≤1 portion of fruit or vegetables a day	1464	**	1.35 (0.91–2.00)	ns	1.47 (0.98–2.20)	ns	2.10 (1.40–3.17)	***	ns	**	M*	D***
Obese (BMI ≥ 30)	1461	ns							ns	O***	ns	D**
Morbidly obese (BMI ≥ 40)	1464	*	1.04 (0.40–2.68)	ns	0.83 (0.28–2.51)	ns	3.02 (1.38–6.62)	**	ns	ns	ns	ns
≤ 2 30 min sessions of exercise/week	1464	ns							I**	O***	F**	D**
Education and employment												
No qualifications (vocational, school, other)	1464	*	1.25 (0.91–1.73)	ns	1.49 (1.06–2.10)	*	1.69 (1.16–2.45)	**	P***	O***	F**	D***
Currently unemployed/on long-term sickness	1438	***	1.20 (0.82–1.74)	ns	2.01 (1.40–2.88)	***	2.94 (2.01–4.31)	***	ns	***	M***	D***

ns, not significant. Letters indicate direction of increasing odds: Y, youngest; O, oldest; W, White British; I, Indian; F, Female; M, Male; D, Deprived. Where there was no clear pattern only significance level is given. BMI, body mass index.

[a]P refers to the overall significance of association between the outcome measure and ACE counts. *<0.05, **<0.01 and ***<0.001.

[b]P refers to the significance of association between the outcome measure and individual ACE categories with 0 ACEs as the reference category.

[c]Gender, ethnicity and age entered as categorical variables and IMD (index of multiple deprivation) as a continuous variable.

[d]Low mental wellbeing was categorized as a score of <23 on the Short Warwick-Edinburgh Mental Wellbeing Scale, low life satisfaction ≤5 on a Likert 10-point scale (see the section Methods).

[e]A drink is a standard UK unit of alcohol equivalent to 10 ml pure alcohol.

However, even accounting for demographics, morbid obesity (BMI ≥40) remained significantly higher in those with 4+ ACEs (Table 4).

Having no qualifications was not associated with ACE counts (Table 2). However, after correcting for demographics, ACE counts of 2–3 and 4+ were associated with increasing odds of having no qualifications (Table 4). Increasing prevalence of current unemployment/long-term sickness was seen with increasing ACEs (Table 2); such increases were maintained in LR but only in those with >1 ACE (Table 4).

For health outcomes, having ever had a sexually transmitted infection (STI) was strongly associated with increasing ACEs (Tables 2 and 5). Having spent ≥1 night in the last 12 months, or 6+ nights ever, in hospital was both associated with having more ACEs (Table 2). After correcting for confounders, the former showed a significant increase only in the 2–3 ACEs category (Table 5), while the latter was associated with ACE counts >1 (Table 5). Similarly, an independent increase in odds of having ever broken a bone was observed with >1 ACE. Diagnoses of cancer and cardiovascular conditions were not associated with ACE count (Table 2) but increased strongly with age (Table 5). Type II diabetes also showed no independent relationship with ACEs (Table 5). However, in bivariate analyses individuals with >1 ACE had higher levels of respiratory and digestive/liver diseases (Table 2). After correcting for confounders only 4+ ACEs remained significant for respiratory disease and a 2–3 ACE count for digestive/liver disease.

Individuals were asked their mother's age at their birth. While 10.3% of those with no ACEs were born to mothers aged <20 years, this rose with ACE count (1 ACE, 13.2%; 2–3 ACEs, 16.7%; 4+ ACEs 20.0%; x^2 = 15.722, P<0.001). This association was maintained after correcting for demographics (as Table 4) with AORs being 1.40 (95% CI: 0.91–2.16), 1.99 (95% CI:1.28–3.09) and 2.55 (95% CI:1.61–4.04) for 1, 2–3 and 4+ ACE categories, respectively.

8.3.1 SPECIALIST SAMPLE

Individuals in the substance use service sample showed a higher prevalence of ACEs than the general population sample (0 ACEs, 4.5%; 1 ACE,

10.4%; 2–3 ACEs 20.9%; 4+ ACEs 64.2%; x^2 = 151.806, P<0.001). Demographics also differed from the general population (see Table 3) by age (50 years 8.5%; x^2 = 22.235, P<0.001), gender (male 73.8%; x^2 = 29.700, P<0.001), deprivation (poorest quintile resident 84.4%; x^2 = 13.554, P<0.001) and ethnicity (White British 92.5%; x^2 = 21.686, P<0.001).

8.4 DISCUSSION

8.4.1 MAIN FINDINGS OF THIS STUDY

Independent of relationships with deprivation, increasing ACE counts are strongly related to adverse behavioural, mental and physical outcomes throughout the life course. Smoking, heavy drinking and cannabis use all increased with ACE counts. Increased heroin or crack cocaine use was also seen in those with 4+ ACEs; consistent with the substance user sample where 64.2% of individuals had 4+ ACEs.

Unlike previous ACE studies, we measured mental wellbeing and life satisfaction; which both reduced rapidly in participants with >1 ACE. Low mental wellbeing and life satisfaction are related to lower investment in health-promoting behaviours and increased uptake of health-harming behaviours. [25,32,33] Here, while low fruit and vegetable consumption and morbid obesity increased in those with 4+ ACEs, ACEs had no impact on obesity or infrequent exercise. However, both these can result from either life-course successes or failures (e.g. sedentary employment, long-term unemployment) confounding relationships with ACEs. [34,35]

The impacts of health-harming behaviours on injury and NCDs are likely to have contributed to the increased hospital stays in those with 4+ ACEs. [36] However, while respiratory and digestive disease showed some increases in prevalence with ACEs, other major causes of premature mortality did not: cancer, cardiovascular conditions and Type II diabetes. Across England and Wales, population size falls by around a third between ages 54 and 70 years,17 and these three causes account for around 70% of deaths in this age group. [37] As those with most ACEs have significantly more risk factors relating to such conditions, premature mortality may have removed many from this population prior to survey.

TABLE 5. Relationships between number of ACEs and behavioural, social and health outcomes.

Outcome measure	n	P[a]	ACE count (reference category: 0 ACEs)						Demographic factors[c]			
			1		2–3		4+		Ethnicity	Age	Gender	IMD
			AOR (95% CI)	P[b]	AOR (95% CI)	P[b]	AOR (95% CI)	P[b]				
Ever broken a bone in your own body	1464	***	1.19 (0.88–1.61)	ns	1.85 (1.35–2.54)	***	2.51 (1.76–3.57)	***	W***	O**	M***	ns
Spent ≥1 night in hospital in last 12 months	1458	*	0.73 (0.45–1.19)	ns	1.63 (1.06–2.50)	*	1.52 (0.94–2.44)	ns	ns	***	F*	D**
Spent ≥6 nights in hospital ever	1460	*	1.25 (0.90–1.73)	ns	1.45 (1.03–2.04)	*	1.77 (1.22–2.57)	**	W***	O***	M*	D***
Ever diagnosed with												
STI	1451	***	8.90 (1.83–43.35)	**	11.14 (2.29–54.27)	**	30.58 (6.89–135.80)	***	ns	Y*	ns	ns
Cancer	1453	ns							ns	O***	F**	ns
Type II diabetes	1457	ns							ns	O***	ns	ns
Cardiovascular conditions[d]	1460	ns							ns	O***	ns	D***
Respiratory disease	1453	*	0.93 (0.50–1.85)	ns	1.21 (0.63–2.33)	ns	2.48 (1.32–4.65)	**	ns	O***	ns	D***
Digestive/liver disease	1460	**	0.99 (0.39–2.55)	ns	3.53 (1.77–7.05)	***	2.27 (0.96–5.37)	ns	ns	O***	ns	ns

ns, not significant. Letters indicate direction of increasing odds: Y, youngest; O, oldest; W, White British; F, Female; M, Male; D, Deprived. Where there was no clear pattern only significance level is given. STI, sexually transmitted infection.

[a]P refers to the overall significance of association between the outcome measure and ACE counts. *<0.05, **<0.01, ***<0.001.

[b]P refers to the significance of association between the outcome measure and individual ACE categories with 0 ACEs as the reference category.

[c]Gender, ethnicity and age entered as categorical variables and IMD (index of multiple deprivation) as a continuous variable.

[d]Including coronary heart disease, myocardial infarction and stroke.

Having had an STI increased even with a single ACE, while nearly a quarter of individuals with 4+ ACEs had/ caused an unintended pregnancy <18 years. Critically unplanned, early pregnancies increase risks of ACEs against resulting children. [38] Consistent with other studies, we identified a link between ACEs and having been born to a mother <20 years. [38,39] Such results are indicative of a cycle where those suffering ACEs take sexual risks, become parents early and raise their children in environments where risks of ACEs are again high. Further our results, like others, [6,40,41] show that individuals with more ACEs are more likely to become victims and perpetrators of violence and be incarcerated in the criminal justice system, again contributing to the next generation's ACEs. Higher ACE counts were also associated with deprivation. Those with 4+ ACEs were more likely to live in deprived areas, be unemployed/on long-term sickness and have no qualifications. These relationships suggest adverse childhoods may inhibit social movement and trap successive family generations in poverty.

8.4.2 WHAT IS ALREADY KNOWN ON THIS TOPIC

Initial ACE studies were undertaken in the USA. Consistent with findings here (Table 4), these studies identified strong links between increasing ACEs and substance use, severe obesity and low mental wellbeing in adulthood. [4,20] The use of recently developed ACE tools is largely limited to the USA with relationships between ACEs and life-course outcomes relatively untested in countries with different approaches to universal health care and child support. However, limited ACE studies have been undertaken elsewhere. Thus, in Canada, as here (Table 5), higher ACEs were linked to poorer adult health and greater health service use. [8] Our findings are also consistent with those from lower income countries with, for example, ACEs having been associated with increased risks of substance use in Nigeria [42] and sexual risk taking and early smoking initiation in the Philippines. [43]

8.4.3 WHAT THIS STUDY ADDS

Although ACEs are more likely to occur in poorer communities, independent of deprivation ACE counts correlate with worse health, criminal justice, employment and educational outcomes over the life course. The impacts of ACEs on criminality, violence, early unplanned pregnancy and retention in poverty means those with ACEs are more likely to propagate a cycle that exposes their own children to ACEs. Population surveys likely underestimate the impact of ACEs on long-term health due to premature mortality removing those with more ACEs from the population.

8.4.4 LIMITATIONS OF THIS STUDY

This first UK ACE study experienced several limitations. For those asked to participate compliance was >70%. Researcher feedback suggested lack of time, not survey content, was the main reason for non-participation. However, with no empirical information on non-participants, bias introduced through selective participation cannot be excluded. Moreover, despite reassurances of anonymity and confidentiality individuals may have deliberately or inadvertently (e.g. poor recall, blocking certain memories) provided incorrect answers. [44] Critically, although we limited our sample to those aged ≤70 years, it is likely that some individuals with high ACE counts will have already died. [45] Longitudinal studies on those with ACEs would avoid this confounder and are urgently needed to map and quantify the full impact of childhood adversity.

8.5 CONCLUSIONS

National and international policy is increasingly focused on the social determinants of long-term health. [46] However, even in deprived communities, residents' behaviours and health outcomes vary considerably. [47] ACEs are a key risk factor for poor outcomes that policy can address. Cost-effective programmes are available that help disadvantaged parents provide safe and supported childhoods (e.g. nurse home visiting, parenting programmes). [48 – 52] Most evaluation of these programmes has been undertaken in the USA. Further work is needed to understand the components of successful programmes necessary elsewhere, especially in countries with universal healthcare systems or limited health assets. However, sufficient evidence is already available for governments to prioritize and invest in ACE-preventing interventions. Too often the focus is on addressing the consequences of ACEs rather than preventing them in the first instance.

REFERENCES

1. Greenfield EA. Child abuse as a life-course social determinant of adult health. Maturitas 2010;66(1):51–5.
2. Maniglio R. The impact of child sexual abuse on health: a systematic review of reviews. Clin Psychol Rev 2009;29(7):647–57.
3. Kessler RC, McLaughlin KA, Green JG et al. Childhood adversities and adult psychopathology in the WHO World Mental Health Surveys. Br J Psychiatry 2010;197(5):378–85.
4. Felitti VJ, Anda RF, Nordenberg D et al. Relationship of childhood abuse and household dysfunction to many of the leading causes of death in adults. The Adverse Childhood Experiences (ACE) Study. Am J Prev Med 1998;14(4):245–58.
5. World Health Organization. Adverse childhood experiences international questionnaire (ACE-IQ). http://www.who.int/violence_ injury_prevention/violence/activities/adverse_childhood_ experiences/en/index.html (19 December 2012, date last accessed).
6. Mair C, Cunradi CB, Todd M. Adverse childhood experiences and intimate partner violence: testing psychosocial mediational pathways among couples. Ann Epidemiol 2012;22(12):832–9.
7. Liu Y, Croft JB, Chapman DP et al. Relationship between adverse childhood experiences and unemployment among adults from five US states. Soc Psychiatry Psychiatr Epidemiol 2012;48(3):357–69.
8. Chartier MJ, Walker JR, Naimark B. Separate and cumulative effects of adverse childhood experiences in predicting adult health and health care utilization. Child Abuse Negl 2010;34(6):454–64.
9. Dube SR, Felitti VJ, Dong M et al. The impact of adverse childhood experiences on health problems: evidence from four birth cohorts dating back to 1900. Prev Med 2003;37(3):268–77.
10. Bellis MA, Hughes K, Perkins C et al. Protecting people, promoting health: a public health approach to violence prevention for England. Liverpool: North West Public Health Observatory, 2012.
11. Anda RF, Butchart A, Felitti VJ et al. Building a framework for global surveillance of the public health implications of adverse childhood experiences. Am J Prev Med 2010;39(1):93–8.
12. World Health Organization Regional Office for Europe. Health 2020: a European policy framework supporting action across government and society for health and well-being. Copenhagen: World Health Organization Regional Office for Europe, 2012.
13. Haatainen KM, Tanskanen A, Kylma J et al. Gender differences in the association of adult hopelessness with adverse childhood experiences. Soc Psychiatry Psychiatr Epidemiol 2003;38(1):12–7.

14. Bentall RP, Wickham S, Shevlin M et al. Do specific early-life adversities lead to specific symptoms of psychosis? A study from the 2007 Adult Psychiatric Morbidity Survey. Schizophr Bull 2012;38(4):734–40.
15. Corcoran P, Gallagher J, Keeley HS et al. Adverse childhood experiences and lifetime suicide ideation: a cross-sectional study in a nonpsychiatric hospital setting. Ir Med J 2006;99(2):42–5.
16. Friestad C, Ase-Bente R, Kjelsberg E. Adverse childhood experiences among women prisoners: relationships to suicide attempts and drug abuse. Int J Soc Psychiatry 2012 [Epub ahead of print].
17. Office for National Statistics. 2011 Census, population and household estimates for England and Wales—unrounded figures for the data published 16 July 2012. http:// www.ons.gov.uk/ons/rel/census/2011-census/population-and-household-estimates-forengland- and-wales—unrounded-figures-for-the-data-published-16- july-2012/ index.html (19 December 2012, date last accessed).
18. Office for National Statistics. Neighbourhood statistics. http:// www.neighbourhood.statistics.gov.uk/dissemination/ (19 December 2012, date last accessed).
19. Department of Health, NHS. Health profiles 2012. http://www. apho.org.uk/default.aspx?QN=P_HEALTH_PROFILES (19 December 2012, date last accessed).
20. Anda RF, Felitti VJ, Bremner JD et al. The enduring effects of abuse and related adverse experiences in childhood. A convergence of evidence from neurobiology and epidemiology. Eur Arch Psychiatry Clin Neurosci 2006;256(3):174–86.
21. Lu W, Mueser KT, Rosenberg SD et al. Correlates of adverse childhood experiences among adults with severe mood disorders. Psychiatr Serv 2008;59(9):1018–26.
22. Frank D, DeBenedetti AF, Volk RJ et al. Effectiveness of the AUDIT-C as a screening test for alcohol misuse in three race/ ethnic groups. J Gen Intern Med 2008;23(6):781–7.
23. Alcohol Learning Centre. AUDIT-C. http://www.alcohollearning centre.org.uk/Topics/Browse/BriefAdvice/?parent=4444&child= 4898 (19 December 2012, date last accessed).
24. Stewart-Brown S, Tennant A, Tennant R et al. Internal construct validity of the Warwick-Edinburgh Mental Well-being Scale (WEMWBS): a Rasch analysis using data from the Scottish Health Education Population Survey. Health Qual Life Outcomes 2009;7:15.
25. Bellis MA, Lowey H, Hughes K et al. Variations in risk and protective factors for life satisfaction and mental wellbeing with deprivation: a cross-sectional study. BMC Public Health 2012;12:492.
26. World Health Organization. Global database on body mass index. http://apps.who.int/bmi/index.jsp (19 December 2012, date last accessed).
27. Department for Communities and Local Government. English indices of deprivation 2010. London: Department for Communities and Local Government, 2011.
28. Royal Mail. Postcode Address File (PAFw). http://www.royalmail. com/marketing-services/address-management-unit/address-dataproducts/ postcode-address-file-paf ?campaignid=paf_redirect (19 December 2012, date last accessed).
29. Hickman M, Taylor C, Chatterjell A et al. Estimating the prevalence of problematic drug use: a review of methods and their application. Bull Narcot 2002;LIV(1/2):15–32.

30. Bellis MA, Hughes K, Wood S et al. National five-year examination of inequalities and trends in emergency hospital admission for violence across England. Inj Prev 2011;17(5):319–25.
31. Kirkwood BR, Sterne JAC. Essential Medical Statistics, 2nd edn. Malden, MA: Blackwell Science Ltd, 2003.
32. Grant N, Wardle J, Steptoe A. The relationship between life satisfaction and health behaviour: a cross-cultural analysis of young adults. Int J Behav Med 2009;16(3):259–68.
33. Hakkarainen R, Partonen T, Haukka J et al. Food and nutrition intake in relation to mental wellbeing. Nutr J 2004;3:14.
34. Church TS, Thomas DM, Tudor-Locke C et al. Trends over 5 decades in U.S. occupation-related physical activity and their associations with obesity. PLoS One 2011;6(5):e19657.
35. Schunck R, Rogge B. Unemployment and its association with health-relevant actions: investigating the role of time perspective with German census data. Int J Public Health 2010;55(4):271–8.
36. World Health Organization. Global health risks: mortality and burden of disease attributable to selected major risks. Geneva: World Health Organization, 2009.
37. Office for National Statistics. Mortality statistics: deaths registered in England and Wales (Series DR), 2011. http://www.ons.gov.uk/ons/ rel/vsob1/mortality-statistics-deaths-registered-in-england-and-walesseries- dr-/index.html (19 December 2012, date last accessed).
38. Sidebotham P, Heron J. Child maltreatment in the 'children of the nineties': a cohort study of risk factors. Child Abuse Negl 2006;30(5):497–522.
39. Stith SM, Liu T, Davies LC et al. Risk factors in child maltreatment: a meta-analytic review of the literature. Aggress Violent Behav 2009;14(1):13–29.
40. Duke NN, Pettingell SL, McMorris BJ et al. Adolescent violence perpetration: associations with multiple types of adverse childhood experiences. Pediatrics 2010;125(4):e778–86.
41. Miller E, Breslau J, Chung WJ et al. Adverse childhood experiences and risk of physical violence in adolescent dating relationships. J Epidemiol Community Health 2011;65(11):1006–13.
42. Oladeji BD, Makanjuola VA, Gureje O. Family-related adverse childhood experiences as risk factors for psychiatric disorders in Nigeria. Br J Psychiatry 2010;196(3):186–91.
43. Ramiro LS, Madrid BJ, Brown DW. Adverse childhood experiences (ACE) and health-risk behaviors among adults in a developing country setting. Child Abuse Neglect 2010;34(11):842–55.
44. Dube SR, Williamson DF, Thompson T et al. Assessing the reliability of retrospective reports of adverse childhood experiences among adult HMO members attending a primary care clinic. Child Abuse Negl 2004;28(7):729–37.
45. Brown DW, Anda RF, Tiemeier H et al. Adverse childhood experiences and the risk of premature mortality. Am J Prev Med 2009;37(5):389–96.
46. Commission on Social Determinants of Health. Closing the gap in a generation: health equity through action on the social determinants of health. Final Report of the

Commission on Social Determinants of Health. Geneva: World Health Organization, 2008.

47. Lakshman R, McConville A, How S et al. Association between arealevel socioeconomic deprivation and a cluster of behavioural risk factors: cross-sectional, population-based study. J Public Health 2011;33(2):234–45.
48. Olds DL, Eckenrode J, Henderson CR Jr et al. Long-term effects of home visitation on maternal life course and child abuse and neglect. Fifteen-year follow-up of a randomized trial. JAMA 1997;278(8):637–43.
49. Hutchings J, Bywater T, Daley D et al. Parenting intervention in Sure Start services for children at risk of developing conduct disorder: pragmatic randomised controlled trial. BMJ 2007;334(7595):678.
50. Aos S, Lieb R, Mayfield J et al. Benefits and costs of prevention and early intervention programs for youth. Olympia, WA: Washington State Institute for Public Policy, 2004.
51. Knapp M, McDaid D, Parsonage E. Mental health promotion and mental illness prevention: the economic case. London: Department of Health, 2011.
52. Edwards RT, O'Ceilleachair A, Bywater T et al. Parenting programme for parents of children at risk of developing conduct disorder: cost effectiveness analysis. BMJ 2007;334(7595):682.

CHAPTER 9

Adverse Childhood Experiences and Adult Smoking, Nebraska, 2011

KRISTIN YEOMAN, THOMAS SAFRANEK, BRYAN BUSS, BETSY L. CADWELL, AND DAVID MANNINO

9.1 INTRODUCTION

Tobacco use is the leading underlying cause of death in the United States (1) and likewise is an important public health problem in Nebraska. During 2010, prevalence of adult smoking in Nebraska was 18.4%, similar to the national average of 19.0% (2,3). Preventing or delaying the onset of tobacco use is a key component in decreasing the occurrence of premature deaths. Understanding the genetic and environmental factors that predispose people to tobacco use is important. One area of study that has received substantial interest involves childhood adverse events. Experiencing childhood sexual and physical abuse and witnessing violence in the home or community substantially increase the risk of tobacco initiation and dependence (4–6).

Investigators are beginning to elucidate the underlying mechanisms by which abuse affects childhood development and subsequent pathology. Changes in hippocampal volume have been demonstrated among people affected by childhood trauma (7). Dysregulation of stress responses among victims of childhood trauma is postulated to increase their subsequent risk for substance abuse (8).

Life course theory (LCT) is an intergenerational approach to health and well-being and posits that health trajectories are developed during each person's lifespan on the basis of genetic, economic, environmental, and social factors (9). LCT promotes broad-based strategies to focus resources on preventing adverse health determinants that occur earlier in the person's life, developing integrated services across the lifespan and reducing risks and fostering protective factors at individual, family, and societal levels (9). Traditionally, public health and medicine have concentrated on disparities within individual disease states rather than on early health determinants. Adverse childhood experiences could be considered early determinants that contribute to adverse health trajectories through increased adoption of unhealthy behaviors.

The 1995 Adverse Childhood Experiences Study demonstrated the effect of childhood maltreatment and household dysfunction on adult smoking, obesity, and excessive alcohol use (10). During 2009, the Centers for Disease Control and Prevention (CDC) added an optional module to the core Behavioral Risk Factor Surveillance System (BRFSS) questions, adapting questions from the Adverse Childhood Experiences Study. That year, 5 states administered the Adverse Childhood Experiences module. An estimated 59% of residents in those states had 1 or more adverse childhood experience (ACE), and approximately 9% had 5 or more (11). Other studies have evaluated individual ACEs as primary exposures and compared outcomes among persons with and without individual ACE exposures; this method has the limitation of different referent groups for each individual ACE analysis, and thus no comparison can be made of the magnitude of associations between outcomes and individual ACEs. Findings from these earlier studies demonstrate a high prevalence of ACEs in a nonrandom selection of states. Establishing the prevalence of ACEs in each state can provide information to help the individual states target local prevention efforts.

Nebraska administered the ACE module during 2011, but the possible associations between ACEs and smoking among Nebraska residents have not been evaluated using these data. A limited number of divisions within Nebraska's Department of Health and Human Services have expressed interest in using ACE data to guide data collection for new childhood maltreatment prevention and intervention programs. The behavioral health and children and family services divisions are focusing on prevention activities in addition to intervention strategies and can use results of state-specific ACE data analysis to assist in program development and education. The maternal and child health division initiated a home visitation program in 2012 and can use results of ACE data analysis to establish appropriate data requirements to monitor program outcomes. We undertook an investigation of ACE prevalence among Nebraska residents and its association with smoking, evaluating ACE data by using a new method adapted from a previous study (12).

9.2 METHODS

We analyzed data from the 2011 Nebraska BRFSS (13). BRFSS is a surveillance system administered by state health departments in conjunction with CDC. Each month, trained interviewers contacted a probability sample of adults in Nebraska to administer a core group of standardized questions regarding health behaviors and practices. A randomly selected subset of the total probability sample completed state-added optional modules, which included the ACE module, designed to obtain information of specific interest to Nebraska. Although the 2011 survey was the first to incorporate respondents with either landline or cellular telephone service, the ACE module did not include respondents with cellular telephones.

Response rates for BRFSS are calculated using standards set by the American Association of Public Opinion Research (AAPOR) Response Rate Formula #4 (www.aapor.org/Standard_Definitions2.htm). The response rate is the number of respondents who completed the survey as a proportion of all eligible and likely eligible persons. The response rate for Nebraska in 2011 was 66%. Detailed information is available in the BRFSS Summary Data Quality Report (14).

The ACE module comprised 11 questions regarding events that respondents experienced before age 18 years. We combined responses to 11 questions into the following ACE categories by adapting category definitions used in other studies as follows (10,11): physical abuse, sexual abuse, verbal abuse, mental illness in a household member, substance abuse in a household member, witnessing abuse, divorce, and incarceration of a household member. BRFSS questions and responses corresponding to individual ACE categories are listed in the Appendix.

We classified these 8 categories into direct and environmental ACEs. We defined direct ACEs as affirmative responses in any of the categories of physical abuse, sexual abuse, or verbal abuse. We defined environmental ACEs as affirmative responses in any of the categories of household mental illness, household substance abuse, witnessing abuse, divorce, or incarceration of a household member.

Definitions and age categories from the initial CDC BRFSS analyses were used to define control variables (11), but we categorized educational attainment into 4 categories (did not complete high school, completed high school, attended some college or technical school, or completed college or technical school), and we added excessive alcohol use as a covariate. We defined respondents as excessive alcohol users if they reported either heavy alcohol intake (≥60 or ≥30 alcoholic drinks for males or females, respectively, in 1 month) or binge drinking (≥5 or ≥4 alcoholic drinks for males or females, respectively, on a single occasion). Marital status and depression were evaluated but not included in the final model because they did not substantially affect the association of ACE status and smoking. The outcome variable of smoking was a self-reported smoker or never smoker. Only 5% (462) respondents were nonwhite, compared with the 2010 Census Bureau estimate for Nebraska of 13.9% nonwhite (15). Preliminary analyses of whites only and all races together reported no substantial differences. Therefore, because of the difficulty of interpreting results for multiple races together and the high probability of bias within the nonwhite sample, subsequent analyses were conducted only for non-Hispanic whites.

We included records with "yes" responses in any individual ACE category within the direct and environmental ACE groups, even in the presence of other missing responses, because inclusion in the direct and environmental groups required the presence of only 1 positive response in any individual ACE within that category. Missing responses in a record that contained "yes" responses would not modify the classification of that record as having a direct or environmental ACE, whereas missing responses in a record with other "no" responses could modify the classification. Therefore, we excluded from analysis records (7.4%) that were missing responses to all variables in either the direct or environmental ACE categories and records with only "no" and missing responses in the direct or environmental ACE categories.

We compared smoking among persons exposed to any of the 3 direct ACE variables with smoking among persons who did not report exposure to any ACE, among persons exposed to any of the 5 environmental ACEs with persons not reporting exposure to any ACE, and among persons exposed to both direct and environmental ACEs with persons not reporting any ACE exposure. We used SAS version 9.3 (SAS Institute Inc, Cary, North Carolina) and SUDAAN version 10.0.1 (RTI International, Research Triangle Park, North Carolina) to account for the complex survey design and weighting methodology used by BRFSS. We calculated prevalence estimates with 95% confidence intervals (CIs). We estimated adjusted relative risk (aRR) with 95% CIs of smoking by ACE status, controlling for age, sex, educational attainment, and excessive alcohol use, by using logistic regression models with predicted margins.

9.3 RESULTS

A total of 10,293 persons participated in the Nebraska BRFSS ACE module. Of these, 3,945 records (38%) were excluded because they were nonwhite, former smokers, or missing 1 or more exposures, control variables, or outcome variables. Of 6,348 remaining records, 49% had no ACEs; 33% had 1 or 2 ACEs; 11% had 3 or 4 ACEs; and 7% had 5 or more ACEs.

Prevalence of environmental ACEs (41.7%; 95% CI, 39.4–44.0) was significantly higher than that of direct ACEs (30.7%; 95% CI, 28.5–32.8) (Table 1). Prevalence of direct ACE exposures within age and education categories ranged from 26.1% (persons aged ≥55 years) to 36.0% (persons aged 25–34 years) and 28.7% (college graduates) to 33.2% (persons not

TABLE 1. Prevalence of Direct[a] and Environmental[b] Adverse Childhood Events by Demographic Characteristic Among Non-Hispanic White Adults in Nebraska, Behavioral Risk Factor Surveillance System, 2011.

Characteristic	Direct		Environmental	
	No. of Respondents	% (95% CI)	No. of Respondents	% (95% CI)
Overall	1,701	30.7 (28.5–32.8)	2,072	41.7 (39.4–44.0)
Sex				
Male	577	28.9 (25.7–32.2)	662	35.5 (31.3–39.7)
Female	1,124	32.3 (29.4–35.1)	1,410	44.2 (41.2–47.2)
Age, y				
18–24	42	24.5 (17.3–31.8)	74	43.7 (35.4–52.0)
25–34	135	36.0 (29.5–42.5)	201	54.3 (47.7–60.9)
35–44	239	33.2 (28.1–38.3)	317	48.4 (42.9–53.8)
45–54	442	35.9 (32.0–39.7)	496	40.3 (36.3–44.3)
≥55	843	26.1 (24.0–28.2)	984	29.9 (27.7–32.1)
Education				
Less than high school diploma	83	33.2 (24.6–41.9)	119	55.0 (45.9–64.1)
High school graduate	549	30.5 (26.5–34.6)	719	42.0 (37.7–46.3)
Some college	543	31.8 (28.0–35.6)	638	42.4 (38.3–46.5)
College graduate	526	28.7 (25.2–32.2)	596	36.9 (32.9–40.8)

Abbreviation: CI, confidence interval.
a Physical, sexual, or verbal abuse.
b Mental illness in a household member, substance abuse in a household member, witnessing abuse, divorce, or incarceration of a household member.

completing high school), respectively. Prevalence of environmental ACE exposures within age and education categories ranged from 29.9% (persons aged ≥55 years) to 54.3% (persons aged 25–34 years) and 36.9% (college graduates) to 55.0% (persons not completing high school), respectively. Prevalence of individual ACEs ranged from 5.9% (household incarceration) to 25.1% (verbal abuse) (Table 2). Among persons with direct ACEs, 81.9% (95% CI, 79.1–84.7) experienced verbal abuse. Among persons with environmental ACEs, 56.7% (95% CI, 52.9–60.5) experienced household substance abuse.

The prevalence of smoking by ACE exposure ranged from 22.2% (direct ACE) to 45.5% (both direct and environmental ACEs) (Table 3). After adjusting for age, sex, education level, and alcohol consumption, direct and environmental ACEs alone and in combination were significantly associated with smoking, with aRRs of 1.5, 1.8, and 2.7 for direct ACEs, environmental ACEs, and both categories, respectively.

TABLE 2. Prevalence of Individual ACE Exposures and Prevalence of Each Individual ACE Category Within Direct[a] and Environmental[b] ACE Categories Among Non-Hispanic White Adults in Nebraska, Behavioral Risk Factor Surveillance System, 2011.

ACE Exposure Category	No. of Respondents	% (95% CI)	Prevalence of Exposure Within ACE Exposure Category[c]
Direct			
Physical abuse	683	13.8 (12.2–15.4)	45.0 (40.8–49.3)
Sexual abuse	514	7.7 (6.7–8.8)	25.3 (22.0–28.6)
Verbal abuse	1,279	25.1 (23.2–27.2)	81.9 (79.1–84.7)
Environmental			
Mental illness in a household member	701	15.5 (13.6–17.3)	37.3 (33.5–41.1)
Substance abuse in a household member	1,172	23.6 (21.5–25.6)	56.7 (52.9–60.5)
Witnessing abuse	653	12.6 (11.0–14.1)	30.5 (27.0–34.0)
Incarceration of a household member	158	5.9 (4.5–7.2)	14.1 (11.1–17.2)
Divorce	734	19.2 (17.2–21.2)	46.1 (42.3–50.0)

Abbreviation: ACE, adverse childhood experience; CI, confidence interval.
a Physical, sexual, or verbal abuse.
b Mental illness in a household member, substance abuse in a household member, witnessing abuse, divorce, or incarceration of a household member.
c Proportions do not sum to 100% because persons might have more than 1 individual ACE within direct or environmental categories.

TABLE 3. Prevalence and Adjusted Relative Risk of Smoking by ACE Exposure Among Non-Hispanic White Adults in Nebraska, Behavioral Risk Factor Surveillance System, 2011.

ACE Exposure	n	Smoking, % (95% CI)	aRR[a] (95% CI)
None	426	14.2 (11.9–16.5)	Reference
Direct[b] only	113	22.2 (16.3–28.1)	1.5 (1.1–2.1)
Environmental[c] only	243	30.3 (25.2–35.5)	1.8 (1.4–2.3)
Both	340	45.5 (40.1–50.9)	2.7 (2.2–3.3)

Abbreviation: ACE, adverse childhood experience; aRR, adjusted relative risk; CI, confidence interval.
a Adjusted for age, sex, education, and alcohol consumption.
b Physical, sexual, or verbal abuse.
c Mental illness in a household member, substance abuse in a household member, witnessing abuse, divorce, or incarceration of a household member.

9.4 DISCUSSION

Our results demonstrate that ACEs are common among Nebraska residents and that the categories of direct and environmental ACEs are both associated with an increased risk for smoking. These results are consistent with previous studies. ACEs have been linked to multiple health behaviors, including smoking (10,16), illicit drug use (10,17,18), alcohol misuse (10,19), obesity (10,20), and adolescent pregnancy (21). Dose-response relationships have been observed between increasing numbers of reported ACEs and smoking persistence among persons with tobacco-related illness (22).

We observed that a higher proportion of residents reported environmental rather than direct ACEs. More environmental than direct ACE categories exist; thus, the potential for experiencing environmental ACEs is likely greater. We demonstrated similar increases in risk for smoking with either direct or environmental ACEs alone. These results suggest that given the higher prevalence of environmental ACEs and its association with increased smoking risk, greater emphasis on preventing environmental ACEs in conjunction with preventing child abuse might decrease smoking among adults.

We evaluated ACEs by using a new method, aggregating individual ACEs into direct and environmental categories. Our method allowed us to compare risk of smoking among persons with direct ACEs, environmental ACEs, and both ACE categories, to persons without any ACEs. This method improves on previous studies comparing outcomes among persons who experienced a specific individual ACE with those of persons without that specific individual ACE, which could potentially diminish the association of the ACE and outcome because persons in the referent group could have ACEs other than the specific ACE under evaluation. For example, persons not experiencing physical abuse could have another individual ACE, such as household mental illness, that is associated with the outcome. Furthermore, comparing outcomes among persons with a specific individual ACE to those of persons without that specific individual ACE limits the ability to compare magnitude of association between 2 individual ACEs (in this example, physical abuse and household mental illness) and the outcome of interest because of differences in referent groups.

Our results using the new method could be useful as a state health department decides the most appropriate strategy to educate the general public about this issue. Explaining 2 categories and demonstrating associations between these categories and adverse outcomes could be useful in improving public knowledge without requiring in-depth explanations of each individual ACE.

ACEs can be considered early health determinants within the framework of LCT. To minimize the effects of ACEs on unhealthy behaviors and negative health outcomes later in life, LCT recommends primary prevention of ACEs through varied strategies aimed at providing the necessary supports throughout childhood development. At the same time, intervention on behalf of children at risk is important, highlighting the need for real-time, actionable surveillance data for each ACE category. Although states have mechanisms to detect and treat child abuse, the full burden of children residing in homes with mental illness, domestic violence, substance abuse, or incarcerated family members is unknown. As a Patient Protection and Affordable Care Act grantee for evidence-based home visiting programs, Nebraska's Maternal and Child Health program is developing indicators for maternal and child well-being and determining appropriate data requirements to establish these indicators. A home visitation program was started during 2012, with the objective of preventing child abuse and neglect, and our study can be used to establish beneficial data collection for this program. Although little evidence exists that nurse home visits directly decrease child abuse and neglect, home visits can improve parenting practices and a child's home environment (23–25). Efforts to improve child well-being in Nebraska can be fostered by providing the state with prevalence estimates of each ACE and with measures of association between ACEs and risk factors for disease. Nebraska stakeholders will be able to develop and modify plans for surveillance and intervention accordingly. These findings can also be used as an example for other states that have received a similar grant and will need to develop their own metrics.

Limitations of this study include the inability to verify self-reported history of ACEs and smoking. Studies evaluating accuracy of responses to questions in adulthood regarding childhood maltreatment demonstrate substantial underreporting but little overreporting (26,27). Thus, we likely provide conservative estimates of the association between smoking and ACEs among Nebraska residents. With a response rate of approximately 66%, differences between responders and nonresponders can introduce bias. Although BRFSS began incorporating cellular telephones into their survey methodology during 2011, the ACE module did not include cellular telephones, potentially underestimating ACE prevalence and associations between ACEs and smoking among persons aged 18–34 years. Finally, our sample did not include a sufficient number of persons of minority race/ethnicity to allow a comparison among different racial/ethnic groups in Nebraska. Strengths of this study include the use of predicted margins in our logistic regression model, enabling us to obtain relative risks rather than odds ratios. Because prevalence of both exposures and outcome were high, odds ratios do not provide an accurate approximation of relative risk. Sample size is another strength of this study, with more than 6,000 subjects in the final data set, which increases the power to detect associations.

ACEs are common in Nebraska and are associated with smoking, a risk factor that contributes to costly and disabling diseases. ACEs can be placed within the context of LCT to strategize methods that promote healthy conditions among all persons regardless of social, economic, and environmental circumstances. Surveillance systems to monitor a substantial number of childhood adverse events do not yet exist. State-specific strategies to monitor adverse events among children and provide interventions might help to decrease smoking among adults.

REFERENCES

1. Mokdad AH, Marks JS, Stroup DF, Gerberding JL. Actual causes of death in the United States, 2000. JAMA 2004;291(10):1238–45. Erratum in JAMA 2005;293(3):293-4; JAMA 2005;293(3):298.
2. Centers for Disease Control and Prevention. Smoking and tobacco use, state highlights, Nebraska. http://www.cdc.gov/tobacco/data_statistics/state_data/state_highlights/2010/states/nebraska/index.htm. Accessed November 6, 2012.
3. Centers for Disease Control and Prevention. Smoking and tobacco use, adult cigarette smoking in the United States: current estimate. http://www.cdc.gov/tobacco/data_statistics/fact_sheets/adult_data/cig_smoking/. Accessed March 28, 2013.
4. Nelson EC, Heath AC, Madden PAF, Cooper ML, Dinwiddie SH, Bucholz KK, et al. Association between self-reported childhood sexual abuse and adverse psychosocial outcomes: results from a twin study. Arch Gen Psychiatry 2002;59(2):139–45.
5. Jun HJ, Rich-Edwards JW, Boynton-Jarrett R, Austin SB, Frazier AL, Wright RJ. Child abuse and smoking among young women: the importance of severity, accumulation, and timing. J Adolesc Health 2008;43(1):55–63.
6. Brady SS. Lifetime community violence exposure and health risk behavior among young adults in college. J Adolesc Health 2006;39(4):610–3.
7. Woon FL, Hedges DW. Hippocampal and amygdala volumes in children and adults with childhood maltreatment-related posttraumatic stress disorder: a meta-analysis. Hippocampus 2008;18(8):729–36.
8. De Bellis MD. Developmental traumatology: a contributory mechanism for alcohol and substance use disorders. Psychoneuroendocrinology 2002;27(1–2):155–70.
9. Halfon N, Hochstein M. Life course health development: an integrated framework for developing health, policy, and research. Milbank Q 2002;80(3):433–79.
10. Felitti VJ, Anda RF, Nordenberg D, Williamson DF, Spitz AM, Edwards V, et al. Relationship of childhood abuse and household dysfunction to many of the leading causes of death in adults. The Adverse Childhood Experiences (ACE) Study. Am J Prev Med 1998;14(4):245–58.
11. Centers for Disease Control and Prevention. Adverse childhood experiences reported by adults—five states, 2009. MMWR Morb Mortal Wkly Rep 2010;59(49):1609–13.
12. Edwards VJ, Holden GW, Felitti VJ, Anda RF. Relationship between multiple forms of childhood maltreatment and adult mental health in community

respondents: results from the Adverse Childhood Experiences Study. Am J Psychiatry 2003;160(8):1453–60.

13. Nebraska Department of Health and Human Services. Nebraska Behavioral Risk Factor Surveillance System. http://dhhs.ne.gov/publichealth/Pages/brfss_index.aspx. Accessed February 25, 2013.
14. US Department of Health and Human Services. CDC. Behavioral Risk Factor Surveillance System 2011 summary data quality report. http://www.cdc.gov/brfss/pdf/2011_Summary_Data_Quality_Report.pdf. Accessed February 26, 2013.
15. United States Census Bureau. 2010 Census interactive population search, Nebraska. http://www.census.gov/2010census/popmap/ipmtext.php?fl=31. Accessed July 31, 2013.
16. Ford ES, Anda RF, Edwards VJ, Perry GS, Zhao G, Li C, et al. Adverse childhood experiences and smoking status in five states. Prev Med 2011;53(3):188–93.
17. Dube SR, Anda RF, Whitfield CL, Brown DW, Felitti VJ, Dong M, et al. Long-term consequences of childhood sexual abuse by gender of victim. Am J Prev Med 2005;28(5):430–8.
18. Fergusson DM, Boden JM, Horwood LJ. The developmental antecedents of illicit drug use: evidence from a 25-year longitudinal study. Drug Alcohol Depend 2008;96(1-2):165–77.
19. Dube SR, Miller JW, Brown DW, Giles WH, Felitti VJ, Dong M, et al. Adverse childhood experiences and the association with ever using alcohol and initiating alcohol use during adolescence. J Adolesc Health 2006;38(4):444.e11–10.
20. Thomas C, Hyppönen E, Power C. Obesity and type 2 diabetes risk in midadult life: the role of childhood adversity. Pediatrics 2008;121(5):e1240–9.
21. Hillis SD, Anda RF, Dube SR, Felitti VJ, Marchbanks PA, Marks JS. The association between adverse childhood experiences and adolescent pregnancy, long-term psychosocial consequences, and fetal death. Pediatrics 2004;113(2):320–7.
22. Edwards VJ, Anda RF, Gu D, Dube SR, Felitti VJ. Adverse childhood experiences and smoking persistence in adults with smoking-related symptoms and illness. Perm J 2007;11(2):5–13.
23. Olds DL, Eckenrode J, Henderson CR Jr, Kitzman H, Powers J, Cole R, et al. Long-term effects of home visitation on maternal life course and child abuse and neglect. Fifteen-year follow-up of a randomized trial. JAMA 1997;278(8):637–43.
24. Duggan A, Caldera D, Rodriguez K, Burrell L, Rohde C, Crowne SS. Impact of a statewide home visiting program to prevent child abuse. Child Abuse Negl 2007;31(8):801–27.
25. Fergusson DM, Grant H, Horwood LJ, Ridder EM. Randomized trial of the Early Start program of home visitation. Pediatrics 2005;116(6):e803–9.
26. Hardt J, Rutter M. Validity of adult retrospective reports of adverse childhood experiences: review of the evidence. J Child Psychol Psychiatry 2004;45(2):260–73.
27. Della Femina D, Yeager CA, Lewis DO. Child abuse: adolescent records vs. adult recall. Child Abuse Negl 1990;14(2):227–31.

There is a supplemental file that is not available in this version of the article. To view this additional information, please use the citation on the first page of this chapter.

CHAPTER 10

The Mediating Sex-Specific Effect of Psychological Distress on the Relationship Between Adverse Childhood Experiences and Current Smoking Among Adults

TARA W. STRINE, VALERIE J. EDWARDS, SHANTA R. DUBE, MORTON WAGENFELD, SATVINDER DHINGRA, ANGELA WITT PREHN, SANDRA RASMUSSEN, LELA MCKNIGHT-EILY, AND JANET B. CROFT

10.1 BACKGROUND

Adverse childhood experiences (ACEs), which can include abuse (emotional, physical, and sexual), neglect (emotional and physical), and household dysfunction, are common among children [1]. In 2010 alone, maltreatment was reported for 695,000 US children (9.2 per 1000 children) [2]. In the largest study of ACEs, over 60% of 17,337 adults reported a history of at least one ACE [3].

Research suggests that ACEs have a long-term impact on the behavioral, emotional, and cognitive development of children [4-6]. This deleterious impact may be due to an unhealthy environment that impedes the resolution of early life development issues [7] as well as actual modifications in brain anatomy and functioning during important developmental periods [8]. These disruptions can lead to adoption of unhealthy coping behaviors throughout the lifespan [9,10] as well as maladaptive psychological functioning or psychological distress [11-14].

Persons who have experienced ACEs and psychological distress may smoke as a method to compensate for deficiencies in social and emotional development as well as a way to self-medicate biological dysregulations produced by abuse or neglect [5,15-18]. Smoking may be viewed as a viable coping option because of its perceived anxiolytic and sedative properties – for example, it's ability to modify mood, manage dysphoria, regulate negative affect, control situational anxiety, and improve concentration [19-23]. As evidence, studies have shown that nicotine reduces anger in both smokers and nonsmokers with high hostility [24,25] and depressive symptoms in both nonsmokers and smokers with depression [26-28].

Psychiatric disorders are one of the most cited risk factors for nicotine dependence [29]. Longitudinal studies have suggested that depression [30-35], behavioral disorders [36], and anxiety [34], particularly PTSD [37], may increase the risk of subsequent smoking. Research has also implicated psychiatric conditions such as schizophrenia [38-41] and ADHD [42-44] as risk factors for smoking.

Several studies have examined the potential mediating effect of mental disorders on the relationship between ACEs and drug use. Studies conducted by Douglas et al. [45] and Lo and Chen [46] suggest that the relationship between childhood abuse and substance dependence may be partially mediated by mood and anxiety disorders. DeWit et al. [47], implicate social phobia as the mediator between adverse life events and chronic stress in childhood and drug dependence in adulthood. According to a literature review conducted by Simpson and Miller [48], psychiatric conditions such as depression and anxiety disorders mediate the relationship between child abuse and substance use disorders in women. Moreover, in a study conducted by White and Widom [49], the authors concluded that PTSD among maltreated girls may increase the risk of subsequent substance use problems.

Despite the fact that smoking continues to be the leading cause of death and disability in the United States [50], the magnitude and complexity of the relationship between ACEs and smoking is only beginning to be understood. Research conducted thus far suggests that ACEs are significantly associated with early smoking initiation, smoking maintenance, heavy smoking, and lifetime smoking across birth cohorts [51-56].

Because of the pervasive effect of ACEs throughout the life course and the deleterious effect of smoking on health, we sought to examine the potential mediating effect of psychological distress on the relationship between ACEs and current adult smoking. Moreover, as current research suggests that child abuse and neglect may affect men and women differently [57] and that stressors leading to smoking initiation and maintenance may vary by sex [58-62], the relationships between ACEs and smoking were further explored by sex. The purpose of this study was threefold: 1. to examine the relationships between ACEs, psychological distress, and adult smoking; 2. to determine if there were sex differences in the relationships between ACEs, psychological distress, and adult smoking, and 3. to determine if psychological distress mediated the relationship between ACEs and adult smoking among males and females.

10.2 METHODS

10.2.1 STUDY SETTING AND PARTICIPANTS

The ACE Study is one of the largest studies to examine childhood trauma as a precursor of adult health in a managed care sample [63]. Data for the current study are based upon Wave II of the ACE Study, which were collected between April and October of 1997. These data were used to examine the relationship between multiple categories of childhood trauma (ACEs) and health and behavioral outcomes later in life. Participants were drawn from adult members of the Kaiser Permanente Medical Care Program in San Diego, California, undergoing a free comprehensive medical examination through the Health Appraisal Clinic (HAC), Department of Preventive Medicine [64].

A total of 13,330 Kaiser Health Plan members completed standardized medical evaluations at the HAC from April through October of 1997. Questionnaires were completed by 8,667 San Diego, California, Kaiser

Permanente Health Maintenance Organization members who agreed to participate in the survey. Among these, 7,210 (83.2%) respondents completed information for the study variables and were included in the analyses (3,895 females and 3,315 males).

10.2.2 SURVEY METHODS AND VARIABLE DEFINITIONS

Prior to the medical examination at the clinic, each Kaiser member attending the San Diego HAC completed a standardized health appraisal questionnaire and the Standard Form-36 (SF-36) questionnaire, which was used to assess functional health and well-being [65,66]. After the physical exam, patients were mailed the study's Family Health History (FHH), a 168-item questionnaire that covers a broad range of childhood exposures and current health behaviors. Participation was voluntary, and patients were assured that the FHH would not become part of their medical record.

Adverse childhood experiences were defined using items from the FHH. The following ten ACE categories were assessed: emotional abuse (2 questions), physical abuse (2 questions), sexual abuse (4 questions), emotional neglect (5 questions), physical neglect (5 questions), witnessing domestic violence against mother or stepmother (4 questions), alcoholic or drug-abusing family members (2 questions), mentally ill household members (2 questions), parents separated or divorced, and incarcerated household members (1 question each) (Table 1). Verbatim ACE study questions can be found at: http://www.cdc.gov/ace/questionnaires.htm webcite. Questions from published surveys were used to construct these ACE items. Questions adapted from the Conflicts Tactics Scale were used to define psychological and physical abuse during childhood and to define violence against the respondent's mother or stepmother [67]. Four questions adapted from the Wyatt Sexual History Questionnaire [68] were used to define sexual abuse during childhood. Questions about exposure to alcohol or drug abuse during childhood were taken from the 1988 National Health Interview Survey [69]. Physical and emotional neglect were assessed by using the Childhood Trauma Questionnaire short form [70].

In addition to examining individual ACEs, an ACE score was constructed to examine the cumulative exposure to the different types of abuse, neglect,

TABLE 1. Definitions of abuse, neglect, and household dysfunction that occurred before age 19 years.

Category	Definitions
Abuse	
Emotional	At least one of the following responses:
	1. Often or very often a parent or other adult in the household swore at you, insulted you, or put you down.
	2. Sometimes, often, or very often they acted in a way that made you think that you might be physically hurt.
Physical	At least one of the following responses:
	1. Sometimes, often, or very often you were pushed, grabbed, slapped, or had something thrown at you.
	2. Sometimes, often, or very often hit so hard that you had marks or were injured.
Sexual	At least one affirmative (yes) response about an adult or a person at least 5 years older:
	1. Ever touched or fondled you in a sexual way.
	2. Had you touch their body in a sexual way.
	3. Attempted oral, anal, or vaginal intercourse with you.
	4. Actually had oral, anal, or vaginal intercourse with you.
Neglect	
Emotional	5 Childhood Trauma Questionnaire (CTQ) questions (Bernstein, et al., 1994) had possible responses of "never true', "rarely true", "sometimes true", "often true", or "very often true". Responses were reverse scored on a Likert scale ranging from 5 to 1, respectively.
	1. There is someone in my family who helped me feel important or special.
	2. I felt loved.
	3. People in my family looked out for each other.
	4. People in my family felt close to each other.
	5. My family was a source of strength and support.
	A total cumulative score of 15 and higher (moderate to extreme on the CTQ clinical scale) defined childhood emotional neglect (Bernstein, et al., 1994).
Physical	5 Childhood Trauma Questionnaire (CTQ) questions (Bernstein, et al., 1994) had possible responses of "never true', "rarely true", "sometimes true", "often true", or "very often true". Responses were scored on a Likert scale ranging from 1 to 5, respectively with items 2 and 5 reverse scored (5 to 1, respectively). :

TABLE 1. CONTINUED.

	1. You did not get enough to eat.
	2. You knew there was someone to take care of you and protect you.
	3. Your parents were too drunk or high to take care of the family.
	4. You had to wear dirty clothes.
	5. There was someone to take you to the doctor if you needed it.
	A total cumulative score of 10 or higher (moderate to extreme on the CTQ clinical scale) defined childhood physical neglect (Bernstein, et al., 1994).
Household dysfunction	
Witnessing domestic violence	At least one affirmative (yes) response to the following about your mother or stepmother:
	1. Sometimes, often, or very often was pushed, grabbed, slapped, or had something thrown at her.
	2. Sometimes, often, or very often was kicked, bitten, hit with a fist, or hit with something hard.
	3. Was ever repeatedly hit over at least a few minutes.
	4. Was ever threatened or hurt by a knife or gun.
Household substance abuse	At least one affirmative (yes) response about living with anyone (before age 18) who:
	1. Was a problem drinker or alcoholic.
	2. Used street drugs.
Household mental illness	At least one affirmative (yes) response about a household member who:
	1. Was depressed or mentally ill.
	2. Attempted suicide.
Parental separation or divorce	Parents were ever separated or divorced.
Incarcerated household member	A household member went to prison.

and household dysfunction [3,52,64,71]. Exposure to any ACE counted as one point, and categories were summed for a total score between 0 and 10 points. The ACE score summarizes the total number of ACEs an adult recalls experiencing as a child or adolescent across the ten categories.

Psychological distress was assessed as a continuous variable and used the Mental Component Summary (MCS) score calculated from the SF-36. The SF-36 is a generic, multipurpose, short-form health survey with 36 questions and eight subscales [66,72]. The eight scales (Physical Functioning, Role Physical, Bodily Pain, General Health, Vitality, Social Functioning, Role Emotional, and Mental Health) form two distinct higher-ordered clusters, designated physical health (PCS) and mental health (MCS), which account for 80%–85% of the variance in the eight scales [73,74]. The reliability estimates of the two summary scales have generally exceeded 0.90 [65]. Predictive studies of validity have linked SF-36 scale scores and the MCS score to the clinical course of depression [75-78]. The MCS score is calculated from a complex set of computer-generated algorithms. All eight scales comprise the MCS score, but three scales (Mental Health, Role Emotion, and Social Functioning) correlate most highly and contribute most to the scoring [65]. Role Physical, Bodily Pain, Vitality, Social Functioning, Role Emotional, and Mental Health all reference the past four weeks. Physical Functioning and General Health reference the respondent's current health and functional status [65]. As the mean MCS score decreases, level of psychological distress increases. The general US population mean MCS norm score for males is 50.73 and for females is 49.33 [65].

Current smoking status was assessed using two questions: a) "Have you smoked at least 100 cigarettes in your entire life?, and b) "Do you smoke cigarettes now?" Persons who had smoked at least 100 cigarettes in their lifetime and smoked at the time of the survey were considered adult current smokers [52,79-81].

10.2.3 STATISTICAL ANALYSIS

Mediation analyses were conducted to identify and explain the relationship between ACEs and adult current smoking based on the inclusion of the MCS score as an indicator for psychological distress [82]. In logistic models that included psychological distress and ACEs (individual or total score) as independent variables and adult current smoking as the dependent variable, psychological distress was treated as a potential mediating variable [82,83].

Several criteria must be satisfied in order for mediation analysis to be valid (Figure 1). First, the independent variable (ACEs) must be significantly associated with the dependent variable (adult current smoking) (c coefficient); the mediating variable (psychological distress) must be significantly associated with the dependent variable (adult current smoking) with the independent variable (ACEs) included in the model (b coefficient); and the independent variable (ACEs) must be significantly associated with the mediating variable (psychological distress) (a coefficient) [84]. Second, the independent variable (ACEs) must be known to cause the mediation variable (psychological distress), which in turn causes the dependent variable (adult current smoking) [84].

The Sobel test was used to determine the significance of the indirect effect of the independent variable (ACEs) on the dependent variable (adult current smoking) through the mediator (psychological distress) [85]. Because the dependent variable (adult current smoking) and the independent variable (ACEs) were dichotomous and the mediating variable (psychological distress) was continuous, the coefficients in the mediation analyses were on two different scales. To make the coefficients compatible, we used techniques developed by MacKinnon and Dwyer [86] to calculate the Sobel statistic.

All models were first examined without being adjusted and were then adjusted for age group (18–34, 35–54, 55–74, and 75 years or older), race/ethnicity (white, black, Hispanic, Asian, Native American, and other), education (no high school diploma, high school or general educational development, some college/technical school, and college graduate), parental smoking during childhood (yes vs. no) to control for familial/genetic tendencies to smoke, and alcohol use in the previous month (yes vs. no) given that alcohol and smoking are highly correlated [87]. All statistical analyses were conducted using SAS 9.2 and Excel. Significance was tested at an alpha level of $p<.05$.

10.3 RESULTS

10.3.1 DESCRIPTIVE CHARACTERISTICS

The sample consisted of 3,895 females (54.0%) and 3,315 males (46.0%). The mean age was 55.9 years; nearly three-quarters of the participants

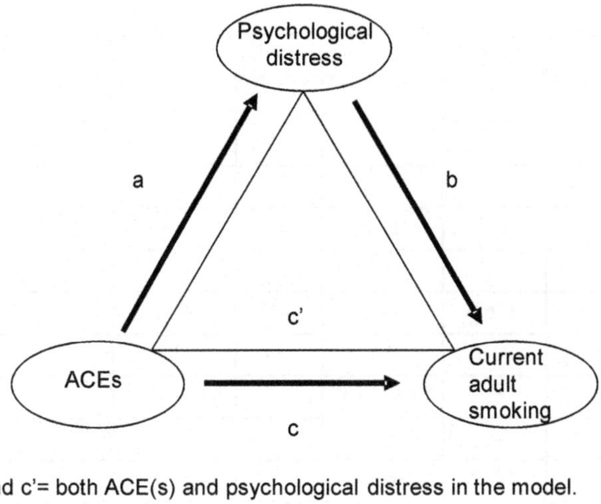

Figure 1. Mediation model.

were white and had at least some college or technical education (Table 2). Because there were different sex by effect interactions in the three primary mediation models, all analyses were stratified by sex.

Approximately 56% of women consumed alcohol in the previous month prior to the survey as did 65% of men. Over 70% of men and women reported that one or more parent smoked during their childhood. Approximately 7.6% of the women in the survey currently smoked as did 8.5% of men. The MCS score was slightly lower for women than men (51.2 versus 53.2).

Women were significantly more likely than men to report childhood emotional abuse (11.7% versus 8.2%), sexual abuse (24.2% versus 16.7%), emotional neglect (16.4% versus 12.2%), parental separation or divorce (25.3% versus 22.4%), mental illness in the household (25.0% versus 14.6%), household substance abuse (29.9% versus 25.5%), and an incarcerated household member (6.9% versus 4.8%) (Table 3). Men were significantly more likely than women to report physical abuse (28.6% versus 24.6%) and neglect (10.5% versus 8.6%).

TABLE 2. Selected characteristics of the population by sex.

Characteristics	Females (n=3,895)		Males (n=3,315)		Chi-square test	
	n %		n %		Value p-value (df)	
Age group (years)						
18-34	440	11.3	234	7.1	52.7 (3)	<0.0001
35-54	1516	38.9	1213	36.6		
55-74	1563	40.1	1481	44.7		
75+	376	9.7	387	11.7		
Mean age (SD)		54.8 (15.4)		57.3 (14.4)		
Race						
White	2874	73.8	2517	75.9	19.3 (5)	0.0017
Black	158	4.1	132	4.0		
Hispanic	428	11.0	340	10.3		
Asian	353	9.1	226	6.8		
Native American	13	0.3	14	0.4		
Other	69	1.8	86	2.6		
Education						
No high school diploma	306	7.9	214	6.5	88.7 (3)	<0.0001
High school/GED	653	16.8	402	12.1		
Some college/ technical	1666	42.8	1280	38.6		
College graduate	1270	32.6	1419	42.8		
Alcohol consumed in past month	2172	55.8	2158	65.1	65.0 (1)	<0.0001
History of parental smoking	2791	71.7	2434	73.4	2.8 (1)	0.0940
Mean MCS score (SD)*		51.2 (9.5)		53.2 (8.2)		
Current smoker	294	7.6	281	8.5	2.1 (1)	0.1470

*Mental Component Summary Score (MCS) based on SF-36.

TABLE 3. ACE characteristics of study sample by sex.

ACE	Females (n=3,895)	Males (n=3,315)	Chi-square test	
	%	%	Value (df)	p-value
Abuse				
Emotional	11.7	8.2	23.8 (1)	<0.0001
Physical	24.6	28.6	14.5 (1)	0.0001
Sexual	24.2	16.7	61.2 (1)	<0.0001
Neglect				
Emotional	16.4	12.2	25.2 (1)	<0.0001
Physical	8.6	10.5	7.7 (1)	0.0054
Household dysfunction				
Witnessing domestic violence	13.6	12.1	3.8 (1)	0.0526
Parental separation or divorce	25.3	22.4	8.6 (1)	0.0034
Mental illness in household	25.0	14.6	119.4 (1)	<0.0001
Household substance abuse	29.9	25.5	17.4 (1)	<0.0001
Incarcerated household member	6.9	4.8	14.6 (1)	0.0001
Total number of ACEs				
0	32.1	34.7	50.2 (4)	<0.0001
1	24.1	26.9		
2	14.7	16.1		
3	10.4	9.3		
4+	18.7	13.0		

10.3.2 RELATIONSHIP BETWEEN ACES AND CURRENT ADULT SMOKING

The unadjusted associations between current adult smoking and ACEs by sex can be found in Figure 2. After adjustment for sociodemographic characteristics, parental smoking during childhood, and alcohol use in the past month, the odds of adult smoking was at least 1.4 times greater among women who have been emotionally or physically abused, physically neglected, or had experienced parental separation or divorce (versus women who had not experienced each of these ACEs) (Table 4). Notably, the odds of smoking was markedly greater among women WHO had an incarcerated household member during childhood (AOR 2.3, 95% CI: 1.6-3.2) (versus women who had not had an incarcerated household member during childhood). While the odds of current adult smoking among women increased as the ACE score rose, this association was not significant after adjustment (Figure 1, c coefficient).

Among men, the prevalence and unadjusted odds of current adult smoking was significant for physical abuse, emotional neglect, parental separation or divorce, living with a family member who abused substances, and having an incarcerated household member. Notably, after adjusting for covariates, none of these associations were significant.

10.3.3 RELATIONSHIP BETWEEN ACES AND PSYCHOLOGICAL DISTRESS

In the unadjusted models, the mean MCS score, an indicator of psychological distress, was lower among those with any ACE compared to those without the given ACE among both women and men (with the exception of incarcerated household member among men), suggesting increased psychological distress (Figure 3). In the adjusted linear regression models among women (Table 5), all associations between the individual ACEs and the psychological distress indicator were significant except for that in which the independent variable was a childhood exposure to incarcerated household members. Among men, all adjusted associations with the psychological distress indicator were significant except for those in which

TABLE 4. Adjusted odds ratios (OR) and 95% confidence intervals for the relationships between ACEs and adult current smoking, by sex.

ACE	Females Adjusted[a]OR (95% CI)	Males Adjusted[a]OR (95% CI)
Abuse		
Emotional		
Yes	1.4 (1.1-2.0)*	1.2 (0.8-1.8)
No	Referent	Referent
Physical		
Yes	1.4 (1.1-1.8)*	1.3 (1.0-1.7)
No	Referent	Referent
Sexual		
Yes	1.2 (0.9-1.6)	0.9 (0.7-1.3)
No	referent	Referent
Neglect		
Emotional		
Yes	1.2 (0.9-1.7)	1.2 (0.9-1.8)
No	Referent	Referent
Physical		
Yes	1.5 (1.1-2.2)*	1.1 (0.7-1.6)
No	Referent	Referent
Household dysfunction		
Witnessing domestic violence		
Yes	1.4 (1.0-1.9)	0.9 (0.6-1.3)
No	Referent	Referent
Parental separation or divorce		
Yes	1.4 (1.1-1.9)*	1.1 (0.8-1.5)
No	Referent	Referent
Mental illness in the household		
Yes	1.1 (0.8-1.4)	1.1 (0.8-1.5)
No	Referent	Referent
Household substance abuse		
Yes	1.0 (0.8-1.3)	1.1 (0.8-1.4)

TABLE 4. CONTINUED.

No	referent	Referent
Incarcerated household member		
Yes	2.3 (1.6-3.2)*	1.1 (0.7-1.8)
No	Referent	Referent
ACE score		
0	Referent	Referent
1	0.7 (0.5-1.0)	1.2 (0.8-1.7)
2	1.3 (0.9-1.8)	1.3 (0.9-2.0)
3	1.3 (0.9-2.0)	0.9 (0.6-1.5)
4+	1.4 (1.0-2.0)	1.2 (0.8-1.7)

[a] Odds ratios (OR) and 95% confidence intervals (CI). Multivariable logistic regression models included age group, race, education, parental smoking during childhood, and alcohol use in past month.

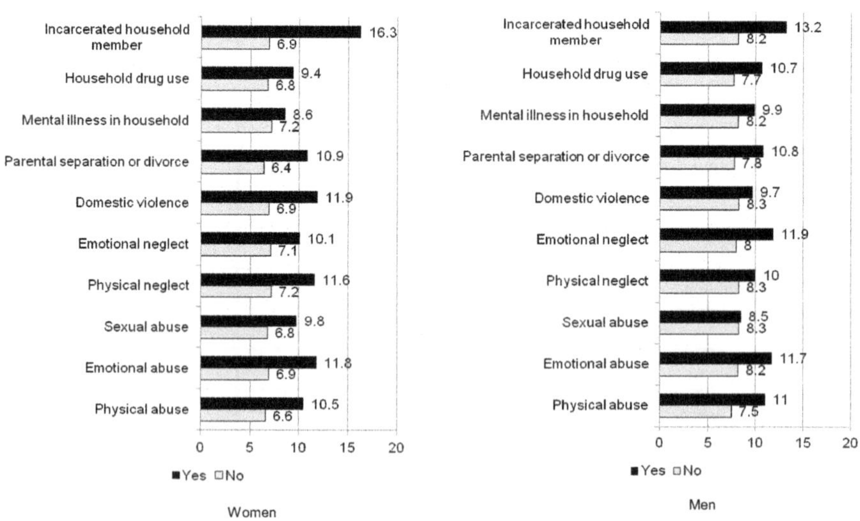

Figure 2. Prevalence of current smoking by ACE status and gender.

the independent variable was parental separation or divorce or incarcerated household member. As the ACE score increased in both adjusted and unadjusted linear regression models, the level of psychological distress also increased (i.e., mean score decreased as number of ACEs increased) (Figure 1, a coefficient).

10.3.4 RELATIONSHIP BETWEEN PSYCHOLOGICAL DISTRESS AND CURRENT ADULT SMOKING

In the models adjusted for sociodemographic characteristics, parental smoking during childhood, and past 30 day consumption of alcohol, the association between psychological distress and current adult smoking was significant for both women (AOR=0.98; 95% CI: 0.97-0.99; Wald chi-square=15.22, DF=1, p-value <0.0001) and men (AOR=0.98; 95% CI: 0.97-1.00; Wald chi-square=5.73, DF=1, p=0.0166). With the addition of

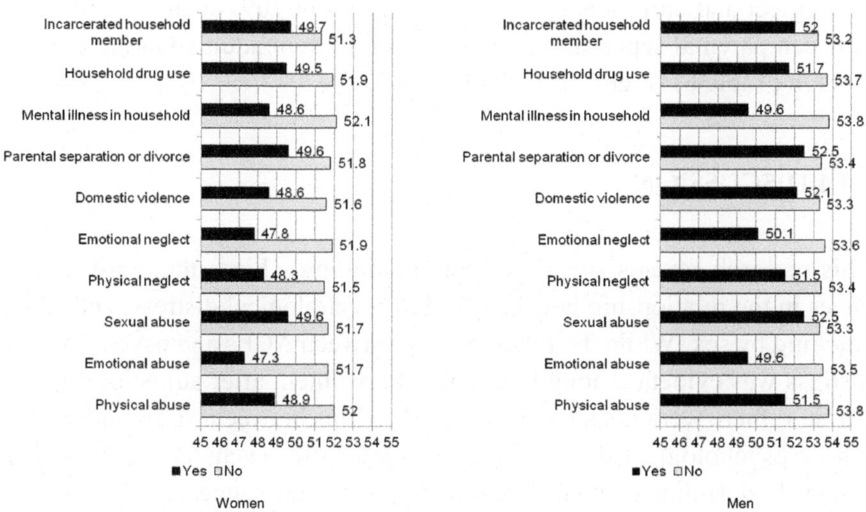

*MCS score is developed from the SF-36. Level of psychological distress increases as the MCS score decreases.

Figure 3. Mean Mental Component Summary (MCS) score by ACE status and gender.

each ACE in the model, the associations remained significant for women (AOR=0.98; 95% CI: 0.97-0.99; p-value range: p=0.0004 for model with mental illness in household to p=0.0014 for model with emotional abuse) but not men (AOR=0.99, 95% CI: 0.87-1.00, p-value range: p=0.0523 for the model with sexual abuse to p=0.0934 for the model with incarcerated household member) (Figure 1, b coefficient).

10.3.5 MEDIATING ROLE OF PSYCHOLOGICAL DISTRESS ON THE RELATIONSHIP BETWEEN ACES AND CURRENT ADULT SMOKING

Given that after adjusting for covariates, there was no significant association between any of the ACEs and smoking or psychological distress and smoking (with ACEs included) among men, mediation analyses were limited to women. After adjusting for covariates, psychological distress mediated 22% of the relationship between emotional abuse and current adult smoking, approximately 17% of the relationship between physical abuse and current adult smoking, 14% of the relationship between physical neglect and current adult smoking, and about 10% of the relationship between parental separation or divorce and current adult smoking among women (Table 6) (Figure 1, c' coefficient).

10.4 DISCUSSION

This research reveals several important findings. First, there are differences in the relationship between ACEs, psychological distress, and adult smoking by sex. While the relationships between ACEs and psychological distress was evident among both men and women, after adjusting for covariates, there were not significant relationships between ACEs and smoking or psychological distress and smoking (after each ACE was added to the model) among men. Second, this research suggests that women, particularly those who have experienced emotional or physical abuse, physical neglect, or parental separation or divorce as children may be at particular risk for smoking in adulthood. In fact, approximately 22% of

TABLE 5. Adjusted coefficientsaand 95% confidence intervals for the relationships between ACEs and psychological distress, by sex.

ACE	Females Adjusted[a] Coefficients (95% CI)	Males Adjusted[a] Coefficients (95% CI)
Abuse		
Emotional	−3.9 (−4.8- -3.0)*	−3.6 (−4.6- -2.6)*
Physical	−2.6 (−3.3- -1.9)*	−2.1 (−2.7- -1.5)*
Sexual	−1.8 (−2.5- -1.1)*	−0.9 (−1.6- -0.1)*
Neglect		
Emotional	−3.7 (−4.5- -2.9)*	−3.4 (−4.2- -2.5)*
Physical	−2.8 (−3.8- -1.7)*	−1.9 (−2.7- -1.0)*
Household dysfunction		
Witnessing domestic violence	−2.4 (−3.2- -1.5)*	−0.9 (−1.7- -0.01)*
Parental separation or divorce	−1.6 (−2.3- -0.9)*	−0.6 (−1.3-0.03)
Mental illness in the household	−3.1 (−3.8- -2.5)*	−4.0 (−4.8- -3.3)*
Household substance abuse	−1.7 (−2.4- -1.0)*	−1.7 (−2.3- -1.1)*
Incarcerated household member	−0.9 (−2.1-0.2)	−0.9 (−2.2-0.4)
ACE score	−1.1 (−1.3- -0.9)*	−1.0 (−1.2- -0.8)*

[a]Multivariable linear regression models included age group, race, education, parental smoking during childhood, and alcohol use in past month.
*$p<0.05$.

the relationship between emotional abuse and adult smoking was mediated though psychological distress as was 17% of the relationship between physical abuse and adults smoking, 14% of the relationship between physical neglect and adult smoking, and 10% of the relationship between parental separation and divorce and adult smoking.

Our findings confirm results of earlier research suggesting sex differences in smoking behavior and pattern. Although negative affect, including depression, is related to smoking among both men and women, the relationship is much stronger for women [88-90]. In fact, recent research suggests that stressful childhood life events may disproportionately influence

TABLE 6. Sobel statistics and percent mediated. Women.

	Sobel Test[a]		% mediated[b]
ACE	Test Statistic (SE)	p-value	
Abuse			
Emotional	−3.36 (0.02)	0.0008	22.0%
Physical	−3.29 (0.02)	0.0010	16.8%
Neglect			
Physical	−3.01 (0.02)	0.0026	14.0%
Household dysfunction			
Parental sep/div	−2.88 (0.01)	0.0040	10.2%

Note. Sobel test and proportion of mediation obtained from linear and logistic regression models adjusted for covariates including age group, race, education, parental smoking during childhood, and alcohol use in past month; P-values drawn from the normal distribution under the assumption of a 2-tailed z-test. The hypothesis is that the mediated effect equals zero.
Excel spreadsheet created by Nathaniel R. Herr (February, 2006), Adopted from Kenny, 2006. Available at: http://nrherr.bol.ucla.edu/Mediation/logmed.html.
[a] Sobel test. http://www.quantpsy.org/sobel/sobel.htm
[b] equation (c-c′)/c.

a women's decision to use drugs [48-57]. This may be due in part to differences in coping styles and socialization [56]; females may develop more passive styles of responding to threats and distressing events as opposed to boys who may engage in a more active coping style [91-95]. Interestingly, women are often less dependent on nicotine then men [60,96-98], they are less likely to be heavy smokers [79], and have lower concentrations of cotinine (a byproduct of nicotine). Notably, however, studies have consistently found that women have lower quit rates than men [61,62,97], have lower confidence in their ability to quit [98,99], and often experience worse withdrawal symptoms during smoking cessation attempts [59,97]. In fact, recent research suggests that the smoking rates for adolescent and adult women may actually be increasing [100].

Our study indicates that women are more likely than men to report emotional and sexual abuse and emotional neglect while men are more likely to report physical abuse and neglect. Literature has consistently indicated that women are more likely than men to report sexual abuse [101] and men are more likely than women to report physical abuse [102]. The authors could find very little research that examined emotional abuse and neglect and physical neglect by sex; specifically research that did not contain the same data used in this study. The one study we did find indicated that women were significantly more likely than men to report emotional abuse and slightly more likely than men to report emotional neglect, although not statistically significantly so [103]. This same study indicated that men were significantly more likely than women to report physical neglect, results consistent with our findings [103].

Much research has already examined potential biases and limitations of the ACE Study data. Research conducted by Felitti et al. [64] determined that respondent and nonrespondent groups were similar with regard to sociodemographic characteristics (e.g., percentages of women, mean years of education, and marital status), self-rated health, engagement in adverse health behaviors (e.g., smoking and other substance abuse), and presence of chronic diseases such as heart attack, stroke, chronic obstructive lung disease, hypertension, and diabetes. Edwards et al. [104] conducted research examining potential response bias and found that persons who did not participate in the ACE Study experienced childhood sexual abuse at the same rate as those who agreed to participate; research made possible by a dichotomous screening question about childhood sexual abuse in the health history survey. Moreover, those who participated in the study who reported sexual abuse had similar levels of current mental and physical health problems as those who did not participate and also reported sexual abuse [104]. Test-retest reliability research conducted by Dube et al. [105], found that childhood sexual, physical, and emotional abuse, as well as forms of household dysfunction (i.e., mental illness in household, substance abuse in household, parental discord or divorce, incarcerated household member, and domestic violence), showed good Cohen's Kappa agreement as defined by Fleiss [106] and Landis and Koch [107] (range=0.46–0.86). Finally, while persons in the ACE Study are older, more educated, and less likely to smoke than the general population,

ACE Study sexual and physical abuse estimates are similar to those derived from adult population-based surveys [108-110].

There are several limitation that warrants further examination. First, the ACE Study data are cross-sectional and do not collect specific information on temporality. Although most current literature suggests that the majority of psychiatric disorders associated with smoking occur prior to smoking initiation [29-44], other pathways have been posited (e.g., bidirectional association, common environmental and genetic factors for both, and smoking initiation prior to psychological distress) [111,112]. Notably, in a study designed to specifically examine the stress-smoking relationship among adolescents, negative life events and negative affect were related to an increase in smoking over time, with no evidence of reverse causation [35]. Additional longitudinal studies are needed to further clarify the relationships between ACEs, psychological distress, and smoking among adults. Second, there is undoubtedly more than one pathway that would lead an adolescent to smoking initiation (e.g., peer pressure). Moreover, there could be a cohort effect because participants in this study likely began to smoke at a time when smoking was more socially acceptable than it is now, and therefore the relative contribution of ACEs and psychological distress may increase or decrease as the rates of smoking decrease over time. Third, at the inception of the study, domestic violence was recognized to primarily occur against women. It is commonly known now that domestic violence occurs to both men and women in the household. Given this, our study has underestimated the prevalence of domestic violence in the household. Fourth, longitudinal follow-up studies of adults with documented childhood abuse suggested that retrospective reports of childhood abuse often underrepresented actual events [113-115]. However, in a recent study by Tourangeau and Yan [116], the authors indicate that respondents are less likely to underreport undesirable events and behaviors when the questions are self-administered and when the data are collected in private. Bias also may be introducted if there are differences in reporting retrospective information about childhood abuse by sex. In an article by Widom and Morris [114], among persons with a history of documented sexual abuse in childhood, fewer men than women later considered the event sexual abuse. Fifth, according to recent research, the joint effect of multiple ACEs on mental disorders are non-additive and often attenuate with age. This, combined with recall failure, often overestimates the effects of summary ACE scales [117]. Given this, as was found in this study, one might not expect to see a dose–response relationship between number of ACEs and psychological distress. Further research is needed to determine an appropriate summary measure for retrospective studies. Sixth, it is not plausible that women would have more exposure to several of the ACEs (eg, household dysfunction) than men. This suggests that women are more sensitive to several of the ACE measures or are more willing to report them. Finally, psychological distress is a non-specific concept that can encompass everything from temporary negative emotion to chronic mental disorders. However, research suggests that the MCS is a good predictor of depressive disorders [76].

This study has important policy implications for public health approaches to smoking cessation. Despite increasingly stronger disincentives to smoking, including higher tobacco taxes and fewer places to smoke, the rate of smoking in the U.S. fell only slightly, from 20.9% in 2005 to 19.3% in 2010. At this slow rate of decline, by 2020 the adult smoking rate will only have fallen to about 17% [118]. Given the strong association between ACEs and smoking, interventions targeted to trauma survivors may enhance the effectiveness of broader-based anti-smoking efforts.

10.5 CONCLUSIONS

Several recent articles have suggested that persons who have experienced ACEs are more likely to smoke, but the exact mechanism linking ACEs with adult current smoking has not been fully elucidated. This research provides preliminary evidence that among women, psychological distress may be a potential intermediate variable in the relationship between ACEs and adult current smoking. As such, when addressing smoking cessation in clinical practice, it may be important to understand not only psychological distress, but the underlying role of childhood trauma. Having knowledge about childhood trauma history in clinical practice may provide the opportunity to integrate trauma focused interventions. Moreover, to create effective intervention and prevention programs, research should be conducted to further elucidate the causes, developmental paths, and critical points that link ACEs to smoking, especially in adolescence [57]. Identifying potential modifiable risk factors for smoking onset in adolescents (e.g., ACEs), as well as building resiliency and positive social support networks for abused children may decrease the prevalence of smoking among children and adolescents exposed to maltreatment. Research examining additional potential covariates, including temporality, intensity, frequency, and duration of maltreatment [119,120]; victim's past and current environmental circumstances; and genetic influences on smoking behavior and mental illness is also warranted [121,122].

REFERENCES

1. Flaherty EG, Thompson R, Litrownik AJ, Zolotor AJ, Dubowitz H, Runyan DK, English DJ, Everson MD: Adverse childhood exposures and reported child health at age 12. Academic Pediatrics 2009, 9:150-156.
2. U.S. Department of Health and Human Services: Administration for Children and Families. Administration on Children, Youth, and Families. Children's Bureau. Child maltreatment. 2010. http://www.acf.hhs.gov/programs/cb/pubs/cm10/cm10.pdf
3. Anda RF, Felitti VJ, Bremner JD, Walker JD, Whitfield C, Perry BD, Dube SR, Giles WH: The enduring effects of abuse and related adverse experiences in childhood. A convergence of evidence from neurobiology and epidemiology. European Archives of Psychiatry and Clinical Neuroscience 2006, 256:174-186.
4. Arias I: The legacy of child maltreatment: long-term health consequences for women. Journal of Womens Health 2004, 13:468-473.
5. Repetti RL, Taylor SE, Seeman TE: Risky families: family social environments and the mental and physical health of offspring. Psychol Bull 2002, 128:330-366.
6. Taylor SE, Lerner JS, Sage RM, Lehman BJ, Seeman TE: Early environment, emotions, responses to stress, and health. J Personal 2004, 72:1365-1393.
7. Sroufe AL, Rutter M: The domain of developmental psychopathology. Child Development 1984, 55:17-29.
8. McEwen BS, Stellar E: Stress and the individual. Mechanisms leading to disease. Arch Intern Med 1993, 153:2093-2101.
9. Leitenberg H, Gibson LE, Novy PL: Individual differences among undergraduate women in methods of coping with stressful events: the impact of cumulative childhood stressors and abuse. Child Abuse and Neglect 2004, 28:181-192.
10. Stevens SL, Colwell B, Smith DW, Robinson J, McMillan C: An exploration of self-reported negative affect by adolescents as a reason for smoking: implications for tobacco prevention and intervention programs. Preventive Medicine 2005, 41:589-596.
11. Boney-McCoy S, Finkelhor D: Psychosocial sequelae of violent victimization in a national youth sample. J Consulting and Clinical Psych 1995, 5:726-736.

12. Edwards VJ, Holden GW, Anda RF, Felitti VJ: Relationship between multiple forms of childhood maltreatment and adult mental health in community respondents: results from the adverse childhood experiences study. Am J Psychiatry 2003, 160:8.
13. Kessler RC, Gillis-Light J, Magee WJ, Kendler KS, Eaves LJ: Childhood adversity and adult psychopathology. In Stress and Adversity Over the Life Course: Trajectories and Turning Points. Edited by Gotlib IH, Wheaton B. New York: Cambridge University Press; 1997:29-49.
14. Ridner SH: Psychological distress: concept analysis. J Adv Nurs 2004, 45:536-545.
15. Balfour DJ, Fagerstrom KO: Pharmacology of nicotine and its therapeutic use in smoking cessation and neurodegenerative disorders. Pharmacol Ther 1996, 72:51-81.
16. Glassman AH, Helzer JE, Covey LS, Cottler LB, Stetner F, Tipp JE, Johnson J: Smoking, smoking cessation, and major depression. JAMA 1990, 264:1546-1549.
17. Lerman C, Audrain J, Orleans CT, Boyd R, Gold K, Main D, Caporaso N: Investigation of mechanisms linking depressed mood to nicotine dependence. Addict Behav 1996, 21:9-19.
18. Penny GN, Robinson JO: Psychological resources and cigarette smoking in adolescents. Br J Psychol 1986, 77(Pt 3):351-357.
19. Escobedo LG, Reddy M, Giovino GA: The relationship between depressive symptoms and cigarette smoking in US adolescents. Addiction 1998, 93(3):433-440.
20. Kassel JD, Stroud LR, Paronis CA: Smoking, stress, and negative affect: correlation, causation, and context across stages of smoking. Psychol Bull 2003, 129(2):270-304.
21. Koval JJ, Pederson LL, Mills CA, McGrady GA, Carvajal SC: Models of the relationship of stress, depression, and other psychosocial factors to smoking behavior: a comparison of a cohort of students in grades 6 and 8. Preventive Medicine 2000, 30(6):463-477.
22. Mermelstein R: Ethnicity, gender and risk factors for smoking initiation: an overview. Nicotine and Tobacco Research 1999, 1(Suppl 2):S39-S43.
23. West R: Beneficial effects of nicotine: fact or fiction? Addiction 1993, 88(5):589-590.
24. Jamner LD, Shapiro D, Jarvik ME: Nicotine reduces the frequency of anger reports in smokers and nonsmokers with high but not low hostility: an ambulatory study. Exp Clin Psychopharmacol 1999, 7(4):454-463.
25. Whalen CK, Jamner LD, Henker B, Delfino RJ: Smoking and moods in adolescents with depressive and aggressive dispositions: evidence from surveys and electronic diaries. Heal Psychol 2001, 20(2):99-111.
26. Covey LS, Glassman AH, Stetner F: Depression and depressive symptoms in smoking cessation. Comprehensive Psychiatry 1990, 31(4):350-354.
27. Covey LS, Glassman AH, Stetner F: Major depression following smoking cessation. Am J Psychiatry 1997, 154(2):263-265.
28. Covey LS, Tam D: Depressive mood, the single-parent home, and adolescent cigarette smoking. Am J Public Health 1990, 80(11):1330-1333.
29. Dierker LC, Donny E: The role of psychiatric disorders in the relationship between cigarette smoking and DSM-IV nicotine dependence among young adults. Nicotine and Tobacco Research 2008, 10:439-446.
30. Breslau N, Peterson EL, Schultz LR, Chilcoat HD, Andreski P: Major depression and stages of smoking. A longitudinal investigation. Arch Gen Psychiatry 1998, 55(2):161-166.

31. Dierker LC, Avenevoli S, Merikangas KR, Flaherty BP, Stolar M: Association between psychiatric disorders and the progression of tobacco use behaviors. Journal of the American Academy of Child and Adolescent Psychiatry 2001, 40(10):1159-1167.
32. Fergusson DM, Goodwin RD, Horwood LJ: Major depression and cigarette smoking: results of a 21-year longitudinal study. Psychol Med 2003, 33(8):1357-1367.
33. Kandel DB, Davies M: Adult sequelae of adolescent depressive symptoms. Arch Gen Psychiatry 1986, 43(3):255-262.
34. Patton GC, Carlin JB, Coffey C, Wolfe R, Hibbert M, Bowes G: Depression, anxiety, and smoking initiation: a prospective study over 3 years. Am J Public Health 1998, 88(10):1518-1522.
35. Wills TA, Sandy JM, Yaeger AM: Stress and smoking in adolescence: a test of directional hypotheses. Heal Psychol 2002, 21(2):122-130.
36. Breslau N: Psychiatric comorbidity of smoking and nicotine dependence. Behav Genet 1995, 25(2):95-101.
37. Feldner MT, Babson KA, Zvolensky MJ: Smoking, traumatic event exposure, and post-traumatic stress: a critical review of the empirical literature. Clin Psychol Rev 2007, 27(1):14-45.
38. de Leon J, Dadvand M, Canuso C, White AO, Stanilla JK, Simpson GM: Schizophrenia and smoking: an epidemiological survey in a state hospital. Am J Psychiatry 1995, 152(3):453-455.
39. Hughes JR, Hatsukami DK, Mitchell JE, Dahlgren LA: Prevalence of smoking among psychiatric outpatients. Am J Psychiatry 1986, 143:993-997.
40. Williams JM, Ziedonis D: Addressing tobacco among individuals with a mental illness or an addiction. Addict Behav 2004, 29(6):1067-1083.
41. Ziedonis DM, Kosten TR, Glazer WM, Frances RJ: Nicotinedependence and schizophrenia. Hospital and Community Psychiatry 1994, 45(3):204-206.
42. Chilcoat HD, Breslau N: Pathways from ADHD to early drug use. Journal of the American Academy of Child and Adolescent Psychiatry 1999, 38(11):1347-1354.
43. Milberger S, Biederman J, Faraone SV, Chen L, Jones J: ADHD is associated with early initiation of cigarette smoking in children and adolescents. Journal of the American Academy of Child and Adolescent Psychiatry 1997, 36(1):37-44.
44. Pomerleau OF, Downey KK, Stelson FW, Pomerleau CS: Cigarette smoking in adult patients diagnosed with attention deficit hyperactivity disorder. J Subst Abus 1995, 7(3):373-378.
45. Douglas KR, Chan G, Gelernter J, Arias AJ, Anton RF, Weiss RD, Brady K, Poling J, Farrer L, Kranzler HR: Adverse childhood events as risk factors for substance dependence: Partial mediation by mood and anxiety disorders. Addict Behav 2010, 35:7-13.
46. Lo CC, Cheng TC: The impact of childhood maltreatment on young adults' substance abuse. American Journal of Drug and Alcohol Abuse 2007, 33:139-146.
47. DeWit DJ, MacDonald K, Offord DR: Childhood stress and symptoms of drug dependence in adolescence and early adulthood: social phobia as a mediator. American Journal of Orthopsychiatry 1999, 69:61-72.
48. Simpson TL, Miller WR: Concomitance between childhood sexual and physical abuse and substance use problems. A review. Clin Psychol Rev 2002, 22:27-77.

49. White HR, Widom CS: Three potential mediators of the effects of child abuse and neglect on adulthood substance use among women. Journal of Studies on Alcohol and Drugs 2008, 69:337-347.
50. Mokdad AH, Marks JS, Stroup DF, Gerberding JL: Actual causes of death in the United States, 2000. JAMA 2004, 291:1238-1245.
51. Acierno RA, Kilpatrick DG, Resnick HS, Saunders BE, Best CL: Violent assault, posttraumatic stress disorder, and depression. Risk factors for cigarette use among adult women. Behav Modif 1996, 20:363-384.
52. Anda RF, Croft JB, Felitti VJ, Nordenberg D, Giles WH, Williamson DF, Giovino GA, et al.: Adverse childhood experiences and smoking during adolescence and adulthood. JAMA 1999, 282:1652-1658.
53. Dube SR, Felitti VJ, Dong M, Giles WH, Anda RF: The impact of adverse childhood experiences on health problems: evidence from four birth cohorts dating back to 1900. Preventive Medicine 2003, 37:268-277.
54. Edwards VJ, Anda RF, Gu D, Dube SR, Felitti VJ: Adverse childhood experiences and smoking persistence in adults with smoke-related symptoms and illness. The Permanente Journal 2007, 11:5-7.
55. Nichols HB, Harlow BL: Childhood abuse and risk of smoking onset. Journal of Epidemiology and Community Health 2004, 58:402-406.
56. Simantov E, Schoen C, Klein JD: Health-compromising behaviors: why do adolescents smoke or drink? identifying underlying risk and protective factors. Archives of Pediatrics and Adolescent Medicine 2000, 154:1025-1033.
57. Widom CS, Marmorstein NR, White HR: Childhood victimization and illicit drug use in middle adulthood. Psychol Addict Behav 2006, 20:394-403.
58. Byrne DG, Mazanov J: Source of adolescent stress, smoking and the use of other drugs. Stress Medicine 1999, 15:215-227.
59. Perkins KA, Donny E, Caggiula AR: Sex differences in nicotine effects and self-administration: review of human and animal evidence. Nicotine and Tobacco Research 1999, 1:301-315.
60. Perkins KA, Jacobs L, Sanders M, Caggiula AR: Sex differences in the subjective and reinforcing effects of cigarette nicotine dose. Psychopharmacology 2002, 163:194-201.
61. Perkins KA, Scott J: Sex differences in long-term smoking cessation rates due to nicotine patch. Nicotine and Tobacco Research 2008, 10:1245-1250.
62. Wetter DW, Kenford SL, Smith SS, Fiore MC, Jorenby DE, Baker TB: Gender differences in smoking cessation. J Consult Clin Psychol 1999, 67:555-562.
63. Edwards VJ, Anda RF, Felitti VJ, Dube SR: Adverse childhood experiences and health-related quality of life as an adult. In Health Consequences of Abuse in the Family: A Clinical Guide for Evidence-Based Practice. Edited by Kendell T. KA Washington, DC: American Psychiatric Association; 2004:81-93. OpenURL
64. Felitti VJ, Anda RF, Nordenberg D, Williamson DF, Spitz AM, Edwards V, Koss MP, Marks JS: Relationship of childhood abuse and household dysfunction to many of the leading causes of death in adults. The Adverse Childhood Experiences (ACE) Study. American Journal of Preventive Medicine 1998, 14:245-258.

65. Ware JE, Kosinski M, Keller SD: SF-36 Physical and Mental Health Summary Scales: A User's Manual. Boston, MA: New England Medical Center, the Health Institute; 1994.
66. Ware JE, Snow KK, Kosinski M, Gandek B: SF-36 Health Survey Manual and Interpretation Guide. Boston, MA: New England Medical Center, The Health Institute; 1993.
67. Straus M: Gelles RJ: Physical violence in American families: Risk factors and adaptation to violence in 8,145 families. New Brunswick: Transaction Press; 1990.
68. Wyatt GE: The sexual abuse of Afro-American and white-American women in childhood. Child Abuse and Neglect 1985, 9:507-519.
69. Schoenborn CA, National Center for Health Statistics: Advanced Data fromVital and Health Statistics, No. 205. Exposure to alcoholism in the family. United States; 1988. http://www.cdc.gov/nchs/data/ad/ad205.pdf.
70. Bernstein DP, Stein JA, Newcomb MD, Walker E, Pogge D, Ahluvalia T, Stokes J, Handelsman L, Medrano M, Desmond D, Zule W: Development and validation of a brief screening version of the Childhood Trauma Questionnaire. Child Abuse and Neglect 2003, 27:169-190.
71. Dong M, Anda RF, Felitti VJ, Dube SR, Williamson DF, Thompson TJ, Loo CM, Giles WH: The interrelatedness of multiple forms of childhood abuse, neglect, and household dysfunction. Child Abuse and Neglect 2004, 28:771-784.
72. Ware JE, Sherbourne CD: The MOS 36-item short-form health survey (SF-36). I. Conceptual framework and item selection. Medical Care 1992, 30:473-483.
73. Fukuhara S, Ware JE, Kosinski M, Wada S, Gandek B: Psychometric and clinical tests of validity of the Japanese SF-36 Health Survey. Journal of Clinical Epidemiology 1998, 51:1045-1053.
74. Ware JE, Gandek B, Group IP: The SF-36 Health Survey: Development and use in mental health research and the IQOLA project. Int J Ment Heal 1994, 23:49-73.
75. Beusterien KM, Steinwald B, Ware JE: Usefulness of the SF-36 Health Survey in measuring health outcomes in the depressed elderly. Journal of Geriatric Psychiatry and Neurology 1996, 9:13-21.
76. Silveira E, Taft C, Sundh V, Waern M, Palsson S, Steen B: Performance of the SF-36 health survey in screening for depressive and anxiety disorders in an elderly female Swedish population. Quality of Life Research 2005, 14:1263-1274.
77. Weinstein MC, Berwick DM, Goldman PA, Murphy JM, Barsky AJ: A comparison of three psychiatric screening tests using receiver operating characteristic (ROC) analysis. Medical Care 1989, 27:593-607.
78. Wells KB, Burnam MA, Rogers W, Hays R, Camp P: The course of depression in adult outpatients. Results from the Medical Outcomes Study. Arch Gen Psychiatry 1992, 49:788-794.
79. Giovino GA, Schooley MW, Zhu BP, Chrismon JH, Tomar SL, Peddicord JP, Merritt RK, Husten CG, Eriksen MP: Surveillance for selected tobacco-use behaviors—United States, 1990–1994. MMWR Morb Mortal Wkly Rep 1994, 43(suppl 3):1-43.
80. Nelson DE, Holtzman D, Bolen J, Stanwyck CA, Mack KA: Reliability and validity of measures from the Behavioral Risk Factor Surveillance System (BRFSS). Social and Preventive Medicine 2001, 46(Suppl 1):S03-S42.

81. Nelson DE, Powell-Griner E, Town M, Kovar MG: A comparison of national estimates from the National Health Interview Survey and the Behavioral Risk Factor Surveillance System. Am J Public Health 2003, 93:1335-1341.
82. Baron RM, Kenny DA: The moderator-mediator variable distinction in social psychological research: conceptual, strategic, and statistical considerations. J Personal Soc Psychol 1986, 51:1173-1182.
83. Kraemer HC, Stice E, Kazdin A, Offord D, Kupfer D: How do risk factors work together? Mediators, moderators, and independent, overlapping, and proxy risk factors. Am J Psychiatry 2001, 158:848-856.
84. MacKinnon DP: Introduction to statistical mediation analysis. New York, NY: Lawrence Erlbaum Assoc; 2008.
85. Sobel ME: Asymptotic intervals for indirect effects in structural equations models. In Sociological methodology. Edited by Leinhart S. San Francisco: Jossey-Bass; 1982:312.
86. MacKinnon DP, Dwyer JH: Estimating mediated effects in prevention studies. Eval Rev 1993, 17:144-158.
87. Jiang N, Ling PM: Reinforcement of smoking and drinking: tobacco marketing strategies linked with alcohol in the United States. Am J Public Health 2011, 101(10):1942-1954.
88. Brandon TH, Baker TB: The Smoking Consequences Questionnaire: The subjective expected utility of smoking in college students. Psychol Assess 1991, 3:484-491.
89. Husky MM, Mazure CM, Paliwal P, McKee SA: Gender differences in the comorbidity of smoking behavior and major depression. Drug and Alcohol Dependence 2008, 93(1–2):176-179.
90. McKee SA, Maciejewski PK, Falba T, Mazure CM: Sex differences in the effects of stressful life events on changes in smoking status. Addiction 2003, 98(6):847-855.
91. Compas BE, Malcarne VL, Fondacaro KM: Coping and stressful events in older children and adolescents. J Consult Clin Psychol 1988, 56:405-411.
92. De Boo GM, Spiering M: Pre-adolescent gender differences in association between temperament, coping, and mood. Clinical Psychology andPsychotherapy 2010, 17(4):313-320.
93. Groe MW, Thomas SP, Shoffner D: Adolescent stress and coping: a longitudinal study. Res Nurs Heal 1992, 15:209-217.
94. Nolen-Hoeksema S, Girgus JS: The emergence of gender differences in depression during adolescence. Psychol Bull 1994, 115:424-443.
95. Peterson AC, Sarigiani PA, Kennedy RE: Adolescent depression: why more girls. Journal of Youth and Adolescence 1991, 20:247-271.
96. Bjornson W, Rand C, Connett JE, Lindgren P, Nides M, Pope F, Buist AS, Hoppe-Ryan C, O'Hara P: Gender differences in smoking cessation after 3 years in the Lung Health Study. Am J Public Health 1995, 85(2):223-230.
97. Royce JM, Corbett K, Sorensen G, Ockene J: Gender, social pressure, and smoking cessations: the Community Intervention Trial for Smoking Cessation (COMMIT) at baseline. Social Science and Medicine 1997, 44(3):359-370.
98. Ward KD, Klesges RC, Zbikowski SM, Bliss RE, Garvey AJ: Gender differences in the outcome of an unaided smoking cessation attempt. Addict Behav 1997, 22(4):521-533.

99. Etter JF, Prokhorov AV, Perneger TV: Gender differences in the psychological determinants of cigarette smoking. Addiction 2002, 97:733-743.
100. De Von Figueroa-Moseley C, Landrine H, Klonoff EA: Sexual abuse and smoking among college student women. Addict Behav 2004, 29(2):245-251.
101. Finkelhor D, Baron L: Risk factors for child sexual abuse. Journal of Interpersonal Violence 1986, 1:43-71.
102. Thompson MP, Kingree JB, Desai S: Gender differences in long-term health consequences of physical abuse of children: data from a nationally representative survey. Am J Public Health 2004, 94(4):599-604.
103. Scher CD, Forde DR, McQuaid JR, Stein MB: Prevalence and demographic correlates of childhood maltreatment in an adult community sample. Child Abuse and Neglect 2004, 28:167-180.
104. Edwards VJ, Anda RF, Nordenberg DF, Felitti VJ, Williamson DF, Wright JA: Bias assessment for child abuse survey: factors affecting probability of response to a survey about childhood abuse. Child Abuse and Neglect 2001, 25:307-312.
105. Dube SR, Williamson DF, Thompson T, Felitti VJ, Anda RF: Assessing the reliability of retrospective reports of adverse childhood experiences among adult HMO members attending a primary care clinic. Child Abuse and Neglect 2004, 28:729-737.
106. Fleiss JL: The measurement of interrater agreement. In Statistical methods for rates and proportions. 2nd edition. ew York: John Wiley and Sons, Inc; 1981:212-236.
107. Landis JR, Koch GG: The measurement of observer agreement for categorical data. Biometrics 1977, 33:159-174.
108. Dong M, Anda RF, Dube SR, Giles WH, Felitti VJ: The relationship of exposure to childhood sexual abuse to other forms of abuse, neglect, and household dysfunction during childhood. Child Abuse and Neglect 2003, 27:625-639.
109. Finkelhor D, Hotaling G, Lewis IA, Smith C: Sexual abuse in a national survey of adult men and women: prevalence, characteristics, and risk factors. Child Abuse and Neglect 1990, 14:19-28.
110. MacMillan HL, Fleming JE, Trocme N, Boyle MH, Wong M, Racine YA, Beardslee WR, Offord DR: Journal of the American Medical Association. 1997, 278:131-135.
111. Costello EJ, Erkanli A, Federman E, Angold A: Development of psychiatric comorbidity with substance abuse in adolescents: effects of timing and sex. Journal of Clinical Child Psychology 1999, 28:298-311.
112. Moolchan ET, Ernst M, Henningfield JE: A review of tobacco smoking in adolescents: treatment implications. Journal of the American Academy of Child and Adolescent Psychiatry 2000, 39:682-693.
113. Hardt J, Rutter M: Validity of adult retrospective reports of adverse childhood experiences: review of the evidence. Journal of Child Psychology and Psychiatry and Allied Disciplines 2004, 45(2):260-273.
114. Widom CS, Morris S: Accuracy of adult recollections of childhood victimization, part 2: childhood sexual abuse. Psychol Assess 1997, 9:34-46.
115. Widom CS, Shepard R: Accuracy of adult recollection of childhood victimization: Part 1. Childhood physical abuse. Psychol Assess 1996, 8:412-421.
116. Tourangeau R, Yan T: Sensitive questions in surveys. Psychol Bull 2007, 133(4):859-883.

117. Green JG, McLaughlin KA, Berglund PA, Gruber MJ, Sampson NA, Zaslavsky AM, Kessler RC: Childhood adversities and adult psychiatric disorders in the National Comorbidity Survey Replication I. Arch Gen Psychiatry 2010, 67(2):113-123.
118. King B, Dube S, Kaufmann R, Shaw L, Pechacek T: Vital signs: cigarette smoking among adults aged ≥18 years – United States, 2005–2010. MMWR Morb Mortal Wkly Rep 2011, 60(35):1207-1212.
119. Cicchetti D, Toth SL: A developmental psychopathology perspective on child abuse and neglect. Journal of the American Academy of Child and Adolescent Psychiatry 1995, 34:541-565.
120. Kaplow JB, Widom CS: Age of onset of child maltreatment predicts long-term mental health outcomes. J Abnorm Psychol 2007, 116:176-187.
121. Batra V, Patkar AA, Berrettini WH, Weinstein SP, Leone FT: The genetic determinants of smoking. Chest 2003, 123:1730-1739.
122. Yoshimasu K, Kiyohara C: Genetic influences on smoking behavior and nicotine dependence: a review. Journal of Epidemiology 2003, 13:183-192.

CHAPTER 11

Adverse Childhood Experiences and Frequent Insufficient Sleep in 5 U.S. States, 2009: A Retrospective Cohort Study

DANIEL P. CHAPMAN, YONG LIU, LETITIA R. PRESLEY-CANTRELL, VALERIE J. EDWARDS, ANNE G. WHEATON, GERALDINE S. PERRY, AND JANET B. CROFT

11.1 BACKGROUND

Adverse childhood experiences (ACEs) have been associated with a variety of negative behavioral and health outcomes in adulthood [1]. Specifically, exposure to ACEs—which are defined as incidents of household abuse or dysfunction during the first 18 years of life—has been linked to the use of illicit drugs [2], depression [3], psychotropic medication use [4], premature mortality [5], and the prevalence of ischemic heart disease (IHD) [6]. The latter finding was judged noteworthy enough for the authors to conclude that psychological factors, such as anger and depressed affect, appear to be more important than traditional risk factors, including smoking and physical inactivity, in mediating the relation of ACEs to the risk of IHD [6]. Thus, ACEs are powerful events with long-lasting consequences

Furthermore, ACEs have been demonstrated to be highly interrelated to each other. Using data obtained from 8,629 members of a managed healthcare plan who completed a survey about exposure to ACEs, Dong et al. [7] found that the presence of one ACE significantly increased the likelihood of reporting exposure to another ACE. These investigators concluded that the number of respondents observed with an elevated total number of ACEs (the ACE score) was much greater than would be expected given the assumptions of independence, thereby demonstrating that ACEs were statistically interrelated [7].

The effects of ACEs continue long after their initial occurrence. Anda et al. [1] examined the association between the ACE score and the risk of 18 subsequent selected outcomes in affective, somatic, substance abuse, memory, sexual, and aggression-related domains. Notably, a strong, graded relationship emerged between the ACE score and the 18 selected outcomes, leading these investigators to conclude that these relationships parallel the cumulative effect of stress exposure to the developing brain [1].

Likewise, sleep is another event posing serious consequences to health and well-being. It has been estimated that 28% of adults suffer from frequent sleep insufficiency—defined as 14 or more days out of the past 30 that the respondent reported that they did not get enough rest or sleep [8]. In addition to increasing the risk of automobile crashes due to drowsy driving [9], insufficient sleep has been associated with increased body mass index (BMI) [10], obesity [11], diabetes [12], mental distress, depressive symptoms, and anxiety [13].

Notably, ACEs have been linked to sleep disturbances among adults. In a retrospective cohort study of health maintenance organization members in California which examined respondents' reports of ever having trouble falling or staying asleep and feeling tired even after a good night's sleep, Chapman et al. [14] found that ACEs were associated with both types of reported sleep disturbances in adulthood, and that the ACE score assumed a graded relationship to them. However, these results were obtained from a large managed care patient population which, while reasonably representative of the demographics of the sample investigated, may nonetheless differ from the population at large. Thus, this investigation examines the relationship between ACEs and frequent insufficient sleep among adults in a more diverse population-based sample.

Both smoking [13,15] and frequent mental distress [13] are associated with insufficient sleep. Therefore, we present models controlling for these variables to better elucidate the relationship between ACEs and sleep and to determine if ACEs could serve, potentially, as indicators promoting the further investigation of sleep sufficiency.

11.2 METHODS

11.2.1 DATA SELECTION

Data were obtained from the 2009 Behavioral Risk Factor Surveillance Survey (BRFSS), a state-based random-digit dialed telephone survey of non-institutionalized U.S. adults aged 18 years and older. Trained interviewers administered standardized questionnaires to a sample of households with landline telephones. Five states (Arkansas, Louisiana, New Mexico, Tennessee, and Washington) administered a supplemental ACE survey question module as part of the BRFSS survey. In the five states investigated, cooperation rates—the proportion of all respondents interviewed—ranged from 70.1% (Washington) to 78.8% (Arkansas) [16]. The BRFSS survey was approved by the Institutional Review Boards of the Centers for Disease Control and Prevention and all participating states' Departments of Health. During the telephone interview, all respondents provided informed consent to participate in the BRFSS survey. Of 29,212 respondents in these 5 states, 25,810 (88.4%) of adults aged 18 years or older completed all questions pertaining to ACEs and perceived number of days of insufficient sleep. We excluded respondents with missing values (6.0%) or refusals (4.2%) on one or more of the ACE questions, as well as respondents with missing values on the question pertaining to sufficient sleep (1.4%).

11.2.2 FREQUENT INSUFFICIENT SLEEP

The outcome variable of interest, frequent insufficient sleep, was defined as a response of ≥14 days to the following question, "During the past 30 days, for about how many days have you felt you did not get enough rest or sleep?"

11.2.3 ADVERSE CHILDHOOD EXPERIENCES

The eleven questions included about ACEs were adopted from a longer set of ACE-related questions featured in a study, conducted jointly by the Kaiser Permanente Health Appraisal Clinic in San Diego, CA and the Centers for Disease Control and Prevention, to assess associations between childhood maltreatment and well-being later in life [17]. Questions comprising the 2009 ACE module on the BRFSS, measured three categories of childhood abuse (verbal, physical, and sexual abuse) and five categories of household dysfunction (household mental illness, incarcerated household members, household substance abuse, parental separation/divorce, and witnessing domestic violence) to which the respondent was exposed during childhood. Alternative responses to the questions were provided by the interviewer to the respondent. Notably, less than 0.5% responded "don't know or not sure" to any one of the ACE questions, which was defined as a negative response for the ACE category referenced [18].

Verbal abuse was defined as a response of "more than once" to the question "How often did a parent or adult in your home ever swear at you, insult you, or put you down?" Physical abuse was defined as a response of either "once" or "more than once" to the question "How often did your parents or adult in your home ever hit, beat, kick, or physically hurt you in any way? Do not include spanking." A response of either "once" or "more than once" to any of the following three questions defined sexual abuse: "How often did anyone at least 5 years older than you or an adult, ever touch you sexually?", "How often did anyone at least 5 years older than you or an adult try to make you touch them sexually?" or "How often did anyone at least 5 years older than you or an adult force you to have sex?"

Affirmative responses to questions about living with a household member who "was depressed, mentally ill, or suicidal" or who "served time or was sentenced to serve time in prison, jail, or other correctional facility" defined two respective household dysfunction variables. Living with a household substance abuser was defined as a "yes" response to at least one of two questions about living with anyone who "was a problem drinker or alcoholic" or "used illegal street drugs or abused prescription medications." Having "parents who were separated or divorced" was defined by a "yes" response to a question asking about that as opposed to answering "no," or "parents not married." A response of "once" or "more than once" to the question "How often did your parents or adults in your home ever slap, hit, kick, punch, or beat each other up" defined witnessing domestic violence [18].

The ACE score was created by summing the total number of ACE categories which elicited positive responses (range: 0-8). ACE scores of 5 or more were combined into one category (≥5) due to small sample sizes. Six categories of ACE score (0, 1, 2, 3, 4, and ≥5) were featured in analyses, with zero experiences serving as the referent. Specifically, ≥5 ACEs were combined into a single category to obtain adequate statistical power and because of the consistently graded relationship observed between frequent insufficient sleep and high (≥5) ACE score (data not shown).

11.2.4 POTENTIAL MEDIATORS

Smoking status was defined as current smokers (smoked ≥100 cigarettes in the past and were smoking every day or some days now), former smokers (smoked ≥100 cigarettes in the past, but were not smoking now), or non-smokers (those who never smoked). Respondents were asked to report their perceived mental health in a question gauging frequent mental distress (FMD). Respondents were considered as having FMD if they answered ≥14 days to the question, "Now thinking about your mental health, which includes stress, depression, and problems with emotions, for how many days during the past 30 days was your mental health not good?"

11.2.5 COVARIATES

Gender, age in years (18-24, 25-34, 35-44, 45-64 and ≥65), race/ethnicity (non-Hispanic white, non-Hispanic black, Hispanic, or other non-Hispanic), education (less than high school graduate, high school diploma or GED, some college, or college graduate), and body mass index in kg/m^2 (BMI <18.5 was defined as underweight, BMI=18.5-24.9 as normal weight, BMI=25.0-29.9 as overweight, and BMI ≥30 as obese) were examined as covariates in the association between ACEs and frequent insufficient sleep.

11.2.6 STATISTICAL ANALYSES

Adjusted odds ratios (AORs) and 95% confidence intervals (CIs) for frequent insufficient sleep by individual ACE and by ACE score were obtained from multivariate logistic regression models adjusting for gender, age, race/ethnicity, education, and BMI, as well as the potential mediators of smoking status or FMD. We assessed whether the relationship between ACEs and days of insufficient sleep was attenuated by smoking status or FMD by measuring the percentage of change in odds ratios evidenced between a model with and a model without the specific mediator = $[(OR_{\text{no mediator}} - OR_{\text{with mediator}})/(OR_{\text{no mediator}} - 1)] * 100$ [19,20]. To be statistically conservative, 10% or more of the percentage change indicated that there was a significant mediation effect [19] only if the following three criteria were met: 1) there was a statistically significant relationship between ACEs and frequent insufficient sleep, 2) there was a significant relationship between ACEs and the mediating variable, and 3) there was a significant relationship between the mediating variable and frequent insufficient sleep [21].

All analyses were conducted using SAS-callable SUDAAN to account for the complex study design, with a statistical significance level of $p<0.05$.

11.3 RESULTS

11.3.1 STUDY POPULATION CHARACTERISTICS

The study population was comprised of 16,474 women (52%) and 9,336 men (48%) from five U.S. states (Table 1). The majority of the study population was non-Hispanic white (77.1%) and had at least some college education (62.9%). Sixty-six percent (66.3%) of respondents were overweight or obese, and 18.8% were current smokers. Frequent mental distress was reported by 10.8% of respondents and 28.8% reported frequent sleep insufficiency.

The majority of respondents reported ≥1 ACE (59.5%) and 8.7% reported ≥5 ACEs. Specifically, the most frequently reported ACEs were having lived with a substance abusing household member (29.1%), parental separation or divorce (26.6%), and exposure to verbal abuse (26.1%) during childhood (Table 1).

11.3.2 FREQUENT INSUFFICIENT SLEEP

As evident in Table 2, a greater percentage of frequent insufficient sleep was reported by women than men (30.6% vs. 26.8%, respectively, $p < 0.05$), among respondents aged 25-34 years relative to those aged ≥65 years (35.4% vs. 15.4%, respectively, $p < 0.05$). Frequent insufficient sleep was likewise more prevalent among those with less than a high school education than among college graduates (35.4% vs. 25.1%, respectively, $p < 0.05$), and among those who were obese than among those of normal weight (33.2% vs. 26.6%, respectively, $p < 0.05$).

11.3.3 RELATIONSHIPS BETWEEN POTENTIAL MEDIATORS AND FREQUENT INSUFFICIENT SLEEP

Frequent insufficient sleep was more prevalent among current smokers than among those who had never smoked (40.3% vs. 25.5%, respectively,

TABLE 1. Selected participant characteristics, including frequent insufficient sleep, individual ACEs, and ACE score among adults aged 18 years and older in 5 states, 2009 BRFSS.

Characteristic	Unweighted sample size	Weighted % (95% CI)
Total	25,810	100.0
Gender		
Men	9,336	48.4 (47.3-49.6)
Women	16,474	51.6 (50.4-52.7)
Age, years		
18-24	750	8.1 (7.3- 8.9)
25-34	2,073	17.2 (16.2-18.2)
35-44	3,354	23.3 (22.1-24.4)
45-54	5,300	19.5 (18.7-20.3)
55-64	6,062	15.1 (14.6-15.7)
≥65	8,140	16.8 (16.2-17.4)
Race/ethnicity		
White, Non-Hispanic	19,485	77.1 (76.2-78.0)
Black, Non-Hispanic	2,599	10.7 (10.0-11.5)
Hispanic	2,179	6.7 (6.3- 7.2)
Non-Hispanic/Others*	1,356	5.4 (4.9- 5.9)
Education attainment		
<High school	2,540	9.0 (8.3- 9.7)
High school graduates or GED	7,236	28.1 (27.0-29.1)
Some college	7,465	30.1 (29.0-31.1)
College graduates	8,541	32.8 (31.9-33.8)
Body Mass Index, kg/m2		
Underweight (<18.5)	407	1.6 (1.3- 1.9)
Normal Weight (18.5-24.9)	8,110	32.1 (31.0-33.1)
Overweight (25.0-29.9)	8,800	35.4 (34.3-36.6)
Obese (≥30)	7,541	30.9 (29.8-32.0)
Smoking status		
Current smokers	4,336	18.8 (17.8-19.7)
Former smokers	7,748	26.2 (25.2-27.2)
Never smoked	13,639	55.0 (53.9-56.1)
Frequent mental distress (≥14 days/the past 30 days)	2,752	10.8 (10.1-11.6)

TABLE 1. CONTINUED.

ACEs before age 18		
Verbal abuse	6,297	26.1 (25.1-27.0)
Physical abuse	3,616	14.8 (14.0-15.6)
Sexual abuse	3,310	12.1 (11.4-12.7)
Substance abusing household member	7,021	29.1 (28.1-30.2)
Household mental illness	4,423	19.5 (18.6-20.4)
Witnessing domestic violence	3,906	16.3 (15.5-17.2)
Incarcerated household member	1,261	7.2 (6.4- 7.9)
Parental separation/divorce	5,583	26.6 (25.6-27.7)
ACE score		
0	11,208	40.5 (39.4-41.6)
1	5,894	22.4 (21.5-23.4)
2	3,221	13.1 (12.3-13.9)
3	2,179	8.8 (8.2- 9.4)
4	1,435	6.5 (5.9- 7.2)
≥5	1,873	8.7 (8.0- 9.3)
Frequent insufficient sleep (≥14 days/the past 30 days)	6,522	28.8 (27.7-29.8)

*Non-Hispanic/others includes persons responding as non-Hipanic and Asian, Native Hawaiian or Pacific Islander, American Indian or Alaska Native, Multiracial, or other race only.

p <0.05). Frequent insufficient sleep was also higher among those reporting FMD than among those who did not (63.2% vs. 24.5%, respectively, p <0.05) (Table 2).

11.3.4 RELATIONSHIPS BETWEEN ADVERSE CHILDHOOD EXPERIENCES AND POTENTIAL MEDIATORS

Current smoking and FMD were significantly higher (p <0.05) among persons with each individual ACE than among those without that ACE (Table

TABLE 2. Prevalence of insufficient sleep (≥14 days/30 days) by selected participant characteristics, individual ACEs and ACE score among adults aged ≥18 years in 5 states, 2009 BRFSS.

Characteristic	% (95% CI)
Total	28.8 (27.7-29.8)
Sex	
Men	26.8 (25.1-28.6)
Women	30.6 (29.4-31.8)
Age, years	
18-24	32.3 (27.6-36.9)
25-34	35.4 (32.2-38.6)
35-44	33.6 (30.8-36.3)
45-54	30.3 (28.3-32.2)
55-64	25.3 (23.5-27.0)
≥65	15.4 (14.2-16.5)
Race/ethnicity	
White, Non-Hispanic	28.4 (27.2-29.6)
Black, Non-Hispanic	31.5 (27.9-35.0)
Hispanic	26.4 (23.4-29.5)
Others	32.6 (28.2-37.1)
Educational attainment	
<high school	35.4 (31.4-39.4)
High school graduates or GED	27.7 (25.7-29.7)
Associate degree	31.9 (29.8-34.0)
College graduates	25.1 (23.5-26.7)
Body Mass Index, kg/m2	
Underweight (<18.5)	33.5 (25.1-41.8)
Normal Weight (18.5-24.9)	26.6 (24.7-28.5)
Overweight (25.0-25.9)	27.0 (25.2-28.8)
Obese (≥30)	33.2 (31.2-35.2)
Heavy drinking	
No	28.6 (27.5-29.7)
Yes	31.7 (27.2-36.3)

TABLE 2. CONTINUED.

Smoking status	
Current smokers	40.3 (37.3-43.2)
Former smokers	27.3 (25.4-29.3)
Never smoked	25.5 (24.2-26.9)
Frequent mental distress (≥14 days/the past 30 days)	
No	24.5 (23.5-25.6)
Yes	63.2 (59.6-66.8)

3). Smoking increased with the ACE score such that the prevalence of current smoking was 37.8% among those with ≥5 ACEs compared to 13.0% among those with no ACEs ($p < 0.05$). FMD also increased with increasing ACE score such that the prevalence of FMD was 27.3% among those with ≥5 ACEs compared to 6.0% among those with no ACEs ($p < 0.05$).

11.3.5 RELATIONSHIPS BETWEEN ADVERSE CHILDHOOD EXPERIENCES AND FREQUENT INSUFFICIENT SLEEP

Respondents reporting each individual ACE had a significantly greater prevalence of frequent sleep insufficiency relative to respondents who indicated they had not been exposed ($p < 0.05$) (Table 4). Similarly, the ACE score assumed a significant graded relationship with the prevalence of frequent sleep insufficiency. Among those indicating no ACEs, 21.3% reported frequent insufficient sleep relative to 47.0% of those with ≥5 ACEs ($p < 0.05$). This association remained significant after adjusting for sex, age, race/ethnicity, education, and categorical BMI (adjusted odds ratio [AOR]=2.53; 95% confidence interval [CI]=2.09-3.06) (Table 4, Model 1).

11.3.6 MEDIATING EFFECTS

The effects of variables potentially mediating the relationship between ACEs and frequent sleep insufficiency are presented in Table 4 (Models 2

TABLE 3. Prevalence of current smoking and frequent mental distress by individual ACEs and ACE score, 2009 BRFSS.

Adverse childhood experience	Current smoking % (95% CI)	Frequent mental distress % (95% CI)
Verbal abuse		
No	16.1 (15.0-17.2)	8.2 (7.4- 9.0)
Yes	26.4 (24.4-28.4)	18.2 (16.5-20.0)
Physical abuse		
No	17.1 (16.1-18.1)	9.1 (8.3- 9.9)
Yes	28.5 (25.8-31.2)	21.1 (18.7-23.4)
Sexual abuse		
No	17.6 (16.6-18.6)	9.4 (8.6-10.2)
Yes	27.4 (24.5-30.3)	21.2 (18.8-23.6)
Substance abusing household member		
No	15.5 (14.5-16.6)	8.3 (7.5- 9.1)
Yes	26.7 (24.6-28.8)	17.0 (15.3-18.7)
Mentally ill household member		
No	17.4 (16.3-18.4)	8.8 (8.0- 9.6)
Yes	24.6 (22.4-26.9)	19.3 (17.3-21.3)
Witnessing domestic violence		
No	17.1 (16.1-18.0)	9.2 (8.4- 9.9)
Yes	27.7 (24.7-30.6)	19.4 (16.9-21.9)
Incarcerated household member		
No	17.3 (16.4-18.3)	9.9 (9.2-10.6)
Yes	37.5 (32.0-43.0)	22.9 (18.4-27.4)
Parental separation/ divorce		
No	15.8 (14.8-16.7)	9.6 (8.8-10.4)
Yes	27.1 (24.7-29.5)	14.2 (12.3-16.1)
ACE score		
0	13.0 (11.7-14.2)	6.0 (5.1- 6.9)
1	17.9 (15.9-19.9)	8.9 (7.2-10.5)
2	19.5 (16.6-22.4)	11.1 (9.3-12.9)

TABLE 3. CONTINUED.

3	21.4 (18.2-24.6)	16.8 (13.5-20.0)
4	27.8 (23.0-32.5)	17.2 (13.8-20.6)
≥5	37.8 (33.7-41.9)	27.3 (23.6-30.9)

and 3). Model 2 adjusts for all covariates included in Model 1 with the addition of smoking status. All of the individual ACEs remained significantly associated with frequent sleep insufficiency, although the relationship between ACEs and sleep insufficiency was slightly attenuated by the addition of smoking status to the model. The ACE score retained a significant graded relationship with frequent insufficient sleep ([AOR (95% CI)=1.25 (1.08-1.45) for 1 ACE and =2.26 (1.86-2.75) for ≥5 ACEs] relative to persons with no ACEs). The attenuation observed suggests that smoking status may be a partial mediator of the relationship between ACEs and frequent sleep insufficiency (Table 4, Model 2).

Similarly, Model 3 includes all covariates featured in Model 1, while additionally adjusting for FMD. Further attenuation of many of the ACEs is observed, which is consistent with partial mediation of the relationship between ACEs and frequent insufficient sleep. However, frequent insufficient sleep was no longer significant for the associations with an incarcerated household member (AOR=1.23[0.95-1.60]), or parental divorce/separation (AOR=1.14[0.99-1.31]) with the addition of FMD to the model. This suggests that FMD exerted a greater effect on frequent sleep insufficiency than these two ACEs. A graded -- albeit further attenuated -- relationship was observed between the ACE score and frequent sleep insufficiency: AOR for 1 ACE=1.21 (1.04-1.41), while AOR for ≥5 ACEs=1.80 (1.46-2.21) compared to persons with no ACEs (Table 4, Model 3).

11.4 DISCUSSION

This investigation indicates that ACEs experienced before age 18 are positively associated with frequent insufficient sleep in adult community

TABLE 4. Crude prevalence and adjusted odds ratio (OR) and 95% confidence interval of frequent insufficient sleep (≥14 days/30 days) by individual ACEs and ACE score, 2009 BRFSS.

ACE	% (95% CI)	Model 1 AOR (95% CI)	Model 2 AOR (95% CI)	Model 3 AOR (95% CI)
Verbal abuse				
No	25.6 (24.4-26.8)	1.00 (referent)	1.00 (referent)	1.00 (referent)
Yes	37.9 (35.8-40.0)	1.59 (1.42-1.79)	1.50 (1.33-1.68)*	1.32 (1.16-1.50)†
Physical abuse				
No	26.7 (25.6-27.8)	1.00 (referent)	1.00 (referent)	1.00 (referent)
Yes	40.9 (38.0-43.8)	1.71 (1.50-1.97)	1.62 (1.41-1.86)*	1.43 (1.23-1.65)**
Sexual abuse				
No	27.1 (26.0-28.3)	1.00 (referent)	1.00 (referent)	1.00 (referent)
Yes	40.9 (37.9-43.8)	1.66 (1.44-1.93)	1.56 (1.35-1.81)*	1.40 (1.19-1.64)**
Substance abusing household member				
No	25.7 (24.5-26.8)	1.00 (referent)	1.00 (referent)	1.00 (referent)
Yes	36.4 (34.3-38.6)	1.47 (1.30-1.65)	1.38 (1.23-1.55)*	1.25 (1.10-1.42)†
Mentally ill Household member				
No	26.0 (24.8-27.1)	1.00 (referent)	1.00 (referent)	1.00 (referent)
Yes	40.4 (37.9-43.0)	1.68 (1.47-1.92)	1.60 (1.40-1.83)*	1.42 (1.23-1.64)**
Witnessing domestic violence				
No	26.8 (25.7-27.9)	1.00 (referent)	1.00 (referent)	1.00 (referent)
Yes	39.1 (36.2-42.0)	1.58 (1.37-1.82)	1.51 (1.31-1.73)*	1.35 (1.16-1.57)**
Incarcerated household member				
No	27.8 (26.7-28.8)	1.00 (referent)	1.00 (referent)	1.00 (referent)
Yes	42.1 (36.7-47.5)	1.54 (1.21-1.95)	1.40 (1.10-1.78)**	1.23 (0.95-1.60)†

TABLE 4. CONTINUED.

Parental separation/ divorce				
No	26.5 (25.4-27.7)	1.00 (referent)	1.00 (referent)	1.00 (referent)
Yes	35.0 (32.6-37.3)	1.23 (1.08-1.40)	1.16 (1.02-1.32)**	1.14 (0.99-1.31)**
ACE score				
0	21.3 (19.8-22.8)	1.00 (referent)	1.00 (referent)	1.00 (referent)
1	27.0 (24.9-29.1)	1.28 (1.11-1.49)	1.25 (1.08-1.45)*	1.21 (1.04-1.41)**
2	34.7 (31.6-37.8)	1.74 (1.46-2.06)	1.68 (1.41-1.99)	1.61 (1.35-1.92)*
3	34.4 (31.0-37.8)	1.68 (1.40-2.02)	1.60 (1.33-1.93)*	1.41 (1.15-1.72)**
4	38.1 (33.0-43.2)	1.91 (1.48-2.46)	1.77 (1.39-2.26)*	1.56 (1.20-2.03)**
≥5	47.0 (42.9-51.0)	2.53 (2.09-3.06)	2.26 (1.86-2.75)*	1.80 (1.46-2.21)†

Model 1: multivariate logistic regression model with sex, age, race/ethnicity, education, and categorical BMI.
Model 2: Model 1 plus smoking status (current smoking vs. former smoker/never smoked).
Model 3: Model 1 plus FMD.
*-10%-<20% percentage change of OR in term of formula=((OR1-OR2(3))/(OR1-1.0))*100.
** 20%-<40% percentage change of OR.
†40%-<60% percentage change of OR.

dwellers. As previously noted, these results are similar to those from prior research examining the association between ACEs and two forms of disturbed sleep in a managed care patient population [14]. The current findings thus extend this association of ACEs with sleep impairment to specifically include frequent insufficient sleep within the domain of a population-based sample.

Although associations between childhood sexual abuse and sleep disturbance have been previously reported [22-24], this research has largely been restricted to investigations featuring relatively brief follow-up intervals [23], or only gauging childhood sexual abuse [22-24]. However, related investigation has found both childhood sexual abuse and childhood physical abuse to be positively associated with difficulties falling asleep, staying asleep, or early awakening among a cohort of individuals with a median age of 47 years [25]. This finding is consistent with the results of previous research revealing these forms of childhood abuse were associated with sleep disturbance decades after their occurrence [14].

In an investigation assessing the frequency of self-reported childhood physical, emotional, and sexual abuse, Greenfield, Lee, Friedman, and Springer [26] analyzed data from 835 respondents in the National Survey of Midlife Development in the United States. Specifically, these investigators examined the association of these three forms of abuse with global sleep pathology, as measured by the Pittsburgh Sleep Quality Inventory, as well as with a variety of specific sleep characteristics, such as subjective sleep quality, sleep duration, and habitual sleep efficiency in adulthood. Consistent with the results of the present investigation, that study reported that all three types of childhood abuse examined were associated with global sleep pathology, as well as with specific sleep problems [26]. Additionally, related investigation has revealed that childhood adversities such as parental divorce, long-term financial difficulties, and frequent fear of a family member were associated with poor self-reported sleep quality in adulthood [27].

Notably, the results of our investigation are similar to those obtained among a clinical sample. Bader, Shafer, Schenkel, Nissen, and Schwander [28] examined the association of ACEs with actigraphic and polysomnographic sleep parameters. These investigators found that patients who reported moderate to severe ACEs exhibited a significantly greater number of both awakenings and movement arousals relative to patients reporting few or no ACEs.

The present study further addressed the effects of smoking and FMD on the associations between ACEs and frequent insufficient sleep. These relationships were slightly attenuated by smoking status and moderately attenuated by FMD. Our study findings are consistent with the results of research indicating that smoking is significantly associated with insufficient sleep [13,15,29]. Further, smoking is associated with short and long sleep durations, both of which have been linked to risk for excess mortality [30].

The attenuation of the association between ACEs and frequent insufficient sleep by FMD is consistent with psychiatric nomenclature featuring sleep disturbance as a criterion for the diagnosis of depression [31]. Early detection of and intervention regarding ACEs thus appear particularly warranted as insomnia symptoms [32] and sleep disturbance [33] have been reported to persist even after depression has improved or remitted. Notably, childhood abuse has also been associated with posttraumatic stress disorder (PTSD) symptoms [34], with recent evidence suggesting that the nightmares and insomnia characteristic of PTSD may compromise the consolidation of fear extinction memory and, ultimately, recovery [35]. This further suggests the potentially lasting impact of ACEs, although PTSD was not assessed in this investigation.

This investigation is subject to several limitations. First, our data on both sleep and ACEs were obtained by self-report, with the former assessed by a single item not corroborated by actigraphy, polysomnography, or medical records, Specifically, relative to data garnered by objective measures, sleep difficulties are frequently overreported [36]. However, previous research examining potential biases in the elicitation of ACEs concluded that retrospective self-reports of childhood abuse or neglect are apt to be conservative [37], thereby biasing the results towards the null. Second, our results are cross-sectional thereby prohibiting any inference of causality. Moreover, the presence of ACEs might also increase the risk of adverse events after age 18 years, which this data set does not permit assessment of. Additonally, given that the definition of FMD describes behavioral characteristics not inconsistent with those associated with ACEs, the association between these phenomena could be circuitous. This study was also limited to participants with landline telephones. Subsequent research has indicated that, relative to adults with landlines, adults with only cell phones are more likely to be binge drinkers and current smokers, to engage in regular physical activity and to have an unmet medical care need due to cost, and to be less likely to be use preventive healthcare services, and to be obese [38]. Finally, the generalizability of our findings may be limited, as data were collected from five states.

11.5 CONCLUSION

In conclusion, the results of the present investigation indicate that ACEs are positively associated with frequent insufficient sleep in U.S. adult community-dwellers. This relationship was attenuated—but generally remained significant—by FMD and smoking. These results suggest that ACEs could be potential indicators fostering further investigation of sleep insufficiency, along with consideration of FMD and smoking.

REFERENCES

1. Anda RF, Felitti VJ, Bremner JD, et al.: The enduring effects of abuse and related adverse experiences in childhood. A convergence of evidence from neurobiology and epidemiology. Eur Arch Psychiatry Clin Neurosci 2006, 256(3):174-186.
2. Dube SR, Felitti VJ, Dong M, Chapman DP, Giles WH, Anda RF: Childhood abuse, neglect, and household dysfunction and the risk of illicit drug use: The adverse childhood experiences study. Pediatrics 2003, 111(3):564-572.
3. Chapman DP, Whitfield CL, Felitti VJ, Dube SR, Edwards VJ, Anda RF: Adverse childhood experiences and the risk of depressive disorders in adulthood. J Affect Disord 2004, 82(2):217-225.
4. Anda RF, Brown DW, Felitti VJ, Bremner JD, Dube SR, Giles WH: Adverse childhood experiences and prescribed psychotropic medications in adults. Am J Prev Med 2007, 32(5):389-394.
5. Brown DW, Anda RF, Tiemeier H, et al.: Adverse childhood experiences and the risk of premature mortality. Am J Prev Med 2009, 37(5):389-396.
6. Dong M, Giles WH, Felitti VJ, Dube SR, et al.: Insights into causal pathways for ischemic heart disease: Adverse childhood experiences study. Circulation 2004, 110(13):1761-1766.
7. Dong M, Giles WH, Felitti VJ, et al.: The interrelatedness of multiple forms of childhood abuse, neglect, and household dysfunction. Child Abuse Negl 2004, 28(7):771-784.
8. McKnight-Eily LR, Liu Y, Perry GS, et al.: Perceived insufficient rest or sleep among adults – United States, 2008. MMWR 2009, 58(42):1175-1179.
9. Millman RP, Working Group on Sleepiness in Adolescents/Young Adults; & AAP Committee on Adolescence: Excessive sleepiness in adolescents and young adults: Causes, consequences, and treatment strategies. Pediatrics 2005, 115(6):1774-1786.
10. Wheaton AG, Perry GS, Chapman DP, McKnight-Eily LR, Presley-Cantrell LR, Croft JB: Relationship between body mass index and perceived insufficient sleep among U.S. adults: An analysis of 2008 BRFSS data. BMC Publ Health 2011, 11:295.

11. Vorona RD, Winn MP, Babineau TW, Eng BP, Feldman HR, Ware JC: Overweight and obese patients in a primary care population report less sleep than patients with a normal body mass index. Arch Intern Med 2005, 165(1):25-30.
12. Shankar A, Syamala S, Kalidindi S: Insufficient rest or sleep and its relation to cardiovascular disease, diabetes, and obesity in a national, multiethnic sample. PLoS One 2010, 5(11):e14189.
13. Strine TW, Chapman DP: Associations of frequent sleep insufficiency with health-related quality of life and health behaviors. Sleep Med 2005, 6(1):23-27.
14. Chapman DP, Wheaton AG, Anda RF, Croft JB, Edwards VJ, Liu Y, et al.: Adverse childhood experiences and sleep disturbances in adults. Sleep Med 2011, 12(8):773-779.
15. Sabanayagam C, Shankar A: The association between active smoking, smokeless tobacco, second-hand smoke exposure and insufficient sleep. Sleep Med 2011, 12(1):7-11.
16. Behavioral Risk Factor Surveillance System 2009 Summary Data Quality Report. (Version#1-Revised 02/18/2011). Available at: http://ftp.cdc.gov/pub/Data/Brfss/2009_Summary_Data_Quality_Report.pdf webcite. Accessed November 21, 2012
17. Felitti VJ, Anda RF, Nordenberg D, et al.: Relationship of childhood abuse and household dysfunction to many of the leading causes of death in adults: The adverse childhood experiences study. Am J Prev Med 1998, 14(4):245-248.
18. Bynum L, Griffin T, Ridings DL, et al.: Adverse childhood experiences reported by adults – five states, 2009. MMWR 2010, 59(49):1609-1613.
19. Rothman K, Greenland S, Lash T: Measures of effect and measures of association. In Modern epidemiology. Philadelphia, PA: Lippincott, Williams, & Wilkins; 2008:51-70.
20. van de Mheen H, Stronks K, Mackenbach J: A lifecourse perspective on socio-economic inequalities in health: The influence of childhood socio-economic conditions as selection process. Sociol Health Illn 1998, 20(5):754-777.
21. Baron R, Kenny D: The moderator-mediator distinction in social psychological research: Conceptual, strategic, and statistical considerations. J Pers Soc Psychol 1986, 51(6):1173-1182.
22. Abrams MP, Mulligan AD, Carleton RN, Asmundson GJG: Prevalence and correlates of sleep paralysis in adults reporting childhood sexual abuse. J Anxiety Disorders 2008, 22(8):1535-1541.
23. Calam R, Horne L, Glasgow D, Cox A: Psychological disturbance and child sexual abuse: A follow-up study. Child Abuse Negl 1998, 22(19):901-913.
24. McNally RJ, Clancy SA: Sleep paralysis in adults reporting repressed, recovered, or continuous memories of childhood sexual abuse. J Anx Disord 2005, 19(5):595-602.
25. Gal G, Levav I, Gross R: Psychopathology among adults abused during childhood or adolescence: Results from the Israel-based world mental health survey. J Nerv Ment Dis 2011, 199(4):222-229.
26. Greenfield EA, Lee C, Friedman EL, Springer KW: Childhood abuse as a risk factor for sleep problems in adulthood: Evidence from a U.S. national study. Ann Behav Med 2011, 42(2):245-256.

27. Koskenvuo K, Hublin C, Partinen M, Paunio T, Koskenvuo M: Childhood adversities and quality of sleep in adulthood: A population-based survey of 26,000 Finns. Sleep Med 2010, 11(1):17-22.
28. Bader K, Schafer V, Schenkel M, Nissen L, Schwander J: Adverse childhood experiences associated with sleep in primary insomnia. J Sleep Res 2007, 16(3):285-296.
29. Kaneita Y, Ohida T, Takemura S, et al.: Relation of smoking and drinking to sleep disturbance among Japanese pregnant women. Prev Med 2005, 41(5–6):877-882.
30. Ryu SY, Kim KS, Han MA: Factors associated with sleep duration in Korean adults: Results of a 2008 community health survey in Gwangju metropolitan city, Korea. J Korean Med Sci 2011, 26(3):1124-1131.
31. American Psychiatric Association: Diagnostic and statistical manual of mental disorders. 4th edition. Washington, DC: American Psychiatric Association; 1994.
32. Pigeon WR, May PE, Perlis ML, Ward EA, Lu N, Talbot NL: The effect of interpersonal psychotherapy for depression on insomnia symptoms in a cohort of women with sexual abuse histories. J Traum Stress 2009, 22(1):634-638.
33. Carney CE, Harris AL, Friedman J, Segal ZV: Residual sleep beliefs and sleep disturbance following cognitive behavioral therapy for major depression. Depress Anx 2011, 28(6):464-470.
34. Van Vorhees EE, Dedert EA, Calhoun PS, et al.: Childhood trauma exposure in Iraq and Afghanistan war era veterans: Implications of posttraumatic stress disorders symptoms and adult functional support. Child Abuse Negl 2012, 36(5):423-432.
35. van Liempt S: Sleep disturbances and PTSD: A perpetual cycle? Eur J Psychotraum 2012., 3 Epub 2012 Oct 3
36. Jackowska M, Dockray S, Hendrickx H, Steptoe A: Psychosocial factors and sleep efficiency: Discrepancies between subjective and objective evaluations of sleep. Psychosom Med 2011, 73(9):810-816.
37. Edwards VJ, Anda RF, Nordenberg DF, Felitti VJ, Williamson DF, Wright JA: Bias assessment for child abuse survey: Factors affecting probability of response to a survey about childhood abuse. Child Abuse Negl 2001, 25(2):307-312.
38. Hu SS, Balluz S, Battaglia MP, Frankel MR: Improving public health surveillance using a dual-frame survey of landline and cell phone numbers.

CHAPTER 12

Suicidal Behaviors Among Adolescents in Juvenile Detention: Role of Adverse Life Experiences

MADHAV P. BHATTA, ERIC JEFFERIS, ANGELA KAVADAS, SONIA A. ALEMAGNO, AND PEGGY SHAFFER-KING

12.1 INTRODUCTION

In 2010, 1,926 adolescents aged 10–19 years died as a result of suicide, making it the third leading cause of death among adolescents in the United States (U.S.) [1]. For every completed suicide many more adolescents seriously think about attempting suicide (suicide ideation), make a plan to attempt suicide (suicide plan), and actually attempt suicide one or more times (suicide attempt) [2]. In addition, there are non-fatal attempts that result in an injury that requires medical attention. Therefore, completed suicides are only a fraction of the larger public health concern of suicide and suicidal behaviors among adolescents.

Suicide is the leading cause of death among adolescents in juvenile detention facilities [3], with rates 3 to 18 times higher than the age-matched general population adolescents [4]. Similarly, rates of suicidal behaviors (ideation, plan and attempt) also tend to be higher among incarcerated adolescents than general population adolescents [5], [6]. Among U.S. adolescents in juvenile detention facilities, the estimates of the lifetime prevalence of suicide ideation range from 22.0% to 58.3% and of a lifetime suicide attempt range from 11.0% to 33.0% [5], [7], [8], [9], [10]. Adolescent suicide and suicidal behaviors, therefore, are of special interest for the juvenile detainee population.

Risk factors for suicide and suicidal behaviors in incarcerated adolescents include: mental disorders (borderline personality disorder traits; affective disorders; substance use disorders; post-traumatic stress disorder; anxiety; social phobia; and attention-deficit hyperactivity disorder) [3],[5], [7], [11],[12], [13], [14], [15], [16], [17], [18, [19]; female gender [5], [6], [8]; race [11], [20]; impulsivity [10], [13]; anger [14], [17]; a tendency to act out [18], [21]; younger age [5]; and perceived negative parenting [16]. Adolescents in juvenile detention often have higher rates of risk factors for suicide including substance abuse, mental disorders, trauma, and stressful life events than the general population youths [22]. Moreover, being in juvenile detention is itself a highly stressful event that may increase the risk of suicide among these adolescents. Therefore, screening at intake to a juvenile justice facility to identify individuals at a high risk of suicide is important for suicide prevention among these vulnerable youths [23].

Only a limited number of studies have assessed the role of adverse life experiences on suicidal behaviors in incarcerated adolescents. In previous studies, sexual abuse, exposure to violence, and housing stress have been reported as potential risk factors for suicide ideation and attempt among incarcerated adolescents [5], [8], [9], [24], [25], [26]. However, major limitations of these studies include the limited adverse life experiences studied and the small sample sizes, especially for females. To our knowledge, this is one of the largest epidemiologic studies to assess the influence of multiple adverse life experiences (sexual abuse, homelessness, running away, and substance abuse in the family) on suicide ideation and suicide attempt among male and female adolescents at an urban juvenile detention facility in the U.S. Understanding the influence of various risk factors on suicide ideation and attempt among adolescents in juvenile justice facilities has implications for developing appropriate screening tools and intervention programs aimed at suicide prevention.

12.2 MATERIALS AND METHODS

12.2.1 ETHICS STATEMENT

This was a voluntary and anonymous survey and sex was the only identifiable demographic information collected. To maintain total anonymity of the participants, requirement for written informed consent/assent was waived. The waiver of written consent/assent and the overall study was approved by the University of Akron Institutional Review Board.

12.2.2 PARTICIPANTS

Participants in the study were adolescents processed at a juvenile detention facility in an urban area in Ohio. The study population and methods for data collection have been previously described [27]. Briefly, during the intake process at the facility between 2003 and 2007, adolescents were asked to participate in a voluntary, anonymous survey of risk and protective factors for adverse health outcomes. Seventy-six percent of the adolescents entering the facility were male. The racial/ethnic distribution of the population included 75.2% African Americans, 20.7% whites, 3.9% Hispanics, 0.1% Asians, and 0.1% others. The age distribution included: 2.6% younger than 12 years, 3.7% aged 12, 7.7% aged 13, 12.8% aged 14, 19.7% aged 15, 25.0% aged 16, and 28.3% aged 17 years. The detention center served a county with a population of 1.3 million and housed both pre- and post-adjudicated youths with various alleged offenses including personal, property, drug, public order, and unruly offenses. The average length of stay in the facility was 12.5 days. A total of 3,156 adolescents agreed to participate and completed all the key questions for the present analysis. The study sample accounted for 80% of all intakes at the detention center during the data collection period.

12.2.3 SURVEY INSTRUMENT ADMINISTRATION

Adolescents self-administered the survey instrument by interacting anonymously with a voice enabled computer that read a set of 100 "yes" or "no" questions related to risk and protective factors that were heard over headphones. Adolescents responded by pressing "Y" or "N" on the computer keyboard. The instrument measured risk in the following domains: problems with alcohol and drug use; alcohol and drug treatment history; mental and physical health problems and treatment history for each; sexual behavior; anger management and physical violence; adverse life experiences; and lack of family support.

12.2.4 PRIMARY OUTCOMES OF INTEREST

The primary outcomes of interest in this study were suicide ideation and suicide attempt. Suicide ideation, defined as ever having thoughts about killing oneself, was measured using a "Yes" or "No" response to the question "Have you ever thought about killing yourself?". Suicide attempt, defined as ever having tried to kill oneself, was measured using a "Yes" or "No" response to the question "Have you ever tried to kill yourself?".

12.2.5 PRIMARY EXPOSURES OF INTEREST

12.2.5.1 ADVERSE LIFE EXPERIENCES

The four adverse life experiences measured included: sexual abuse (anyone had ever touched them or done anything to them in a sexual way that they did not want to have done); drug or alcohol abuse by a member of the household (anyone in their home drink or use drugs enough to embarrass or upset them); running away from home (had ever stayed away from home for more than two nights because they didn't want their family to know about something or they were afraid to go home), and homelessness (had ever lived on the street or in a shelter). The independent and joint effects of each adverse life experience with suicide ideation and suicide attempt were assessed.

12.2.6 SECONDARY EXPOSURES OF INTEREST

12.2.6.1 OTHER INDIVIDUAL AND FAMILY RELATED RISK FACTORS

Physical health symptoms were measured using six items that asked the adolescents of any of the following symptoms currently: night sweats, diarrhea, swollen glands, loss of weight without intention, coughing blood, or shortness of breath. Recent medical problems were measured using the following three items: had experienced any serious medical problems in the past year; currently under the care of a physician; or taking medication for a health problem. Family support was measured using three items: when something went wrong, their family was there to help them; they could depend on their family; and their family helped them to be the person that they wanted to be. Risky sexual behavior was measured by four items: first sexual experience younger than age 13; ever had unprotected sex; sex while drunk or high; and ever having exchanged sex for anything (e.g., drugs, money).

12.2.6.2 SUBSTANCE ABUSE RISK FACTORS.

Drug use, measured by eight items, addressed the use of drugs at least once a month during the preceding six months: used [marijuana; powder or crack cocaine; LSD (acid); heroin; inhalants (huffing or sniffing things like glue, paint thinner, gasoline, etc.); uppers (speed, amphetamines, meth, crystal meth, crank); downers (valium, librium, Xanax, barbs, barbiturates); or other substances] at least once a month for the past 6 months. Problem with alcohol use was measured using eight items: drank more than one drink of alcohol just about every day; when drinking, drank four or more drinks during that day; drinking ever kept them from doing things they were supposed to do; was hard to stop drinking once they started;

ever wanted to keep drinking after their friends have had enough; ever drank secretly or when alone; ever gotten into a fight when drinking; and people nagged them or complained about their drinking. History of substance abuse treatment was measured using two items: ever gone to treatment, a counselor, or a doctor because of alcohol use; and ever gone to treatment, a counselor, or a doctor because of drugs use.

12.2.6.3 MENTAL HEALTH RISK FACTORS.

History of mental health treatment was measured using four items: had ever seen or were currently seeing a counselor or psychologist because of school, family or personal problems; had ever been hospitalized for mental health or emotional problems; and taking prescription medication for mental health problems. Symptoms of depression was measured using six items: lost interest in things that they usually did at home, at school or with their friends; felt sad or tired most of the time; felt like their life was a mess and will never get better; felt like they are unimportant or worthless; hard to concentrate at school or work; and thought about death a lot. Anger management issue was measured using four items: had a bad temper that they couldn't control sometimes; got into physical fights at school or at home that they regretted later; have had arguments at home where they threatened to hurt each other; and have had physical fights in their home where they hurt each other.

For each of the secondary exposure of interest, an index score was created for the variable by summing the response to each question in the category. The score was dichotomized as an adolescent reporting no history of exposure (score = 0) or any history of exposure (score ≥1) for that particular variable.

12.2.7 STATISTICAL ANALYSES

The differences in the outcomes and exposure variables of interest between males and females were assessed using the $\chi 2$-test. To assess the individual relationship of adverse life experiences and other exposures/potential risk factors with suicide ideation and suicide planning, univariable logistic regression analyses were performed and crude odds ratio (OR) and the associated 95% confidence intervals (CI) are reported. Multivariable logistic regression analyses were performed to assess the independent effect of the primary exposure variables with suicide ideation and suicide attempt, respectively, while controlling for the potential confounders. The final logistic regression models included all the variables significantly associated with the outcomes at $\alpha = 0.05$ in the univariable analyses. The combined effects of multiple adverse life experiences were computed by exponentiation of the sum of logistic regression coefficient for independent effects. Multivariable logistic regression analyses stratified by gender were performed and the OR and associated 95% CI are reported. All the data analyses were performed using SAS® 9.3.1 (SAS Institute, Cary, NC).

12.3 RESULTS

Of the total 3,156 adolescents participating in the study, 694 (22.0%) were females and 2,462 (78.0%) were males. Overall, 42.7% of the adolescents reported at least one of the four adverse life experiences, with 24.5%, 12.7%, and 5.5% respectively reporting 1, 2, and 3 or 4 adverse life experiences. Table 1 presents the overall and sex stratified prevalence of specific adverse life experience and other potential risk factors for suicide ideation and attempt among the adolescents in the study. Females were significantly more likely to report experiencing each of the four adverse life events than males ($p<0.0001$). Females also significantly reported higher levels of risky sexual behaviors, experiencing physical health symptoms, receiving medical care for a health problem in the past year, and mental health related problems than males. Additionally, females reported a significantly lower level of family support than males. There was no significant difference in the substance abuse risk factors between male and female adolescents in this study.

12.3.1 SUICIDE IDEATION AND SUICIDE ATTEMPT

Overall 601 (19.0%) of the adolescents reported suicide ideation and 376 (11.9%) reported suicide attempt. Female adolescents were significantly more likely to report suicide ideation (36.6% versus 14.1%; $p<0.001$) and suicide attempt (25.4% versus 8.1%; $p<0.001$) than males (Table 1).

Table 2 presents the unadjusted and adjusted odds of suicide ideation and suicide attempt for adverse life experiences and other risk factors. In the multivariable logistic regression analyses, experiencing sexual abuse (OR = 2.75; 95% C.I. = 2.08–3.63) and homelessness (1.51; 1.17–1.94) were associated with an increased odds of suicide ideation, while sexual abuse (3.01; 2.22–4.08), homelessness (1.49; 1.12–1.98), and running away from home (1.38; 1.06–1.81) were associated with increased odds of suicide attempt among adolescents. In addition, other factors significantly associated with both suicide ideation and suicide attempt included: being female; having physical health symptoms; having had or receiving medical care for a serious health problem in the past year; problem with alcohol abuse; having problems with anger management; having any symptoms of depression; and a history of mental health treatment (Table 2).

Table 3 presents the results of the stratified analyses of the risk factors for suicide ideation and suicide attempt by sex. It is interesting to note that risky sexual behaviors was not associated with either suicide ideation (OR = 1.00) or suicide attempt (OR = 0.99) in the overall analyses. However, risky sexual behaviors was positively associated (2.19; 1.28–3.76) with suicide ideation among females and, while not statistically significant, negatively associated (0.77; 0.57–1.05) among males.

12.3.2 INDEPENDENT AND COMBINED EFFECTS OF ADVERSE LIFE EXPERIENCES

Table 4 presents the independent and combined effects of sexual abuse and other adverse experiences on the odds of suicide ideation and suicide attempt while controlling for other potential risk factors. Sexual abuse is the strongest adverse life experience predictor for both suicide ideation and suicide attempt. With an increasing number of adverse life experiences the odds of suicide attempts increased, indicating a positive dose-response relationship. An individual who experienced all four adverse events was 7.81 times more likely (95% C.I.: 2.41–25.37) to have ever attempted suicide than one who experienced none of the adverse events.

TABLE 1. Suicidal Behaviors and Potential Risk Factors by Sex Among Adolescents in an Urban Juvenile Detention Center in Ohio, 2003–2007.

	All (N = 3,156)	Male (n = 2,462)	Female (n = 694)	
	Proportion (95% CI)*	Proportion (95% CI)*	Proportion (95% CI)*	p-value[a]
Suicide Ideation and Attempt (Yes)				
Ever thought about suicide	19.0 (17.7–20.4)	14.1 (12.7–15.5)	36.6 (33.0–40.2)	<.0001
Ever attempted suicide	11.9 (10.8–13.1)	8.1 (7.0–9.2)	25.4 (22.2–28.6)	<.0001
Adverse Life Experiences				
Any	42.7 (41.0–44.5)	36.1 (30.3–38.1)	66.0 (62.5–69.5	<.0001
Sexual abuse	12.2 (11.1–13.3)	4.6 (3.7–5.4)	39.5 (35.8–43.1)	
Homelessness	16.9 (15.6–18.2)	15.4 (14.0–16.9)	21.9 (18.2–25.0)	
Running away from home	26.0 (24.5–27.6)	21.5 (19.9–23.1)	42.1 (38.4–45.8)	
Drug use in the family	12.6 (11.4–13.7)	11.2 (10.0–12.5)	17.3 (14.5–20.1)	
Other Individual and Family Related Factors (Index score ≥1)[b]				
Risky sexual behaviors	74.5 (72.9–76.1)	73.2 (71.4–74.9)	79.1 (76.1–82.1)	0.0016
Physical health symptoms	33.8 (32.2–35.5)	30.0 (28.2–31.8)	47.4 (43.7–51.1)	<.0001
Recent medical problems	43.9 (42.2–45.7)	40.3 (38.5–42.3)	56.9 (53.1–60.6)	<.0001
Family support	89.1 (88.0–90.2)	90.8 (89.6–91.9)	83.1 (80.4–85.9)	<.0001

TABLE 1. CONTINUED.

Substance Abuse Factors (Index score ≥1)[b]				
Drug use in the prior 6 months	40.0 (39.2–38.2)	39.7 (37.7–41.6)	40.8 (37.1–44.5)	0.6030
History of substance abuse treatment	17.5 (16.2–18.9)	17.5 (16.0–19.2)	17.6 (14.8–20.4)	0.9445
Problems with alcohol use	33.9 (32.3–35.6)	33.6 (31.8–35.5)	35.0 (31.5–38.6)	0.4967
Mental Health Factors (Index score ≥1)[b]				
Symptoms of depression	69.3 (67.7–70.9)	67.3 (65.4–69.1)	76.7 (73.5–79.8)	<.0001
Problem with anger management	71.9 (70.5–73.4)	69.1 (67.2–70.9)	81.7 (78.8–84.6)	<.0001
History of mental health treatment	62.2 (60.5–63.9)	57.8 (55.8–59.7)	78.1 (75.0–81.2)	<.0001

* 95% Confidence Interval

[a] x^2-Test; 2-sided p-value 1

[b] Index score range: Risky sexual behaviors: 0–4; Physical health symptoms: 0–7; Medical care: 0–3; Family support: 0–3; Drug use in the prior 6 months: 0–8; Problems with substance use: 0–4; History of substance abuse treatment: 0–2; Problems with alcohol use: 0–8; Depression: 0–6; Problem with anger management: 0–4; History of mental health treatment: 0–6.

TABLE 2. Logistic Regression Analyses of Risk Factors for Suicide Ideation and Suicide Attempt Among Adolescents in an Urban Juvenile Detention Center in Ohio, 2003–2007.

Risk Factor	Suicide Ideation		Suicide Attempt	
	Unadjusted OR (95% CI)*	Adjusted OR (95% CI)*	Unadjusted OR (95% CI)*	Adjusted OR (95% CI)*
Female	3.50 (3.00–4.26)	1.72 (1.35–2.19)	3.85 (3.08–4.81)	1.65 (1.24–2.18)
Adverse Life Experiences				
Sexual abuse	6.70 (5.34–8.40)	2.75 (2.08–3.63)	7.62 (5.96–9.74)	3.01 (2.22–4.08)
Homelessness	2.83 (2.30–3.48)	1.51 (1.17–1.94)	3.04 (2.39–3.85)	1.49 (1.12–1.98)
Running away from home	3.08 (2.55–3.70)	1.20 (0.95–1.51)	3.61 (2.90–4.51)	1.38 (1.06–1.81)
Drug use in the family	1.94 (1.53–2.46)	1.05 (0.79–1.39)	2.32 (1.77–3.03)	1.26 (0.92–1.73)
Other Individual and Family Related Factors (Index score ≥1 vs. 0)[a]				
Risky sexual behaviors	1.34 (1.24–1.45)	1.00 (0.77–1.30)	1.41 (1.28–1.55)	0.99 (0.72–1.36)
Physical health symptoms	1.87 (1.70–2.05)	1.55 (1.26–1.92)	1.84 (1.66–2.02)	1.35 (1.05–1.75)
Recent medical problems	1.77 (1.62–1.95)	1.60 (1.30–1.98)	1.82 (1.63–2.03)	1.72 (1.33–2.22)
Family support	0.77 (0.71–0.83)	0.99 (0.73–1.35)	0.77 (0.70–0.85)	0.89 (0.63–1.26)

TABLE 2. CONTINUED.

Substance Abuse Factors (index score ≥1 vs. 0)[a]				
Drug use in the prior 6 months	1.61 (1.43–1.82)	1.13 (0.90–1.41)	1.61 (1.41–1.83)	1.08 (0.83–1.42)
History of substance abuse treatment	1.52 (1.31–1.76)	0.99 (0.77–1.30)	1.59 (1.35–1.88)	1.10 (0.81–1.48)
Problem with alcohol use	1.27 (1.21–1.34)	1.43 (1.13–1.80)	1.27 (1.20–1.34)	1.46 (1.11–1.93)
Mental Health Factors (index score ≥1 vs. 0)[a]				
Symptoms of Depression	1.76 (1.67–1.86)	2.63 (1.93–3.58)	1.66 (1.56–1.76)	1.47 (1.03–2.09)
Problem with anger management	1.77 (1.65–1.90)	1.75 (1.30–2.35)	1.82 (1.67–1.98)	2.40 (1.59–3.61)
History of mental health treatment	2.56 (2.34–2.78)	3.50 (2.61–4.69)	2.80 (2.54–3.09)	4.68 (3.06–7.16)

*OR (95% CI): Odds Ratio (95% Confidence Interval).

[a] Index score range: Risky sexual behaviors: 0–4; Physical health symptoms: 0–7; Medical care: 0–3; Family support: 0–3; Drug use in the prior 6 months: 0–8; Problems with substance use: 0–4; History of substance abuse treatment: 0–2; Problems with alcohol use: 0–8; Depression: 0–6; Problem with anger management: 0–4; History of mental health treatment: 0–6.

TABLE 3. Multivariable Logistic Regression Analyses by Sex of Risk Factors for Suicidal Ideation and Suicide Attempt Among Adolescents in an Urban Juvenile Detention Center in Ohio, 2003–2007.

	Suicide Ideation		Suicide Attempt	
	Male	Female	Male	Female
	Adjusted OR (95% CI)*	Adjusted OR (95% CI)*	Adjusted OR (95% CI)*	Adjusted OR (95% CI)*
Adverse Life Experiences				
Sexual abuse	3.09 (2.00–4.76)	2.43 (1.67–3.53)	4.03 (2.54–6.38)	2.39 (1.59–3.60)
Homelessness	1.55 (1.13–2.12)	1.51 (0.98–2.33)	1.37 (0.93–2.01)	1.63 (1.04–2.55)
Running away from home	1.25 (0.93–1.67)	1.05 (0.71–1.56)	1.43 (1.00–2.03)	1.39 (0.90–2.12)
Drug use in the family	1.20 (0.84–1.69)	0.85 (0.53–1.37)	1.31 (0.86–1.97)	1.21 (0.74–1.99)
Other Individual and Family Related Factors (Index score ≥1 vs. 0)[a]				
Risky sexual behaviors	0.77 (0.57–1.05)	2.19 (1.28–3.76)	0.94 (0.64–1.39)	1.29 (0.72–2.30)
Physical health symptoms	1.55 (1.20–2.02)	1.57 (1.07–2.28)	1.47 (1.06–2.04)	1.16 (0.76–1.77)
Recent medical problems	1.53 (1.18–1.98)	1.63 (1.12–2.38)	1.79 (1.28–2.50)	1.53 (1.01–2.32)

TABLE 3. CONTINUED.

Family support	0.89 (0.60–1.33)	1.29 (0.79–2.10)	0.83 (0.52–1.34)	0.97 (0.58–1.61)
Substance Abuse Factors (index score ≥1 vs. 0)[a]				
Drug use in the prior 6 months	1.08 (0.82–1.42)	1.15 (0.77–1.73)	0.90 (0.64–1.27)	1.42 (0.91–2.21)
History of substance abuse treatment	1.02 (0.75–1.40)	0.87 (0.54–1.41)	0.98 (0.67–1.44)	1.36 (0.83–2.14)
Problem with alcohol use	1.28 (0.97–1.70)	1.88 (1.22–2.91)	1.54 (1.08–2.18)	1.33 (0.83–2.14)
Mental Health Factors (index score ≥1 vs. 0)[a]				
Symptoms of depression	2.98 (2.01–4.43)	2.08 (1.24–3.50)	1.72 (1.16–2.50)	1.11 (0.63–1.95)
Problem with anger management	1.95 (1.35–2.81)	1.44 (0.85–2.44)	2.37 (1.41–3.98)	2.52 (1.29–4.96)
History of mental health treatment	4.02 (2.81–5.75)	2.50 (1.48–4.23)	4.81 (2.85–8.11)	4.35 (2.08–9.12)

*OR (95% CI): Odds Ratio (95% Confidence Interval).

[a] Index score range: Risky sexual behaviors: 0–4; Physical health symptoms: 0–7; Medical care: 0–3; Family support: 0–3; Drug use in the prior 6 months: 0–8; Problems with substance use: 0–4; History of substance abuse treatment: 0–2; Problems with alcohol use: 0–8; Symptoms of depression: 0–6; Problem with anger management: 0–4; History of mental health treatment: 0–6.

TABLE 4. Association of Multiple Adverse Life Experiences with Suicide Ideation and Suicide Attempt Among Adolescents in an Urban Juvenile Detention Center in Ohio, 2003–2007.

Risk Factors	Suicide Ideation	Suicide Attempt
	Adjusted[a] OR (95% CI)*	Adjusted[a] OR (95% CI)*
Sexual abuse only versus none	2.75 (2.08–3.63)	3.01 (2.22–4.08)
Sexual abuse and homelessness versus neither	4.54 (2.67–7.70)	4.48 (2.48–8.09)
Sexual abuse, homelessness, and running away from home versus none	5.45 (2.55–11.66)	6.19 (2.62–14.66)
Sexual abuse, homelessness, running away from home, and drug use in the family versus none	5.72 (2.02–16.21)	7.81 (2.41–25.37)

[a] Adjusted for sex, family support, drug and alcohol use, sexual risk behaviors, physical health symptoms, recent medical problems, history of mental health treatment, symptoms of depression, and anger management problems.
* OR (95% CI): Odds Ratio (95% Confidence Interval).

12.4 DISCUSSION

The findings of this large epidemiologic study of suicide ideation and attempt among male and female adolescents in an urban U.S. juvenile detention center have implications for prevention, intervention, policy, and research. The present study adds to the existing knowledge about the risk factors for suicidal behaviors in male and female adolescents in juvenile detention facilities by assessing the independent and joint influence of multiple adverse life experiences. The key findings of this study were that a history of sexual abuse, homelessness, and running away from home were independently significantly associated with ever attempting suicide. In addition, we observed a dose-response relationship between the number of adverse life experiences and suicidal behaviors, particularly suicide attempt. An individual experiencing all four adverse events was 5.7 and 7.8 times more likely to report suicide ideation and suicide attempt, respectively, than someone experiencing none. Considering the substantial prevalence of adverse life experiences observed among adolescents in this study, these risk factors are likely to have significant impact on future suicidal behaviors in this population.

Adolescents entering the juvenile detention facility in this study were at a substantial and elevated risk of suicide ideation (19.0%) and suicide attempts (11.9%). These results are similar to a previous comparable study that reported a prevalence of 11.0% for ever attempted suicide in 1,829 adolescents surveyed at intake to a detention center in Chicago [8]. We also observed a significant difference in the prevalence of suicidal behaviors among males and females, which also is consistent with previous findings in both the general population and adolescents in the juvenile justice system [5], [6].

In terms of individual adverse life experiences, a history of sexual abuse was the strongest independent predictor for both suicide ideation (OR = 3.0) and suicide attempt (OR = 2.8), which is consistent with findings of a previous study of incarcerated adolescents in the U.S [5]. Sexual abuse, as operationalized in this study, encompasses a broad definition without specificity in terms of type, frequency, age at occurrence, duration, or the characteristics of the perpetrator [28]. Using this broad definition of this measure is likely to underestimate the true effect due to possible non-differential misclassification of the exposure. Therefore, the association between sexual abuse and suicide ideation and suicide attempt may be even stronger than the association observed in this study.

A history of sexual abuse has a stronger association in males with both suicide ideation (OR = 3.1 vs. 2.4) and suicide attempt (OR = 4.0 vs. 2.4) than females but the observed difference was not statistically significant. With a prevalence of 39.5%, females, however, were 8.5 times more likely than males to report a history of sexual abuse. This observed difference in the prevalence of sexual abuse between male and female adolescents is consistent with that observed in the general population of adolescents [29]. Moreover, female detainees in this study were also significantly more likely to report experiencing other adverse life experiences than males. Adverse life experiences, including sexual abuse, are likely to result in a greater impact on suicidal behaviors in females than males due to a higher level of exposure.

Significant gender differences in self-reported suicidal behaviors and adverse life experiences highlight the need for a gender specific screening tool and programming for suicide prevention among detained adolescents. It should be noted that while females generally report higher rates of suicide ideation and attempt, they typically have lower suicide completion rates [1], [6]. As such, rates of completed suicides should not be used in isolation to guide practice and policy because this single indicator would likely mask the seriousness of the issue in female detainees. The difference in the levels of adverse life experiences among males and females may partly explain the difference in suicidal behaviors by gender. Suicide screening tools at intake and during the period of detention, therefore, should include questions on the history of adverse life experiences to identify high-risk adolescents. Moreover, intervention programs should include methods to address the effects of adverse life experiences, especially in females.

We also observed a significant association of suicidal behaviors with currently experiencing poor physical health symptoms and a history of serious medical condition. To the best of our knowledge, no previous studies have examined these factors in incarcerated youth. However, in the general population of high school aged adolescents, those with physical disabilities or long-term health problems report higher risk of suicide ideation (OR = 2.7) and suicide attempt (OR = 3.2) than those without disabilities or health problems [30]. We also observed a statistically significant association of suicidal behaviors with mental health risk factors including self-reported history of any symptoms of depression, mental health treatment and anger management issues. These observations are consistent with previous studies which found an association between mental health issues and suicidal behaviors among adolescents in the juvenile justice system [11], [12], [13], [14], [15] [16], [17], [18, [19].

Although screening of all adolescents within the first 24 hours of intake at a facility reduces the odds of suicide attempts, the screening protocols for juvenile facilities vary in terms of adolescents screened, timing of screening, screening tools used, and the qualification of the screeners [23]. Routine suicide screening protocols for all adolescents would be a prudent practice at detention center intake and periodically during the period of detention. The findings of this study point to the need to take into consideration gender, the history of adverse life experience and current physical health status as well as mental health and anger management issues in a potential suicide screening tool, prevention and intervention efforts. Consequently, detention facilities should have the capacity to evaluate and monitor these risk factors, which is not always the case. Ideally, psychological screenings conducted at intake that point to an elevated risk of suicide would be followed up by appropriate gender specific intervention programming to reduce the risk of suicide among adolescents in the juvenile justice system.

This study has several strengths and limitations, thus the findings have to be interpreted accordingly. With a sample size of 3,156, it is one of the largest studies conducted among adolescents in juvenile detention to assess the influence of adverse life experiences in suicidal behaviors by gender. We were able to control for the potential confounding effects of many known risk factors for suicidal behaviors including substance abuse and a history of mental health problems to assess the independent effect of adverse life experiences. The Computer-Assisted anonymous self-administered questionnaire likely enabled the participants to respond to the questions more honestly, thus reducing information bias. Because we did not have information on the non-participants, we were unable to assess any potential differences between the study sample and the non-participants to evaluate selection bias. However, the high response rate likely minimized the selection bias, if any. Moreover, the study sample reflected the underlying population in terms of gender distribution, which indicates the overall representativeness of the study sample.

This study is based on cross-sectional data, thus, we simply do not know the temporal sequencing of the risk factors explored and the self-reported life-time suicidal behaviors. Clearly, it is important to study the timing of suicidal behaviors in the context of risk factors, especially in trying to establish a causal relation. However, for the purpose of screening to identify high-risk individuals, this may not be as important a limitation. Although the underlying population was predominantly African-American and aged 13–17 years, the information on the age and race/ethnicity of the individual participants was not collected. While limiting personal identifying information increased anonymity for participants and likely reduced information bias, we could not assess the confounding effect of these variables. Similarly, we were unable to assess the influence of other underlying risk factors such as socioeconomic status and sexual orientation in this study. Additionally, we did not assess impact of other adverse and traumatic life experiences such as peer bullying, physical abuse, family instability, and community violence. Further research should focus on assessing the influence of these adverse life experiences in order to gain a comprehensive understanding of their effect on suicidal behaviors on adolescents in juvenile detention.

Another limitation of the study is that we did not specifically measure various types of mental disorders, including depression, which have previously shown to be associated with suicidal behaviors [11], [12], [13], [14], [15] [16], [17], [18, [19]. Having any symptoms associated with depression, as defined in this study, is not a specific measure of depression. Therefore, this study did not assess the influence of specific mental health disorders including depression on suicidal behaviors. However, a history of having ever received treatment for mental health issues was measured in the study. Although the prevalence of having any symptoms of depression seems high (69%), the fact that 62% of the adolescents reported having ever received a mental health treatment points to a significant prevalence of mental health issues in this population. Finally, secondary risk factors assessed in this study may be mediators rather than being confounders in the association between adverse life experiences and suicidal behaviors [31]. Future studies should assess the potential mediation of the relationship, particularly by the history of mental health problems.

Understanding the risk factors for suicidal behaviors among detained adolescents is essential for intervention programs for suicide prevention within juvenile correctional facilities. The detained adolescents will eventually be released into the general public and continue to be at high risk for suicide. Therefore, health professionals within and outside the juvenile justice system who care for these adolescents must be aware of the impact of adverse life experiences on suicidal behaviors for effective therapy and intervention for suicide prevention in this high-risk population.

REFERENCES

1. Centers for Disease Control and Prevention (2013) Web-based Injury Statistics Query and Reporting System (WISQARS). Available: http://www.cdc.gov/injury/wisqars/index.html. Accessed July 15, 2013.

2. American Association of Suicidology (2013) USA Suicide: 2010 Official Final Data. Available: http://www.suicidology.org/c/document_library/get_file?folderId=262&name=DLFE-636.pdf. Accessed July 15, 2013.
3. Gallagher CA, Dobrin A (2006) Deaths in juvenile justice residential facilities. J Adolesc Health 38(6): 662–668. doi: 10.1016/j.jadohealth.2005.01.002
4. Fazel S, Benning R, Danesh J (2003) Suicide in male prisoners in England and Wales, 1978–2003. Lancet 366: 1301–1302. doi: 10.1016/s0140-6736(05)67325-4
5. Morris RE, Harrison EA, Knox GW, Tromanhauser E, Marquis DK, et al. (1995) Health risk behavioral survey from 39 juvenile correctional facilities in the United States. J Adolesc Health 17(6): 334–344. doi: 10.1016/1054-139x(95)00098-d
6. Centers for Disease Control and Prevention (2012) Youth Risk Behavior Surveillance – United States, 2011. MMWR Morb Mortal Wkly Rep 61(No. SS-4): 1–161.
7. Freedenthal S, Vaughn MG, Jenson JM, Howard MO (2007) Inhalant use among incarcerated youth. Drug Alcohol Depend 90(1): 81–88. doi: 10.1016/j.drugalcdep.2007.02.021
8. Abram KM, Choe JY, Washburn JJ, Telpin LA, King DC, et al. (2008) Suicidal ideation and behaviors among youths in juvenile detention. J Am Acad Child Adolesc Psychiatry 47(3): 291–300. doi: 10.1097/chi.0b013e318160b3ce
9. Esposito CL, Clum GA (2002) Social support and problem-solving as moderators of the relationship between childhood abuse and suicidality: Applications to a delinquent population. J Trauma Stress 15(2): 137–146. doi: 10.1023/a:1014860024980
10. Sanislow CA, Grilo CM, Fehon DC, Axelrod SR, McGlashan TH (2003) Correlates of suicide risk in juvenile detainees and adolescent inpatients. J Am Acad Child Adolesc Psychiatry 42(2): 234–240. doi: 10.1097/00004583-200302000-00018
11. Alessi NE, McManus M, Brickman A, Grapentine L (1984) Suicidal behavior among serious juvenile offenders. Am J Psychiatry 141(2): 286–287.
12. Plattner B, The SS, Kraemer HC, Williams RP, Bauer SM, et al. (2007) Suicidality, psychopathology, and gender in incarcerated adolescents in Austria. J Clin Psychiatry 68(10): 1593–1600. doi: 10.4088/jcp.v68n1019
13. Rohde P, Seeley JR, Mace DE (1997) Correlates of suicidal behavior in a juvenile detention population. Suicide Life Threat Behav 27(2): 164–175.
14. Penn JV, Esposito CL, Schaeffer LE, Fritz GK, Spirito A (2003) Suicide attempts and self-mutilative behavior in a juvenile correctional facility. J Am Acad Child Adolesc Psychiatry 42(7): 762–769. doi: 10.1097/01.chi.0000046869.56865.46
15. Chapman JF, Ford JD (2008) Relationships between suicide risk, traumatic experiences, and substance use among juvenile detainees. Arch Suicide Res 12: 50–61. doi: 10.1080/13811110701800830
16. Ruchkin VV, Schwab-Stone M, Koposov RA, Vermeiren K, King RA (2003) Suicidal ideations and attempts in juvenile delinquents. J Child Psychol Psychiatry 44: 1058–1066. doi: 10.1111/1469-7610.00190
17. Putnins AL (2005) Correlates and predictors of self-reported suicide attempts among incarcerated youths. Int J Offender Ther Comp Criminol 49(2): 143–157. doi: 10.1177/0306624x04269412
18. Miller ML, Chiles JA, Barnes VE (1982) Suicide attempters within a delinquent population. J Consult Clin Psychol 50(4): 491–498. doi: 10.1037/0022-006x.50.4.491

19. Harris TE, Lennings CJ (1993) Suicide and adolescence. Int J Offender Ther Comp Criminol 37(3): 263–270. doi: 10.1177/0306624x9303700307
20. Kempton T, Forehand R (1992) Suicide attempts among juvenile delinquents: The contribution of mental health factors. Behav Res Ther 30(5): 537–541. doi: 10.1016/0005-7967(92)90038-i
21. Suk E, Mill JV, Vermeiren R, Ruchkin V, Schwab-Stone M, et al. (2009) Adolescent suicidal ideation: A comparison of incarcerated and school-based samples. Eur Child Adolesc Psychiatry 18: 377–383. doi: 10.1007/s00787-009-0740-1
22. Hayes LM (2004) Juvenile Suicide in Confinement: A National Survey. Mansfield, MA: National Center on Institutions and Alternatives.
23. Gallagher CA, Dobrin A (2005) The association between suicide screening practices and attempts requiring emergency care in juvenile justice facilities. J Am Acad Child Adolesc Psychiatry 44(5): 485–493. doi: 10.1097/01.chi.0000156281.07858.52
24. Morgan J, Hawton K (2004) Self-reported suicidal behavior in juvenile offenders in custody: Prevalence and associated factors. Crisis 25(1): 8–11. doi: 10.1027/0227-5910.25.1.8
25. Howard J, Lennings CJ, Copeland J (2003) Suicidal behavior in a young offender population. Crisis 24(3): 98–104. doi: 10.1027//0227-5910.24.3.98
26. Matsumoto T, Tsutsumi A, Izutsu T, Imamura F, Chiba Y, et al. (2009) Comparative study of the prevalence of suicidal behavior and sexual abuse history in delinquent and non-delinquent adolescents. Psychiatry Clin Neurosci 63(2): 238–240. doi: 10.1111/j.1440-1819.2009.01929.x
27. Alemagno SA, Stephens P, Shaffer-King P, Teasdale B (2009) Prescription drug abuse among adolescent arrestees: correlates and implications. J Correct Health Care 15(1): 35–46. doi: 10.1177/1078345808326620
28. Andrews G, Corry J, Armstrong GL, Hutin YJF (2005) Child sexual abuse. In: Ezzati M, Lopez AD, Rodgers A, Murray CJL, editors. Comparative quantification of health risks: Global and regional burden of disease attributable to selected major risk factors. Vol. I. Geneva: WHO. 1851.
29. Bolen RM, Scannapieco M (1999) Prevalence of child sexual abuse: A corrective meta-analysis. Social Service Review 73(3): 281–313. doi: 10.1086/514425
30. Everett Jones S, Lollar DJ (2008) Relationship between physical disabilities or long-term health problems and health risk behaviors or conditions among US high school students. J Sch Health 78(5): 252–7. doi: 10.1111/j.1746-1561.2008.00297.x
31. Johnson JG, Cohen P, Gould MS, Kasen S, Brown J, et al. (2002) Childhood adversities, interpersonal difficulties, and risk for suicide attempts during late adolescence and early adulthood. Arch Gen Psychiatry 59(8): 741–749. doi: 10.1001/archpsyc.59.8.741

PART III

EARLY TRAUMA AND EPIGENETICS

CHAPTER 13

The Link Between Child Abuse and Psychopathology: A Review of Neurobiological and Genetic Research

EAMON MCCRORY, STEPHANE A. DE BRITO, AND ESSI VIDING

13.1 THE IMPACT OF ABUSE ON BRAIN DEVELOPMENT

A growing body of research has investigated how stress, and specifically different forms of childhood abuse, is associated with neuroendocrine function as well as structural and functional differences at the level of the brain. [1] This research is in part motivated by the need to delineate biological mechanisms that may account for the heightened risk of psychological, social and health problems known to be associated with early adversity, including long-term consequences for adult economic wellbeing. [2,3] This paper selectively reviews recent human research related to early stress, maltreatment and their relationship to psychopathology; a number of earlier seminal studies are also included where these help set the research context. We primarily focus on studies of children who have experienced abuse but we also consider several studies of adults with documented histories of early adversity. We begin by briefly considering the evidence for an association between maltreatment or abuse and atypical development of the hypothalamic-pituitary-adrenal (HPA) axis stress response. We then provide a concise overview of neuroimaging studies that have sought to identify differences in regional brain structure and function associated with childhood abuse. We conclude by considering the possible clinical implications of this research.

13.2 METHODS

This review was based on a selection of peer-reviewed articles in English obtained from PubMed that were published from 1995 to the present day; articles related to the study of maltreatment and adversity with a focus on HPA functioning, functional and structural imaging, and behavioural genetic paradigms.

13.2.1 CHILD ABUSE AND THE HPA SYSTEM

The HPA axis represents one of the body's core stress response systems. Exposure to stress triggers release of corticotrophin-releasing hormone (CRH) and arginine vasopressin (AVP) from the paraventricular nucleus of the hypothalamus, which in turn stimulate secretion of adrenocorticotrophic hormone (ACTH) that acts on the adrenal cortex to synthesize cortisol. Feedback loops at several levels ensure that the system is returned to homeostasis since chronically elevated cortisol levels can have deleterious effects on health. [4]

Despite several decades of research, findings from studies investigating HPA axis activity in children and adolescents with a history of maltreatment are mixed. [5] Several studies have reported elevated basal cortisol levels (e.g. Cicchetti and Rogosch [6]) while others have reported no differences. [7] One explanation for these apparently contradictory findings is that elevation is associated with the presence of a concurrent affective disorder; [5] equally, it is possible that different maltreatment experiences that vary in onset and duration lead to differential patterns of adaptation. For example, ongoing exposure to early adversity may be associated with stress habituation over time leading to reduced cortisol levels as observed in some maltreated children with antisocial behaviour. [8] Together these findings suggest that childhood abuse is associated with atypical HPA axis functioning in a substantial minority of abused children and that this may, in turn, be associated with difficulties in emotional and behavioural regulation.

Studies of adults with childhood histories of maltreatment or adversity also report atypical patterns of responsivity in the HPA axis, which may be associated with an increased vulnerability for psychopathology. There is some evidence that HPA hypoactivity tends to characterize adults presenting with post-traumatic stress disorder (PTSD) [9] while hyperactivity of the HPA system tends to characterize adults presenting with depression. [10] Again, these divergent patterns of activity may reflect adaptations of the HPA axis that occur in response to different forms of childhood adversity that vary in onset and chronicity.

Overall, there is a strong case that early stress may lead to an ongoing dysregulation of the HPA axis, which in turn predisposes to psychiatric vulnerability in later life. While there is consensus around this general principle, the putative mechanisms of how the HPA axis might mediate the link between stress and psychopathology and the precise nature of any interaction remain less clear. More studies, especially longitudinal ones, are needed to shed light on these issues.

13.2.2 STRUCTURAL DIFFERENCES

13.2.2.1 SUBCORTICAL STRUCTURES: HIPPOCAMPUS AND AMYGDALA

Animal research has shown that the hippocampus plays a central role in learning and various aspects of memory and that these functions are impaired when animals are exposed to chronic stress. Studies of adults with PTSD who have histories of childhood maltreatment consistently report that these individuals have smaller hippocampal volumes. It is surprising then that structural magnetic resonance imaging (sMRI) studies of children and adolescents with abuse-related PTSD consistently fail to detect decreased hippocampal volume. [11] One possibility is that the impact of stress is delayed and becomes manifest only later in development.

The amygdala, another key subcortical structure, plays a central role in evaluating potentially threatening information, fear conditioning, emotional processing and memory. Given that experiences of abuse typically occur in family environments characterized by unpredictability and threat it might be expected that children growing up in such contexts would show increased amygdala volume, comparable to that found in stress-exposed animals who show increased dendritic arborisation. [12] Until very recently there was a consensus that maltreatment was not associated with differences in amygdala volume. [13] However, in contrast to the existing studies, two recent sMRI investigations that focused on children and adolescents who had experienced prolonged institutional rearing in orphanages in their first two years of life have reported an increase in amygdala volume in maltreated children [14] suggesting that such effects may only be manifest in children who have experienced severe early sensory deprivation. It is noteworthy that the effects of such extreme early adversity on the brain were observed even many years after the adversity had ceased, which is in line with evidence from animal research. [14]

13.2.2.2 CORTICAL STRUCTURES: PREFRONTAL CORTEX AND CEREBELLUM

The prefrontal cortex (PFC) plays a major role in the control of many aspects of behaviour, regulating cognitive and emotional processes through extensive interconnections with other cortical and subcortical regions.

There are mixed findings from studies comparing PFC volume of children with maltreatment-related PTSD and non-maltreated children. Some studies have reported smaller prefrontal volume associated with the experience of maltreatment, [15] and less prefrontal white matter, while other studies have reported larger grey matter volume of the middle-inferior and ventral regions of the PFC in maltreated groups. There are several possible reasons for these inconsistent findings and it is likely that methodological differences across studies, including the use of different imaging techniques and age groups of children, might at least partly account for these reported differences. [1] It is also possible that there are regionally specific windows of vulnerability in brain development. For example, in a unique cross-sectional study, Andersen et al. [16] found that grey matter volume of the frontal cortex was maximally affected by abuse at ages 14–16 years, while the hippocampus and corpus callosum were maximally affected at ages 3–5 years and 9–10 years, respectively, indicating that the frontal cortex in this sample was particularly susceptible to structural change following abuse during the adolescent period. Unfortunately, most brain imaging studies have not systematically considered the age at which different kinds of abuse have occurred. From a clinical perspective it would be helpful for further research to systematically investigate the relative susceptibility of different brain regions at different ages to different forms of early adversity.

The cerebellum plays a crucial role in emotion processing and fear conditioning via its connection with limbic structures and the HPA axis. [17] Decreased volume of the cerebellum in children and adolescents with a history of maltreatment has been a consistent finding in the literature. [1]

13.2.2.3 CORPUS CALLOSUM AND OTHER WHITE MATTER TRACTS

The corpus callosum (CC) is the largest white matter structure in the brain and controls inter-hemispheric communication of a host of processes, including, but not limited to, arousal, emotion, and higher cognitive abilities. With the exception of one study, decreases in CC volume have consistently been reported in maltreated children and adolescents compared to non-maltreated peers. [1] Recent studies that have employed diffusion tensor imaging (DTI) have found decreased fractional anisotropy values (indicative of decreased white matter fibre tracts coherence or lower density of white matter fibre tracts) in maltreated children in frontal and temporal white matter regions, including the uncinate fasciculus which connects the orbitofrontal cortex to the anterior temporal lobe, including the amygdala. [18] The reduction in fractional anisotropy observed was associated with longer periods within an orphanage and may underlie some of the socioemotional and cognitive impairments exhibited by maltreated children. [18]

13.3 FUNCTIONAL DIFFERENCES

In contrast to the number of studies examining structural brain differences, only a few have so far investigated possible functional correlates associated with abuse and maltreatment using brain imaging techniques such as functional MRI (fMRI) or electrophysiological techniques.

13.3.1 FMRI STUDIES

To date, five fMRI studies have compared maltreated or previously institutionalised children to typically developing peers. Building on the experimental evidence that maltreated children show hypervigilance to threatening facial cues two fMRI studies have examined the neural correlates of face processing in a related population. These studies have reported that previously institutionalised children are characterized by increased amygdala response to threatening cues in comparison to non-maltreated children. [19] This adds to evidence from sMRI studies suggesting amygdala abnormality in children exposed to early adversity. Two other studies assessed response inhibition and observed increased activation in the anterior cingulate cortex (ACC) in maltreated youths as compared to controls. These results suggest impaired cognitive control in maltreated youths, which, in turn, could confer risk for psychopathology, [20] especially in the context of heightened subcortical responses such as that observed during affective processing. The fifth study used a verbal declarative memory task and compared youths with posttraumatic stress symptoms (PTSS) secondary to maltreatment with healthy controls. [21] During the retrieval component of the task, the youths with PTSS exhibited reduced right hippocampal activity, whichwas associated with greater severity of avoidance and numbing symptoms.

13.3.2 EVENT-RELATED POTENTIAL (ERP) STUDIES

Much of the existing ERP research has compared the pattern of brain response of adversely treated children and healthy children when processing facial expressions, an ability that is usually mastered by the preschool years. When compared with non-institutionalized peers, institutionalized children who have experienced severe social deprivation showed a pattern of cortical hypoactivation when viewing emotional facial expressions, and familiar and unfamiliar faces. [22] In contrast, a second set of important studies has provided convincing evidence that school-aged children who had been exposed to physical abuse show increases in brain activity specific to angry faces and require more attentional resources to disengage from such stimuli (see Pollak et al. [23]). These ERP findings are consistent with recent fMRI evidence and suggest that some maltreated children are allocating more resources and remain hyper-vigilant to potential social threat in their environment, likely to be at the cost of other developmental processes.

13.4 THE ROLE OF GENETIC INFLUENCES

It is a common but often striking clinical experience to find that two children who have experienced very similar patterns of early adversity have very different outcomes. While this may be partly due to specific environmental or psychological factors characterizing one child, but not the other, there is increasing evidence that such differential outcome may in part at least be due to genetic differences. [24]

We now know that many of the psychiatric outcomes that are associated with maltreatment, such as PTSD, depression and antisocial behaviour, are partly heritable. However, it is incorrect to think that there are particular genes for these disorders. Rather, we are learning that there are a wide number of genetic variants that may subtly alter the structure and functioning of neural circuitry and hormonal systems that are crucial in calibrating our individual response to social affective cues, and in regulating our stress response. [24] In recent years, researchers have focused in particular on the way in which such genetic variants and adverse environments may interact. Such gene by environment interaction (GxE) research has demonstrated that for a range of genetic variants (known as polymorphisms) childhood abuse can increase the risk of later psychopathology for some children more than others. For example Caspi and colleagues [25] were the first to report on an interaction of a measured genotype (monoamine oxidase A, MAOA) and environment (abuse) for a psychiatric outcome and demonstrated that individuals who are carriers for the low-activity allele (MAOA-l) were at an increased risk for antisocial behaviour disorders following maltreatment. Imaging genetic studies have found that the risk genotype, MAOA-l, is related to hyperresponsivity of the brain's threat detection system and reduced activation in emotion regulation circuits. This work suggests a neural mechanism by which MAOA genotype engenders vulnerability to reactive aggression following maltreatment. [26]

In other words, GxE research suggests that a child's genotype may partly determine their level of risk and resilience for adult psychiatric outcomes, including depression and PTSD following childhood maltreatment (e.g. Kaufman et al. [27]). It is important to bear in mind, however, that positive environmental influences, such as social support, can promote resiliency, even in those children carrying 'risk' polymorphisms exposed to maltreatment. [27] This finding illustrates the important point that when considering a GxE interaction, positive environmental influences (such as contact with a supportive attachment figure), are as relevant to consider as negative environmental influences such as maltreatment. Future research will investigate the influence of clinical interventions as a positive environmental factor that may serve to moderate environmental and genetic risk.

13.5 CLINICAL IMPLICATIONS

Developmental neuroscience research is just one small part of a wider societal endeavour to better understand the complex repercussions of child maltreatment, so that as clinicians working with children we become better at early intervention and prevention. [28] This review has highlighted the accumulating evidence pointing to a variety of neurobiological changes associated with child abuse and early adversity. Such changes can, on the one hand, be viewed as a cascade of deleterious effects that are harmful for the child; however, a more evolutionary and developmentally informed view would suggest that such changes are in fact adaptive responses to an early environment characterized by threat. If a child is to respond optimally to the challenges posed by their surroundings then early stress-induced changes in neurobiological systems can be seen as 'programming' or calibrating those systems to match the demands of a hostile environment. From a clinical perspective, such adaptation may heighten vulnerability to psychopathology, partly due to the changes in how emotional and cognitive systems mediate social interaction. [29] For example, early-established patterns of hypervigilance, while adaptive in an unpredictable home environment, may be maladaptive in other settings increasing vulnerability for behavioural, emotional and social difficulties.

While most of the neurobiological research to date has focused on the pathological impact of maltreatment, there is awelcome and growing interest in exploring the concept of resilience and those factors that may promote or enhance neurobiological mechanisms important for emotional regulation and coping. For example, there is emerging genetic and neurobiological evidence supporting the importance of a reliable adult caregiver, and the role they can play in helping to scaffold the vulnerable child's ability to regulate stress. [27,30] There is also work in progress within our own lab to identify possible neural correlates of resilience in children referred to social services for suspected maltreatment or neglect. In our view it is as important to understand the neurobiological functioning of those children who show few ill-effects, despite experiences of adversity, as it is to study those who present with difficulties.

Over the next decade we are likely to see an increasingly rich research agenda addressing why early adversity acts as a generic risk factor for such an arrayof pooroutcomes. While the evidence reviewed here remains preliminary, it points to an interplay between genetic risk and environmental adversity that becomes manifest at the neural level. Specifically, child abuse may lead to atypical development in basic neurocognitive mechanisms for emotional and behavioural regulation in genetically at-risk children. Over time, such 'adaptations' bear a cost in compromising a child's neurocognitive potential to negotiate the everyday social and academic demands of childhood.

REFERENCES

1. McCrory E, De Brito SA, Viding E. Research review: The neurobiology and genetics of maltreatment and adversity. J Child Psychol Psychiatry 2010;51:1079–95
2. Gilbert R, Widom CS, Browne K, et al. Burden and consequences of child maltreatment in high-income countries. Lancet 2009;373:68–81
3. Currie J, Widom CS. Long-term consequences of child abuse and neglect on adult economic well-being. Child Maltreat 2010;15:111–20
4. Lupien SJ, De Leon M, De Santi S, et al. Cortisol levels during human aging predict hippocampal atrophy and memory deficits. Nat Neurosci 1998;1:69–73
5. Tarullo AR, Gunnar MR. Child maltreatment and the developing HPA axis. Horm Behav 2006;50:632–9
6. Cicchetti D, Rogosch FA. The impact of child maltreatment and psychopathology on neuroendocrine functioning. Dev Psychopathol 2001;13:783–804
7. Hart J, Gunnar M, Cicchetti D. Salivary cortisol in maltreated children: Evidence of relations between neuroendocrine activity and social competence. Dev Psychopathol 1995;7:11–26
8. van Goozen SHM, Fairchild G. How can the study of biological processes help design new interventions for children with severe antisocial behavior? Dev Psychopathol 2008;20:941–73
9. Yehuda R, Golier JA, Kaufman S. Circadian rhythm of salivary cortisol in Holocaust survivors with and without PTSD. Am J Psychiatry 2005;162:998–1000
10. Heim C, Mletzko T, Purselle D, Musselman DL, Nemeroff CB. The dexamethasone/corticotropin-releasing factor test in men with major depression: Role of childhood trauma. Biol Psychiatry 2008;63:398–405
11. Jackowski AP, De Arau′ jo CM, De Lacerda ALT, De Jesus Mari J, Kaufman J. Neurostructural imaging findings in children with post-traumatic stress disorder: Brief review. Psychiatry and Clinical Neurosciences 2009;63:1–8
12. Lupien SJ, McEwen BS, Gunnar MR, Heim C. Effects of stress throughout the lifespan on the brain, behaviour and cognition. Nature Reviews Neuroscience 2009;10:434–45
13. Woon FL, Hedges DW. Hippocampal and amygdala volumes in children and adults with childhood maltreatment-related posttraumatic stress disorder: A meta-analysis. Hippocampus 2008;18:729–36
14. Tottenham N, Hare TA, Quinn BT, et al. Prolonged institutional rearing is associated with atypically large amygdala volume and difficulties in emotion regulation. Dev Sci 2010;13:46–61
15. Carrion VG, Weems CF, Richert K, Hoffman BC, Reiss AL. Decreased prefrontal cortical volume associated with increased bedtime cortisol in traumatized youth. Biol Psychiatry 2010;68:491–3
16. Andersen SL, Tomada A, Vincow ES, et al. Preliminary evidence for sensitive periods in the effect of childhood sexual abuse on regional brain development. J Neuropsychiatry Clin Neurosci 2008;20:292–301
17. Schutter DJLG, van Honk J. The cerebellum on the rise in human emotion. The Cerebellum 2005;4:290–4

18. Govindan RM, Behen ME, Helder E, Makki MI, Chugani HT. Altered water diffusivity in cortical association tracts in children with early deprivation identified with tract-based spatial statistics (TBSS). Cereb Cortex 2010;20:561–9
19. Tottenham N, Hare T, Millner A, et al. Elevated amygdala response to faces following early deprivation. Dev Sci (in press)
20. Mueller SC, Maheu FS, Dozier M, et al. Early-life stress is associated with impairment in cognitive control in adolescence: An fMRI study. Neuropsychologia 2010;48:3037–44
21. Carrion VG, HaasBW, Garrett A, Song S, Reiss AL. Reduced hippocampal activity in youth with posttraumatic stress symptoms: An fMRI study. J Pediatr Psychol 2010;35:559–69
22. Parker SW, Nelson CA, Zeanah CH, et al. An event-related potential study of the impact of institutional rearing on face recognition. Dev Psychopathol 2005;17:621–39
23. Pollak SD, Tolley-Schell SA. Selective attention to facial emotion in physically abused children. J Abnorm Psychol 2003;112:323–38
24. Caspi A, McClay J, Moffitt T, et al. Role of genotype in the cycle of violence in maltreated children. Science 2002;297:851–4
25. Viding E, Williamson DE, Hariri AR. Developmental imaging genetics: Challenges and promises for translational research. Dev Psychopathol 2006;18:877–92
26. Viding E, Frith U. Genes for susceptibility to violence lurk in the brain. Proc Natl Acad Sci U S A 2006;103:6085–6
27. Kaufman J, Yang BZ, Douglas-Palumberi H, et al. Brain-derived neurotrophic factor-5-HTTLPR gene interactions and environmental modifiers of depression in children. Biol Psychiatry 2006;59:673–80
28. MacMillan HL,Wathen CN, Barlow J, et al. Interventions to prevent child maltreatment and associated impairment. The Lancet 2009;373:250–66
29. Pollak SD. Mechanisms linking early experience and the emergence of emotions: Illustrations from the study of maltreated children. Curr Dir Psychol Sci 2008;17:370–5
30. Dozier M, Peloso E, Lewis E, Laurenceau JP, Levine S. Effects of an attachment-based intervention on the cortisol production of infants and toddlers in foster care. Dev Psychopathol 2008;20:845–59

CHAPTER 14

Childhood Abuse Is Associated with Methylation of Multiple Loci in Adult DNA

MATTHEW SUDERMAN, NADA BORGHOL, JANE J. PAPPAS, SNEHAL M PINTO PEREIRA, MARCUS PEMBREY, CLYDE HERTZMAN, CHRIS POWER, AND MOSHE SZYF

14.1 BACKGROUND

Abuse in childhood, encompassing physical, sexual or emotional abuse, is a key component of a broader spectrum of child maltreatment [1]. Lifelong consequences of child abuse have been identified, including a greater risk of violence and delinquency, as well as adult depression and attempted suicide [1]. Hazardous behaviors, such as smoking and alcoholism, have also been found to be associated with abuse in childhood [2-4] along with later disease risk factors, including obesity [1,5], poorer immune function [1,6-8] earlier menarche [9-11] and outcomes such as ischemic heart disease [6,12,13] and chronic obstructive lung disease [13,14]. Explanations including biological mechanisms for long-term outcomes of child abuse have yet to be fully explored.

DNA methylation and histone modification play crucial roles in development, adaptation and response to environmental signals [15]. Methylation of cytosine bases occurs at CpG sites and, in gene promoters, usually results in gene silencing, whereas loss of methylation is associated with activity. MicroRNAs that repress the expression of their often numerous target genes are also part of epigenetic regulation [16]. MicroRNAs can down regulate key players in the epigenetic regulation machinery, but can also be silenced themselves by DNA methylation [17]. Whilst epigenetic regulation, by definition, does not alter DNA sequence, DNA variants can influence methylation levels. However, DNA methylation associated with early adversity (prenatal famine) was found to be independent of that associated with genetic variation [18]. Evidence to date suggests that stable changes in DNA methylation in the hippocampus of humans [19] and rats [20,21] are triggered by maltreatment in early life.

Much DNA methylation is tissue specific [22] but most tissues are unavailable for population studies of living individuals. Given the multiple outcomes for childhood abuse, we hypothesize that DNA methylation associated with childhood abuse is system-wide [23]. Several recent studies have supported the possibility of differential DNA methylation associations with social adversity in peripheral blood cells. For example, Borghol et al., demonstrated association of DNA methylation profiles with early life socioeconomic position in blood cells [24]. Provencal et al., showed that differential maternal rearing is associated with differential DNA methylation profiles in both prefrontal cortex and blood T cells [25]. Klengel et al., demonstrated childhood trauma-dependent DNA demethylation in functional glucocorticoid response elements of FKBP5 in blood cells [26]. Mehta et al., have delineated recently DNA methylation signatures of child trauma and posttraumatic stress disorder in blood cells [27]. Although blood cells turn over, they are derived from stem cells and progenitors that stay with us for a life long. Thus, it is plausible that a DNA methylation event in a stem cell population that is introduced in early life remains into adulthood.

We therefore aimed to establish whether childhood abuse is associated with adult gene promoter methylation in a genome-wide investigation of peripheral blood cells [24]. We studied 40 adult males enrolled in the 1958 British Birth Cohort who have been found to have substantial variation in promoter methylation in over 6,000 genes, with a distinct methylation profile associated with socio-economic position [24]. Those with childhood abuse in this cohort have been shown to have long-term associations with negative health outcomes, specifically, a greater prevalence of obesity among those who reported physical abuse in childhood [28].

14.2 METHODS

14.2.1 ETHICS STATEMENT

All participants provided written consent and a blood sample for DNA analysis; ethical approval for a 45y biomedical survey and data analysis was given by the South-East Multi-Centre Research Ethics Committee(ref. 01/1/44) and the Joint UCL/UCLH Committees on the Ethnics of Human Research (Committee A) (ref. 08/H0714/40).

14.2.2 STUDY POPULATION

The selection of 40 adult males from the 1958 cohort [29] has been described previously [24] and are detailed in the Additional files. In brief, 17,638 participants were enrolled, all born in England, Scotland and Wales, during a single week in March 1958. At 45y, 4,177 males provided written consent and a blood sample for DNA analysis; ethical approval was given by the South-East Multi-Centre Research Ethics Committee. After exclusions (e.g. cancer or elevated C-reactive protein levels, immigrants), 3,362 white males were classified by socioeconomic position (SEP) and childhood abuse. Forty males were selected from extremes of SEP, including 12 who reported abuse (7 low and 5 high child SEP; 7 low and 5 high adult SEP). With exclusion of immigrants, the 1958 cohort shows little genetic population stratification [30].

Abuse was identified through participants' reports in a confidential questionnaire at 45y on the following experiences to age 16y: [1] "I was verbally abused by a parent"; [2] "I suffered humiliation, ridicule, bullying or mental cruelty from a parent"; [3] "I was physically abused by a parent

–punched, kicked or hit or beaten with an object, or needed medical treatment"; [4] "I was sexually abused by a parent". A report of any of these was scored as abuse. These questions were from the PATH Through Life Project including items derived from the Parental Bonding Instrument, the British National Survey of Health and Development and the US National Comorbidity Survey [31].

14.2.3 MEASUREMENT OF RELATIVE DNA METHYLATION LEVELS

DNA sample preparation, methylated DNA immunoprecipitation (MeDIP) and microarray hybridization, scanning and data extraction were performed as described previously [24]. Briefly, DNA was extracted from whole blood collected in EDTA at 45 years using an in-house, manual guanidine hydrochloride and ethanol precipitation method. DNA promoter methylation data from 20,533 genes and 489 microRNAs for the 40 participants were generated using MeDIP with an antibody that recognizes and binds 5-methylcytosine (DNA methylation) to isolate methylated DNA fragments. These fragments were then hybridized to custom-designed, high-density oligonucleotide microarrays, covering approximately 1000 bp upstream to 250 bp downstream at 100 bp spacing from the transcription start sites (TSS) in Ensembl (version 44). Microarray data files used in this study can be downloaded from the Gene Expression Omnibus (accession number: GSE31713). Three replicate microarrays were generated per individual and demonstrated adequate reproducibility [24]. Both hierarchical clustering and principal components analysis applied to the 500 most variable probes across all microarrays showed that the three replicates clustered. Furthermore, >70% of the variance in these probes was explained by individual variation.

14.2.4 MICROARRAY STATISTICAL ANALYSIS

The steps taken in the microarray statistical analysis are shown in Additional file 1: Figure S1 and justification for our approach is given in

Additional files. Quality control involved generating MvA plots (i.e. plots of log(Cy5/Cy3) vs log(Cy5 × Cy3)) to identify those with severe dye biases or low signal. Microarrays deemed unacceptable were repeated, so no sample was excluded by quality control. Unsupervised clustering failed to identify batch effects related to hybridization date. Normalization of the final set of microarrays proceeded by computing log ratios of the bound (Cy5) and input (Cy3) microarray channel intensities for each microarray and then microarrays were normalized to one another using quantile normalization under the assumption that all samples have identical overall methylation levels. A probe was called differentially methylated if the modified t-statistic from 'limma' [32] of Bioconductor [33] was significant ($p<0.05$) and the log2 fold-difference of the mean group probe intensities was ≥0.25. A promoter was called differentially methylated if it contained a probe called differentially methylated and if it contained probes for which modified t-statistics were significantly higher or lower than the average probe on the microarray. Significance for the latter was determined by applying the Wilcoxon rank-sum test and then calculating a corresponding false discovery rate (FDR) [34] using the method of Benjamini and Hochberg [35]. Promoters with FDR<20% were called differentially methylated. This false discovery rate (FDR) was designed to test the chances of an overall false discovery among a series of related results. It is particularly useful for an exploratory analysis concerned with making general inferences from among a set of 'discoveries', rather than guarding against one or more individual false positives. The FDR threshold of 20% used here indicates that the expected proportion of promoters incorrectly called differentially methylated is around 20%. We find this threshold acceptable because this preliminary study is not meant to definitively characterise the epigenetic signatures of childhood abuse. In Figure 1, we present a heatmap showing probe methylation scores averaged across triplicate microarrays. Clustering was performed using Ward's hierarchical clustering algorithm with Pearson correlation distance as the distance metric.

All bioinformatic functional analysis was based on gene sets from GO [36], KEGG [37] and mSigDB [38]. Enrichment for differential methylation was determined by applying the hypergeometric test to the overlap between known gene sets and those found in our study to be differentially

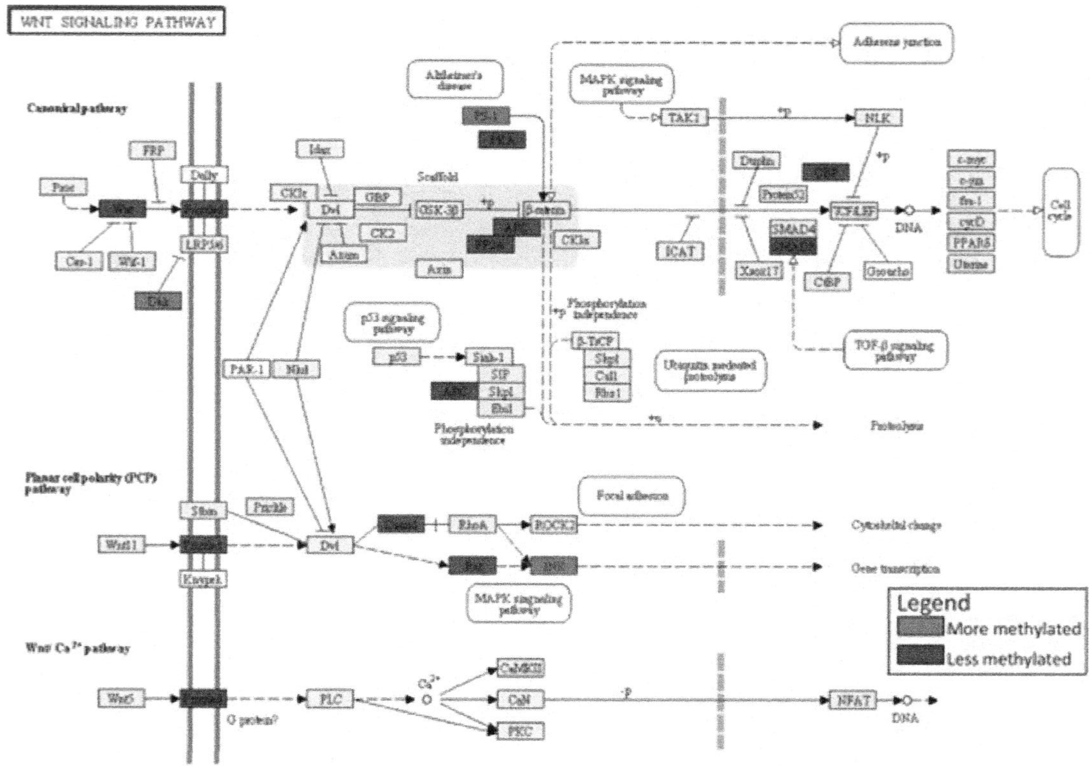

Figure 1. Promoter methylation associated with childhood abuse. Heatmap showing MeDIP probe values from the 997 differentially methylated promoters (rows) across all 40 participants (columns). Each promoter is represented by the probe most associated with childhood abuse. Blackened squares above the columns denote non-abuse males, white squares denote those with childhood abuse. Other covariates included are childhood and adulthood socio-economic position (white=low, gray=high). Neither appears to explain the main sample clusters.

methylated. FDR values were obtained by adjusting these significance levels over all gene sets and pathways considered. The differentially methylated gene set was then subjected to pathway analysis using Ingenuity Pathway Analysis software (http://ingenuity.com/products/pathways_analysis.html).

In assessing megabase regions of the genome, methylation patterns were obtained by computing the mean methylation score difference between abuse and non-abuse groups for each probe, generating a UCSC wiggle track file from these differences and then uploading it for display on the UCSC genome browser (http://genome.ucsc.edu/).

14.2.5 VALIDATION AND FURTHER METHYLATION ANALYSIS

First, we validated the microarray calls, selecting 11 genes with the strongest methylation association with abuse (Additional file 2: Figure S2). Validation was performed using quantitative PCR (qPCR) of bound and input fractions of MeDIP with primers flanking the differentially methylated regions (Additional file 3: Table S1). Second, we validated two of these 11 genes, SLC17A3 and PM20D1, hypermethylated in association with abuse on MeDIP, by bisulfite pyrosequencing (in participants with sufficient DNA), as an independent method that measures methylation at specific sites [39]. Next, bisulfite pyrosequencing analysis of PM20D1 was repeated on an additional 27 males selected using the same criteria as the original [40] group. Details of pyrosequencing conditions, including optimization of PCR amplification using 0, 50 and 100% methylation controls are provided in Additional files.

Cell type ratios in blood are known to fluctuate so certain methylation differences between individuals could be caused by different cell ratios, particularly in promoters of genes with cell-type specific methylation. To rule out this possibility in our analysis, we compared our results to published MeDIP [40], expression [41] and Illumina 450 K [42] profiles of purified blood cell types. In each published dataset, we identified all differentially methylated or expressed genes or probes (as appropriate) between all pairs of available blood cell type profiles and then compared those lists of differences to the list of differentially methylated genes or probes between the abused and non-abused individuals in our study. If variation in blood cell type ratios explains the methylation differences in our analysis, then we would expect to see at least one larger-than-expected intersection. In each case, however, hypergeometric tests failed to identify larger-than-expected intersections ($p > 0.4$ in each case). For the published MeDIP dataset [40], the microarray design used was similar to our design so we were able to construct a 1-1 mapping between over half of the probes across our respective designs. Probes were paired if they were closest and within 150 bp. Unfortunately, this MeDIP dataset only contained profiles for B and T cell purified cell types. We therefore expanded our analysis to include an expression dataset [41] with profiles for CD33+ (myeloid), CD34+, CD71+ (early erythroid), CD4+, CD8+, CD14+ (monocyte), CD19+ (B) and CD56 (natural killer) cells. We also included a recent Illumina 450 K dataset [42] with profiles for granulocytes, neutrophils, eosinophils, CD4+, CD8+, CD14+, CD19+ and CD56+ cells. For both these datasets, results were compared at the gene level.

14.3 RESULTS AND DISCUSSION

Physical, cognitive and emotional characteristics and biomarkers are listed for participants in Table 1. As expected, the abuse group showed more adverse characteristics than the non-abuse group, but differences did not reach conventional p-values in this small sample.

14.3.1 HUNDREDS OF PROMOTERS ARE DIFFERENTIALLY METHYLATED IN ASSOCIATION WITH CHILD ABUSE

In total, 997 gene promoters were differentially methylated in association with childhood abuse, affecting 1141 different genes (Additional files). Of these promoters, 311 were hypermethylated and 686 were hypomethylated in abused compared to non-abused males. Figure 1 shows a heatmap depicting the relative methylation levels for all differentially

TABLE 1. Characteristics of the 40 male study participants.

	Age (y)	No abuse n=28	Abuse n=12	p*
Birthweight, g, mean±SD#	0	3577.35 (574.91)	3338.21 (590.25)	0.24
Height, cm, mean±SD#$	7	1.24 (0.07)	1.21 (0.07)	0.27
Maths score, mean±SD#$	16	14.82 (7.32)	12.29 (7.95)	0.44
Reading score, median (Q1, Q3)#$	16	27 (21, 31)	31 (12, 32)	0.70
Socio-emotional adjustment number~median (Q1-Q3)#$	7	4 (1, 12)	8.5 (2, 13)	0.47
Alcohol drinks daily, n (%)#	42	7 (25.93)	2 (16.67)	0.53
Smokers, n (%)#	42	7 (25.93)	4 (33.33)	0.64
Height, cm, mean±SD#	42	1.78 (0.09)	1.76 (0.06)	0.52
BMI, kg/m2, mean±SD	45	26.63 (3.99)	28.69 (4.39)	0.16
Waist circumference, cm, mean±SD	45	97.43 (10.24)	102 (12.02)	0.23
Diastolic blood pressure, mmHg, mean±SD	45	82.77 (11.71)	85.53 (12.72)	0.51
Systolic blood pressure, mmHg, mean±SD	45	132.92 (18.61)	134.72 (18.90)	0.78
Fev1†, mean±SD#	45	3.84 (0.65)	3.70 (0.63)	0.53

†FEV1 =one-second forced expiratory volume; best test of three spirometry readings.
#N for non-abuse <28 (range 22 to 27).
$N for abuse <12 (range 7 to 10).
~higher score=poorer adjustment.
*p-value from t-test, except for median (IQR), when Two-sample Wilcoxon rank-sum test was used.

methylated promoters and how they cluster within study participants. Even at more stringent thresholds ($p<0.01$ and $q<0.05$, see Methods), there were still 34 differentially methylated promoters corresponding to 58 different genes with similar proportions hypermethylated to hypomethylated. These cluster the study participants very similarly to the larger set of differentially methylated promoters (Additional file 4: Figure S3). To assess whether the broad methylation signature of childhood abuse was affected by the numerical imbalance of abused versus non-abused (N = 12 vs 28), we conducted a permutation analysis. We found that 997 differentially methylated promoters between abused and non-abused was larger than the number of differences associated with 82% of random partitions (410 of 500) of the participants with partition size ratios corresponding to 12 vs 28. To address any concern that the abuse associated methylation differences were reflecting differences in blood cell type ratios, we compared our results with recently published expression and methylation profiles of purified cell types [40-42]. We found no evidence of statistically significant overlaps between our results for abuse and cell-type specific methylation and expression patterns ($p > 0.4$, hypergeometric test; see Methods for details).

In 11 genes selected for validation, the direction of abuse associated methylation differences was confirmed using qPCR of bound and input MeDIP fractions (Additional file 2: Figure S2). We also confirmed abuse associated hypermethylation by pyrosequencing of sites in the promoter of SLC17A3 and the first exon of PM20D1 in the original samples (Figure 2A) and in an additional 27 males for PM20D1 (Figure 2B), and with SNP rs11540014 showing no association with methylation levels (data not shown). However, the associations in the promoter of SLC17A3 were not replicated in the additional 27 males.

14.3.2 ABUSE-ASSOCIATED METHYLATION CLUSTERS BY BIOLOGICAL FUNCTION

Full results of functional analysis are given in Additional files. Differentially methylated gene promoters in abused males (1141 genes) were enriched in regulatory (169 genes) and developmental (230 genes) functions (Table 2). Central to both of these functions is the KEGG WNT signaling pathway; enriched for genes [15] for which promoters are hypomethylated in abused individuals, consistent with activation of this pathway in blood cells of the abuse group (Figure 3). No other KEGG pathway was enriched with differentially methylated genes at $p < 0.05$ (uncorrected for multiple testing). Of the differentially methylated genes that perform some regulatory function, most (134 of 169) are hypomethylated in abused males.

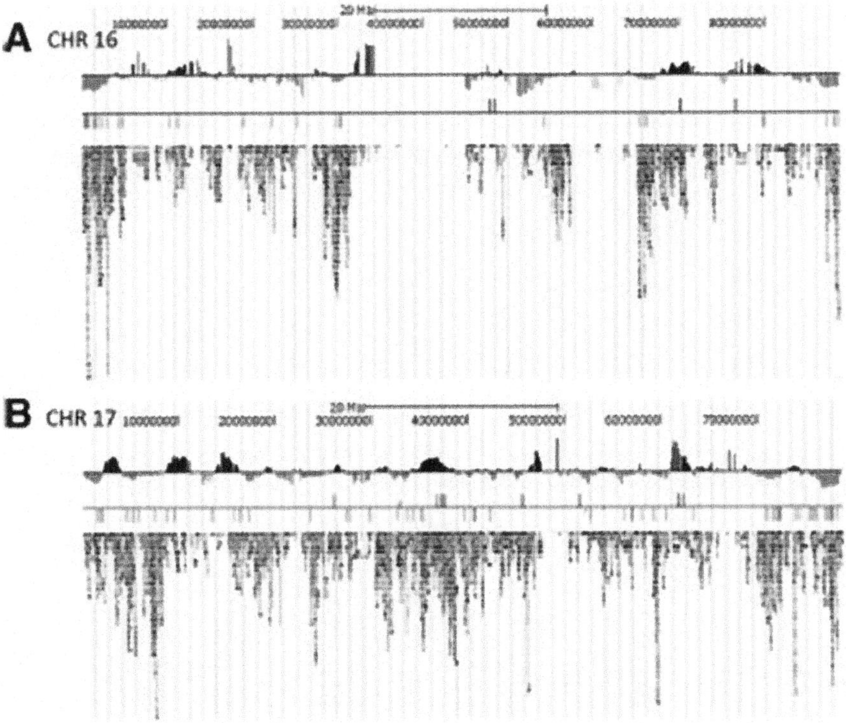

Figure 2. Validation of MeDIP results. A. Quantification of methylation differences in the abuse and non-abuse groups by bisulfite pyrosequencing analysis of the SLC17A3 promoter and the PM20D1 first exon and intron. DNA methylation at 14 CpG sites in the SLC17A3 promoter and 12 and 1 CpG sites in the PM20D1 first exon and first intron, respectively, among the abuse and non-abuse groups is shown (N = 10 vs. 26 for SLC17A3; N = 9 vs 23 for PM20D1). One-sided t-tests were applied to each CpG site to test for association of methylation levels with childhood abuse, and false discovery rates were calculated for the resulting p-values in order to correct for multiple testing. All false discovery rates (FDR) were less than 0.1, indicating significant association between CpG methylation levels and childhood abuse. **: FDR < 0.025; *: FDR < 0.05; ++: FDR < 0.1; +: FDR < 0.2. The bars represent average methylation for all subjects in a group and error bars indicate the standard error of the mean. Physical maps of the regions analyzed are presented above the charts where CpG positions are indicated by balloons. The transcription start site (TSS) is indicated by a hook arrow. The positions of the primers used for pyrosequencing (Additional file 3: Table S2) are indicated by arrows. B. Replication of the quantification of the differences in methylation at PM20D1 between the abuse and non-abuse groups in an additional 27 males that were not profiled using MeDIP (N = 7 vs. 20). Pyrosequencing was applied to measure the methylation levels of 13 CpG sites in the first exon and intron of PM20D1.

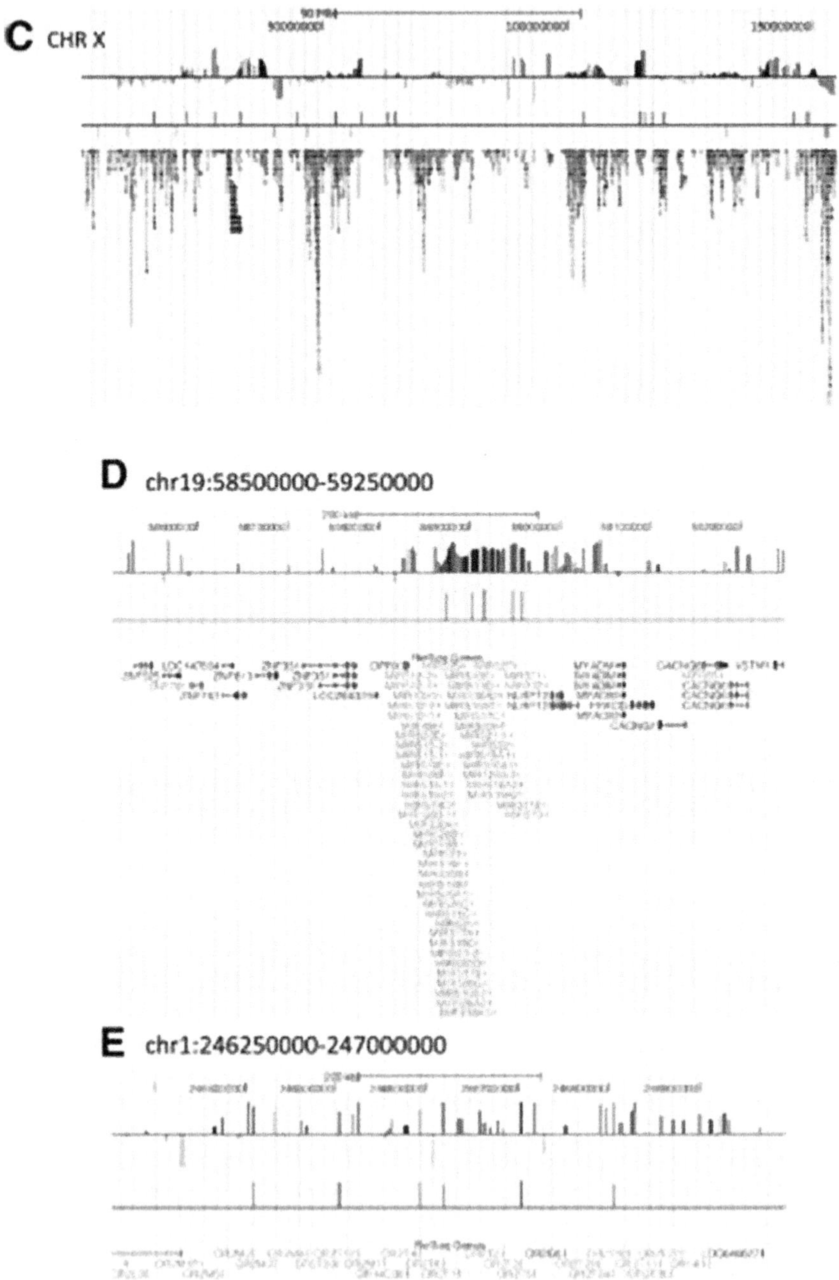

Figure 2. CONTINUED.

The regulation mainly affects transcription as indicated by enrichment of these genes in functional categories such as chromatin modification (28 genes), histone modification (11 genes) and transcription factor binding (35 genes). Similarly, most of the 230 developmental genes are hypomethylated in abused males (172 genes), best characterized by the general gene ontology category "multicellular organismal development" (163 genes). More specific subcategories do not show significant enrichment.

Differentially hypermethylated gene promoters in abused males are enriched in few functional categories. One of these, "cell surface receptor linked signal transduction", contains 125 genes with differentially methylated promoters of which 46 are hypermethylated in abused individuals. An Ingenuity functional analysis of the differentially methylated genes revealed similar molecular and cellular functions associated with transcriptional control (Additional file 5: Figure S4).

14.3.3 ABUSE-ASSOCIATED METHYLATION CONSISTENT WITH MICRORNA TARGETING

MicroRNA genes are, like DNA methylation, known to repress the expression of target genes. However, unlike an individual methylation mark which typically targets a single nearby gene, each microRNA is associated with a specific set of a few hundred target genes [43]. We discovered an association of microRNA DNA hypermethylation with abuse. Of 489 microRNAs analysed, 39 were differentially methylated, of which 31 were hypermethylated in association with abuse. The target genes of six of these included a highly non-random proportion of genes with decreased promoter methylation in abused males (Table 3).

14.3.4 ABUSE-ASSOCIATED HYPOMETHYLATION AND CPG DENSITY

DNA methylation in regions of relatively high CpG frequency, known as CpG islands, plays an important regulatory role in the otherwise CpG-depleted (≤40% of that expected) mammalian genome [44,45].

TABLE 2. Selected functional analysis of abuse associated hypo- and hypermethylation.

Pathway/ function	Number of genes in pathway/function	Differentially methylated		Hypo-methylated			Hyper-methylated		
		n	p	n	p	fdr	n	p	fdr
WNT signaling pathway	142	19	0.0013	15	0.0020	0.53	4	0.22	1
Regulation	2330	169	0.017	134	0.0018	0.51	33	0.88	1
- Chromatin modification	273	32	0.0004	28	0.00005	0.09	4	0.68	1
- Histone modification	105	13	0.013	11	0.008	0.94	2	0.53	1
- Transcription factor binding	493	41	0.034	35	0.006	0.84	6	0.84	1
Development	3054	230	0.0007	172	0.00096	0.40	58	0.17	1
- Multicellular organismal development	2838	213	0.0012	163	0.0006	0.32	50	0.32	1
Cell surface receptor linked signal transduction	1778	125	0.071	79	0.60	1	46	0.002	0.53

'n' is the number of genes in the relevant pathway that are differentially methylated in association with abuse.
'p' was calculated using the hypergeometric test, it indicates the statistical significance of the enrichment.
'fdr' the false discovery rate (FDR) corresponding to the p-value.

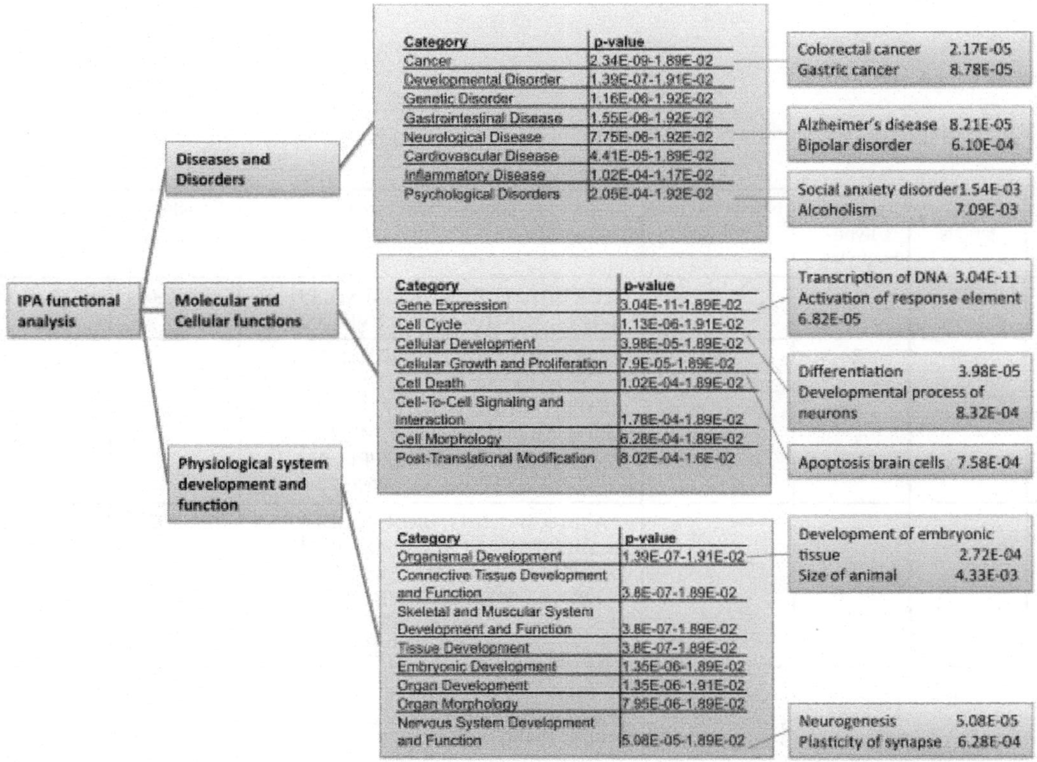

Figure 3. Differential methylation in the WNT signaling pathway. The KEGG (http://www.genome.jp/kegg/mapper.html) depiction of the WNT signaling pathway is shown with hypermethylated gene promoters (more methylated in the group with childhood abuse) colored red and the hypomethylated gene promoters colored blue.

TABLE 3. Methylation of microRNAs and their target genes.

MicroRNA	Number of targets	Number hypo-methylated	Number hyper-methylated	Hypomethylated targets	Enrichment p-value	MicroRNA methylation
mir-514	49	10	1	AFF4, BAALC, BRWD1, CARM1, ENAH, KLF13, MYO1B, NR3C1, SVIL, TCF12	5.71E-05	hypermethylated
let-7d	320	26	6	ATP2A2, BACH1, BRWD1, CDV3, CHD4, CPSF4, DCUN1D2, DOCK3, DOT1L, EFHD2, EZH2, GGA3, LIMD2, LRIG1, MECP2, MGAT4A, MIB1, MLL5, PARD6B, PBX3, PRTG, PTPRU, RDH10, SOCS1, UNC5A, WDR37	0.0030	hypermethylated
mir-520c	274	23	3	ASF1B, BCL2L11, BRP44L, DDHD1, DPYSL5, FLT1, FNDC3B, INHBB, KCNMA1, KLF13, MAP3K14, MECP2, MKNK2, MTUS1, ORMDL3, PBX3, PFN2, RGL1, SMAD2, UBE2Q2, WDR37, ZFP36L2, ZFPM2	0.0035	hypermethylated

mir-215	37	6	0	ARFGEF1, FNDC3B, GRHL1, KLHDC5, LRRFIP1, MECP2	0.0060	hypermethylated
mir-519a	377	28	4	AFF4, BRWD1, BTG3, CELSR2, DNAJB6, LRIG1, MAP3K5, MAP4, MASTL, MCM7, MECP2, MIB1, NPAS2, OBFC2A, PARD6B, PFN2, PTHLH, RAPGEF4, RASD1, SCAMP2, SFRS2, SMOC2, TMEM64, VGLL3, WHSC1, YES1, ZFPM2, ZFYVE9	0.0074	hypermethylated
mir-519e	104	11	2	ARHGEF12, ARL4C, BCOR, CCNG2, CTDSPL2, DLL1, DPYSL5, EFNB3, NEDD4L, NPAS2, RAB35	0.0075	hypermethylated
mir-203	239	20	3	AFF4, BCL7A, CNTFR, CTDSPL2, DNMT3B, EGR1, FALZ, INSIG1, KCTD9, LASP1, MECP2, PLD2, PPM1B, RAP-GEF4, SLC12A2, SMAD1, SPEN, SPIRE1, TCF12, YWHAQ	0.0064	hypomethylated

MicroRNAs are listed that have statistically significant MeDIP differences between abuse and non-abuse groups whose predicted gene targets are enriched for gene promoters that are also differentially methylated between abuse and non-abuse groups. In each case, enrichment is for targets with lower methylation in the abused group.
"enrichment p-value" indicates the level of enrichment for hypomethylated targets.
"microRNA methylation" indicates whether the data predicts significantly higher ("hypermethylated") or lower ("hypomethylated") methylation levels in the abuse group.

In spite of the fact that MeDIP is known to enrich for methylation differences away from CpG islands [46], we observed unusually high CpG frequencies in promoters with reduced methylation levels in abused individuals. This frequency (0.86) is significantly higher than that observed in the average promoter (frequency=0.42; $p<1.4 \times 10^{-285}$) as well as promoters with increased methylation levels in abused individuals (frequency=0.38; $p<4 \times 10^{-138}$; Additional file 6: Figure S5). This frequency (0.86) is even higher than the 0.6 threshold used to define CpG islands.

14.3.3 ABUSE-ASSOCIATED METHYLATION CLUSTERS BY GENOMIC LOCATION

Differentially methylated DNA loci associated with early life environments tend to cluster in the genome [24,47]. Chromosome-wide views of our data reveal megabase-sized regions significantly enriched for differentially methylated promoters (Figure 4). At the chromosomal level, chromosomes 16 and 17 were significantly enriched for hypomethylated promoters in abused individuals, whereas chromosome X was significantly enriched for hypermethylated promoters. At the megabase level, three regions were significantly enriched for differentially methylated promoters ($p<0.05$). All were hypermethylated in abused individuals: chr1:246250000-247000000, chr14:100250000-101000000 and chr19:58500000-59250000 (genome assembly hg18), but only the regions on chromosomes 1 and 19 passed multiple testing correction with FDR below 0.2 (FDR<0.006 and 0.0001, respectively; Figure 4D,E). The regions on chromosomes 14 and 19 each contain a cluster of microRNAs in which promoters account for all of their statistically significant site-specific differential methylation.

Clustering of differential promoter methylation, up to 2 Mb apart, was detectable across the entire genome (Additional file 7: Figure S6).

14.3.4 SOCIO-ECONOMIC POSITION (SEP) AND ABUSE

Previously, we identified 1252 gene promoters associated with childhood SEP and 545 associated with adulthood SEP [24]. Only 73 of 1252 (5.8%)

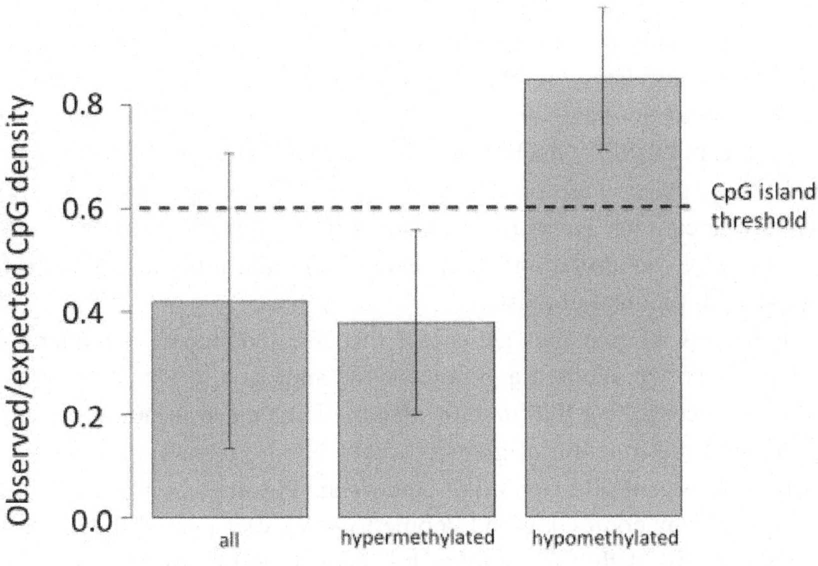

Figure 4. Megabase regions enriched with methylation differences. Promoter MeDIP differences across chromosomes 16 (A), 17 (B) and X (C) and across two smaller genomic regions (D) and (E) are shown using images obtained from the UCSC Genome Browser. The top track depicts average differences of log abuse – log non-abuse. Each bar in the middle track identifies a significant difference. Bars above or below the horizontal line identify sites with higher or lower methylation in the abused group. The bottom track indicates relative gene abundance across the chromosome.

and 19 of 545 (3.5%) gene promoters were also differentially methylated in association with childhood abuse. Just three (CTAGE5, GNG4, MYO1B) were differentially methylated in association with all three characteristics (childhood and adult SEP and childhood abuse). The association for PM20D1 was specific to abuse.

14.4 CONCLUSIONS

Blood DNA of 45y old males revealed differentially methylated gene promoters associated with abuse that occurred three decades earlier in childhood. There were several novel findings from our study. First, hundreds of specific promoter associations were uncovered, with approximately two-thirds hypomethylated in the abused group. Second, replication confirmed that hypermethylation in PM20D1 is associated with childhood abuse. Third, microRNA gene targets tended to be hypomethylated, particularly when the microRNA itself was hypermethylated. Fourth, differentially methylated genes were clustered in discrete functional pathways and in genomic locations. These findings support the hypothesis that the differences in DNA methylation we observed were non-random and reflect an organized biological process.

It is now known that genes act through functional and interacting pathways, so we adopted a genome-wide approach to DNA methylation analysis, recognizing that modest epigenetic changes in numerous genes could reset the function of gene networks having phenotypic effects. We found enrichment of differentially methylated promoters in the WNT signaling pathway complex with hypomethylation of 15 genes in the abused. Elsewhere this pathway complex has been found to play a key role in embryonic development and cellular proliferation [48], and is deregulated in some chronic health conditions such as obesity [49-51], diabetes [52-54], metabolic syndrome [55], cancer [56-59] and inflammatory processes [56-58]. Whilst recognizing that our findings do not provide evidence for causal links between child abuse and later outcomes, they nonetheless raise the prospect of mediation by epigenetic modifications.

Of particular note was hypermethylation of PM20D1 in association with abuse, given a previous study showing a variably methylated region at this metalloproteinase gene was hypermethylated in association with obesity [60]. This association persisted over 10 years of follow-up in an elderly population. Interestingly, child abuse has been shown to be associated with adult obesity in the full 1958 cohort [5] and is suggested by our Table 1. It is perhaps surprising to note that both our association with childhood abuse and the association with obesity were observed in blood DNA when PM20D1 has its highest expression levels in the brain and lowest expression levels in blood [41]. Given that it is highly conserved from yeast to human, it likely plays a key though little understood role in the cell. By contrast, SLC17A3 is like most of the genes differentially methylated in childhood abuse, most highly expressed in blood and a few specific brain regions (hypothalamus, prefrontal cortex, pituitary) [41]. It appears conserved in fewer species, mainly the higher mammals, and the expressed protein acts as a voltage-driven transporter in blood. Given this basic role, it is likely essential at nearly all stages of life.

Further support for epigenetic regulation working through interacting pathways comes from the striking enrichment in the abuse group of hypermethylated microRNAs combined with hypomethylation of their respective gene targets across the genome. It implies that during typical development, active transcription of these microRNAs is combined with synergistic target methylation to create a double layer of repression of these target genes; a repression that is lifted in association with child abuse.

Intriguingly, hypomethylated gene promoters in abused individuals typically contained sequences with very high CpG frequency. Demethylation of such CpG-rich promoters in abused males suggests that abuse leads to increased activity of key basic cellular functions, such as gene regulation and development, as found in pathway analysis. Another genomic feature associated with abuse was the clustering of differential promoter methylation detectable across the entire genome, providing further evidence of genome-wide as well as gene-specific organization of epigenetic profiles.

Previously we observed genome-wide clustering in association with SEP, but importantly, the "methylation signature" for abuse differed, such that <10% of the differentially methylated regions overlapped with childhood SEP [24]. Also, the differentially methylated genes were enriched in different functional pathways, notably, MAP kinase for SEP and WNT for child abuse. Further, the abuse associated differential methylation of microRNAs and their target genes was not seen for SEP. Whilst not ruling out generic associations with early life adversities, our findings suggest that different adversities are associated with different epigenetic changes to the genome.

Several methodological considerations arise here. First, reliable measurement of the frequency and severity of child abuse is not straightforward1. Child abuse was identified through participant's report at 45y and was primarily emotional and physical abuse – only rarely sexual abuse. All measures have biases and inconsistencies yet retrospective reports are an accepted method of ascertainment in population studies [1]. Furthermore, prospective identification of abuse is not feasible in large studies and likely to be unrepresentative. By contrast, retrospective self-report, used here, is feasible though it is likely to underestimate true levels of abuse. Second, given the scale of assessing methylation at all promoters, we could only study a small but selected sample. Whilst our study is imbalanced with respect to abuse (12 vs 28) it has the benefit of control for SEP. Third, we used DNA from whole blood to test our hypothesis, currently the only practical option for population based studies. We cannot know the extent to which our results relate to gene expression. Use of whole blood also raises the possibility that abuse-associated differences in B-to-T cell ratios might account for some of our observations. We have partly addressed this by noting that B-cell and T-cell expression and methylation profiles [40,41] do not differ for many genes with abuse-associated methylation levels. Fourth, those abused in childhood might represent a distinct genetic group, but genetic differences alone are unlikely to account for all methylation differences observed here. Given the possibility of differences in epigenetic response due to genetic variation, future integrated studies of the epigenome and whole genome sequencing are an important next step. Fifth, our study is imbalanced including 28 controls compared to only 12 with childhood abuse resulting in reduced power to identify methylation differences. Nonetheless, this preliminary study was able to discover hundreds of differentially methylated promoters so future studies with better balance are likely discover many more. Finally, there is currently no 'gold standard' for measuring the methylome, yet MeDIP is a well-established genome-wide method that has been evaluated [46,61-65] and we confirmed all the micro-array calls in the top 11 methylation differences. Current genome-wide methods are more complementary than interchangeable and each has its strengths and weaknesses. Our analyses included triplicate arrays and methylation differences were confirmed in selected genes using other gene-specific methods both here and previously [24]. In using an analytic approach that was sensitive to subtle methylation associations across gene networks necessarily results in some false positives (for justification see Additional files). However, the non-random organization of methylation differences throughout the genome supports our main hypothesis that childhood abuse is associated with DNA methylation changes in adult blood.

In sum, the pattern of changes associated with child abuse detected in peripheral blood cells of 45 year-olds suggest that there is a system-wide readjustment of the epigenome to signals triggered by early life abuse. Our study does not demonstrate causality, nor can it demonstrate a temporal relationship between child abuse and DNA methylation levels in adulthood. It does, however, provide a justification for a range of studies addressing epigenetic responses to child abuse and their mediating role with later phenotypic outcomes.

REFERENCES

1. Gilbert R, Widom CS, Browne K, Fergusson D, Webb E, Janson S: Burden and consequences of child maltreatment in high-income countries. Lancet 2009, 373(9657):68-81.
2. Anda RF, Croft JB, Felitti VJ, Nordenberg D, Giles WH, Williamson DF, Giovino GA: Adverse childhood experiences and smoking during adolescence and adulthood. JAMA 1999, 282(17):1652-1658.
3. Anda RF, Whitfield CL, Felitti VJ, Chapman D, Edwards VJ, Dube SR, Williamson DF: Adverse childhood experiences, alcoholic parents, and later risk of alcoholism and depression. Psychiatr Serv 2002, 53(8):1001-1009.
4. Dube SR, Miller JW, Brown DW, Giles WH, Felitti VJ, Dong M, Anda RF: Adverse childhood experiences and the association with ever using alcohol and initiating alcohol use during adolescence. J Adolesc Health 2006, 38(4):444. e441-410
5. Felitti VJ, Anda RF, Nordenberg D, Williamson DF, Spitz AM, Edwards V, Koss MP, Marks JS: Relationship of childhood abuse and household dysfunction to many of the leading causes of death in adults. The Adverse Childhood Experiences (ACE) study. Am J Prev Med 1998, 14(4):245-258.
6. Dong M, Giles WH, Felitti VJ, Dube SR, Williams JE, Chapman DP, Anda RF: Insights into causal pathways for ischemic heart disease: adverse childhood experiences study. Circulation 2004, 110(13):1761-1766.
7. Lehman BJ, Taylor SE, Kiefe CI, Seeman TE: Relation of childhood socioeconomic status and family environment to adult metabolic functioning in the CARDIA study. Psychosom Med 2005, 67(6):846-854.
8. Sumanen M, Koskenvuo M, Sillanmaki L, Mattila K: Childhood adversities experienced by working-aged coronary heart disease patients. J Psychosom Res 2005, 59(5):331-335.
9. Wise LA, Palmer JR, Rothman EF, Rosenberg L: Childhood abuse and early menarche: findings from the black women's health study. Am J Publ Health 2009, 99(Suppl 2):S460-S466.
10. Zabin LS, Emerson MR, Rowland DL: Childhood sexual abuse and early menarche: the direction of their relationship and its implications. J Adolesc Health 2005, 36(5):393-400.

11. Vigil JM, Geary DC, Byrd-Craven J: A life history assessment of early childhood sexual abuse in women. Dev Psychol 2005, 41(3):553-561.
12. Fuller-Thomson E, Brennenstuhl S, Frank J: The association between childhood physical abuse and heart disease in adulthood: findings from a representative community sample. Child Abuse Negl 2010, 34(9):689-698.
13. Goodwin RD, Stein MB: Association between childhood trauma and physical disorders among adults in the United States. Psychol Med 2004, 34(3):509-520.
14. Springer KW: Childhood physical abuse and midlife physical health: testing a multipathway life course model. Soc Sci Med 2009, 69(1):138-146.
15. Jaenisch R, Bird A: Epigenetic regulation of gene expression: how the genome integrates intrinsic and environmental signals. Nat Genet 2003, 33(Suppl):245-254.
16. Chuang JC, Jones PA: Epigenetics and microRNAs. Pediatr Res 2007, 61(5 Pt 2):24R-29R.
17. Baer C, Claus R, Frenzel LP, Zucknick M, Park YJ, Gu L, Weichenhan D, Fischer M, Pallasch CP, Herpel E, Rehli M, Byrd JC, Wendtner CM, Plass C: Extensive promoter DNA hypermethylation and hypomethylation is associated with aberrant microRNA expression in chronic lymphocytic leukemia. Canc Res 2012, 72(15):3775-3785.
18. Tobi EW, Slagboom PE, van Dongen J, Kremer D, Stein AD, Putter H, Heijmans BT, Lumey LH: Prenatal famine and genetic variation are independently and additively associated with DNA methylation at regulatory loci within IGF2/H19. PloS One 2012, 7(5):e37933.
19. McGowan PO, Sasaki A, D'Alessio AC, Dymov S, Labonte B, Szyf M, Turecki G, Meaney MJ: Epigenetic regulation of the glucocorticoid receptor in human brain associates with childhood abuse. Nat Neurosci 2009, 12(3):342-348.
20. Roth TL, Lubin FD, Funk AJ, Sweatt JD: Lasting epigenetic influence of early-life adversity on the BDNF gene. Biol Psychiatr 2009, 65(9):760-769.
21. Weaver IC, Cervoni N, Champagne FA, D'Alessio AC, Sharma S, Seckl JR, Dymov S, Szyf M, Meaney MJ: Epigenetic programming by maternal behavior. Nat Neurosci 2004, 7(8):847-854.
22. Razin A, Szyf M: DNA methylation patterns. Formation and function. Biochim Biophys Acta 1984, 782(4):331-342.
23. Szyf M: How do environments talk to genes? Nat Neurosci 2013, 16(1):2-4.
24. Borghol N, Suderman M, McArdle W, Racine A, Hallett M, Pembrey M, Hertzman C, Power C, Szyf M: Associations with early-life socio-economic position in adult DNA methylation. Int J Epidemiol 2012, 41(1):62-74.
25. Provencal N, Suderman MJ, Guillemin C, Massart R, Ruggiero A, Wang D, Bennett AJ, Pierre PJ, Friedman DP, Cote SM, Hallett M, Tremblay RE, Suomi SJ, Szyf M: The signature of maternal rearing in the methylome in rhesus macaque prefrontal cortex and T cells. J Neurosci Offic J Soc Neurosci 2012, 32(44):15626-15642.
26. Klengel T, Mehta D, Anacker C, Rex-Haffner M, Pruessner JC, Pariante CM, Pace TW, Mercer KB, Mayberg HS, Bradley B, Nemeroff CB, Holsboer F, Heim CM, Ressler KJ, Rein T, Binder EB: Allele-specific FKBP5 DNA demethylation mediates gene-childhood trauma interactions. Nat Neurosci 2013, 16(1):33-41.
27. Mehta D, Klengel T, Conneely KN, Smith AK, Altmann A, Pace TW, Rex-Haffner M, Loeschner A, Gonik M, Mercer KB, Bradley B, Muller-Myhsok B, Ressler KJ, Binder EB: Childhood maltreatment is associated with distinct genomic and

epigenetic profiles in posttraumatic stress disorder. Proc Natl Acad Sci U S A 2013, 110(20):8302-8307.
28. Thomas C, Hypponen E, Power C: Obesity and type 2 diabetes risk in midadult life: the role of childhood adversity. Pediatrics 2008, 121(5):e1240-e1249.
29. Power C, Elliott J: Cohort profile: 1958 British birth cohort (National Child Development Study). Int J Epidemiol 2006, 35(1):34-41.
30. Genome-wide association study of 14,000 cases of seven common diseases and 3,000 shared controls Nature 2007, 447(7145):661-678.
31. Rosenman S, Rodgers B: Childhood adversity in an Australian population. Soc Psychiatry Psychiatr Epidemiol 2004, 39(9):695-702.
32. Smyth GK: Limma: linear models for microarray data. In Bioinformatics and Computational Biology Solutions using R and Bioconductor, Volume 1. Edited by Gentleman VC R, Dudoit S, Irizarry R, Huber W. New York: Springer; 2005:397-420.
33. Gentleman RC, Carey VJ, Bates DM, Bolstad B, Dettling M, Dudoit S, Ellis B, Gautier L, Ge Y, Gentry J, Hornik K, Hothorn T, Huber W, Iacus S, Irizarry R, Leisch F, Li C, Maechler M, Rossini AJ, Sawitzki G, Smith C, Smyth G, Tierney L, Yang JY, Zhang J: Bioconductor: open software development for computational biology and bioinformatics. Genome Biol 2004, 5(10):R80.
34. Soric B: Statistical "discoveries" and effect-size estimation. J Am Stat Assoc 1989, 84(406):608-610.
35. Benjamini Y, Hochberg Y: Controlling the false discovery rate - a practical and powerful approach to multiple testing. J Roy Stat Soc B Met 1995, 57(1):289-300.
36. Ashburner M, Ball CA, Blake JA, Botstein D, Butler H, Cherry JM, Davis AP, Dolinski K, Dwight SS, Eppig JT, Harris MA, Hill DP, Issel-Tarver L, Kasarskis A, Lewis S, Matese JC, Richardson JE, Ringwald M, Rubin GM, Sherlock G: Gene ontology: tool for the unification of biology. Nat Genet 2000, 25(1):25-29.
37. Kanehisa M, Goto S: KEGG: kyoto encyclopedia of genes and genomes. Nucleic Acids Res 2000, 28(1):27-30.
38. Subramanian A, Tamayo P, Mootha VK, Mukherjee S, Ebert BL, Gillette MA, Paulovich A, Pomeroy SL, Golub TR, Lander ES, Mesirov JP: Gene set enrichment analysis: a knowledge-based approach for interpreting genome-wide expression profiles. Proc Natl Acad Sci USA 2005, 102(43):15545-15550.
39. Colella S, Shen L, Baggerly KA, Issa JP, Krahe R: Sensitive and quantitative universal Pyrosequencing methylation analysis of CpG sites. Biotechniques 2003, 35(1):146-150.
40. Rakyan VK, Down TA, Thorne NP, Flicek P, Kulesha E, Graf S, Tomazou EM, Backdahl L, Johnson N, Herberth M, Howe KL, Jackson DK, Miretti MM, Fiegler H, Marioni JC, Birney E, Hubbard TJ, Carter NP, Tavare S, Beck S: An integrated resource for genome-wide identification and analysis of human tissue-specific differentially methylated regions (tDMRs). Genome Res 2008, 18(9):1518-1529.
41. Su AI, Wiltshire T, Batalov S, Lapp H, Ching KA, Block D, Zhang J, Soden R, Hayakawa M, Kreiman G, Cooke MP, Walker JR, Hogenesch JB: A gene atlas of the mouse and human protein-encoding transcriptomes. Proc Natl Acad Sci U S A 2004, 101(16):6062-6067.
42. Reinius LE, Acevedo N, Joerink M, Pershagen G, Dahlen SE, Greco D, Soderhall C, Scheynius A, Kere J: Differential DNA methylation in purified human blood cells:

implications for cell lineage and studies on disease susceptibility. PloS One 2012, 7(7):e41361.

43. Lewis BP, Burge CB, Bartel DP: Conserved seed pairing, often flanked by adenosines, indicates that thousands of human genes are microRNA targets. Cell 2005, 120(1):15-20.
44. Bird AP: CpG-rich islands and the function of DNA methylation. Nature 1986, 321(6067):209-213.
45. Aissani B, Bernardi G: CpG islands: features and distribution in the genomes of vertebrates. Gene 1991, 106(2):173-183.
46. Nair SS, Coolen MW, Stirzaker C, Song JZ, Statham AL, Strbenac D, Robinson MW, Clark SJ: Comparison of methyl-DNA immunoprecipitation (MeDIP) and methyl-CpG binding domain (MBD) protein capture for genome-wide DNA methylation analysis reveal CpG sequence coverage bias. Epigenetics 2011, 6(1):34-44.
47. McGowan PO, Suderman M, Sasaki A, Huang TC, Hallett M, Meaney MJ, Szyf M: Broad epigenetic signature of maternal care in the brain of adult rats. PloS One 2011, 6(2):e14739.
48. Clevers H, van de Wetering M: TCF/LEF factor earn their wings. Trends Genet 1997, 13(12):485-489.
49. Oh DY, Olefsky JM: Medicine. Wnt fans the flames in obesity. Science 329(5990):397-398.
50. Ouchi N, Higuchi A, Ohashi K, Oshima Y, Gokce N, Shibata R, Akasaki Y, Shimono A, Walsh K: Sfrp5 is an anti-inflammatory adipokine that modulates metabolic dysfunction in obesity. Science 2010, 329(5990):454-457.
51. Prestwich TC, Macdougald OA: Wnt/beta-catenin signaling in adipogenesis and metabolism. Curr Opin Cell Biol 2007, 19(6):612-617.
52. Hattersley AT: Prime suspect: the TCF7L2 gene and type 2 diabetes risk. J Clin Invest 2007, 117(8):2077-2079.
53. Cauchi S, Froguel P: TCF7L2 genetic defect and type 2 diabetes. Curr Diab Rep 2008, 8(2):149-155.
54. Jin T: The WNT, signalling pathway and diabetes mellitus. Diabetologia 2008, 51(10):1771-1780.
55. Schinner S: Wnt-signalling and the metabolic syndrome. Horm Metab Res 2009, 41(2):159-163.
56. Pereira CP, Bachli EB, Schoedon G: The wnt pathway: a macrophage effector molecule that triggers inflammation. Curr Atheroscler Rep 2009, 11(3):236-242.
57. Schett G, Zwerina J, David JP: The role of Wnt proteins in arthritis. Nat Clin Pract Rheumatol 2008, 4(9):473-480.
58. Takahashi-Yanaga F, Sasaguri T: The Wnt/beta-catenin signaling pathway as a target in drug discovery. J Pharmacol Sci 2007, 104(4):293-302.
59. Waltzer L, Bienz M: The control of beta-catenin and TCF during embryonic development and cancer. Canc Metastasis Rev 1999, 18(2):231-246.
60. Feinberg AP, Irizarry RA, Fradin D, Aryee MJ, Murakami P, Aspelund T, Eiriksdottir G, Harris TB, Launer L, Gudnason V, Fallin MD: Personalized epigenomic signatures that are stable over time and covary with body mass index. Sci Transl Med 2010, 2(49):49ra67.

61. Irizarry RA, Ladd-Acosta C, Carvalho B, Wu H, Brandenburg SA, Jeddeloh JA, Wen B, Feinberg AP: Comprehensive high-throughput arrays for relative methylation (CHARM). Genome Res 2008, 18(5):780-790.
62. Jia J, Pekowska A, Jaeger S, Benoukraf T, Ferrier P, Spicuglia S: Assessing the efficiency and significance of Methylated DNA Immunoprecipitation (MeDIP) assays in using in vitro methylated genomic DNA. BMC Res Notes 2010, 3:240.
63. Jin SG, Kadam S, Pfeifer GP: Examination of the specificity of DNA methylation profiling techniques towards 5-methylcytosine and 5-hydroxymethylcytosine. Nucleic Acids Res 2010, 38(11):e125.
64. Rajendram R, Ferreira JC, Grafodatskaya D, Choufani S, Chiang T, Pu S, Butcher DT, Wodak SJ, Weksberg R: Assessment of methylation level prediction accuracy in methyl-DNA immunoprecipitation and sodium bisulfite based microarray platforms. Epigenetics 2011, 6(4):410-415.
65. Robinson MD, Stirzaker C, Statham AL, Coolen MW, Song JZ, Nair SS, Strbenac D, Speed TP, Clark SJ: Evaluation of affinity-based genome-wide DNA methylation data: effects of CpG density, amplification bias, and copy number variation. Genome Res 2010, 20(12):1719-1729.

There are several supplemental files that are not available in this version of the article. To view this additional information, please use the citation on the first page of this chapter.

CHAPTER 15

Epigenomic Mechanisms of Early Adversity and HPA Dysfunction: Considerations for PTSD Research

PATRICK O. MCGOWAN

15.1 INTRODUCTION

Childhood adversity can have life-long consequences for the response to stressful events later in life (1). Repeated exposure to trauma alters neurodevelopment (2), enhances the activity of endocrine mechanisms involved in the stress response (3, 4) and increases the risk of multiple forms of psychopathology (5, 6). For example, the risk of suicide is strongly linked to childhood sexual and physical abuse or severe neglect (7–9). Sexual and physical abuse or severe neglect in childhood are also well-known risk factors for adult forms of post-traumatic stress disorder (PTSD), at least in part via changes in neural systems mediating the endocrine response to stress (10). The hypothalamic-pituitary-adrenal (HPA) axis shapes the endocrine response to stress in addition to its role in many other physiological processes, including immune and metabolic function. As such, the HPA axis plays an adaptive role by maintaining allostasis (i.e., stability amid change) in the face of challenging environmental conditions. Part of the explanation for the enhanced impact of adversity in early life is thought to lie in the relatively high degree of plasticity during this period, when environmental factors exert pervasive effects on a number of health trajectories (11, 12). Accumulating evidence indicates that this phenomenon, sometimes called "biological embedding," involves persistent changes in gene regulation via epigenetic mechanisms (13). The goal of this review is to highlight research on epigenetic mechanisms of early life adversity and parental care – prime mediators of offspring neurodevelopment (11) – that addresses several critical issues for research in this rapidly evolving area. We conclude by providing examples of the ways in which research in this area may provide insights for PTSD researchers on the epigenetic impacts of early adversity and highlight challenges for the field going forward.

15.2 EPIGENETIC MECHANISMS: STABILITY AND CHANGE

A first critical issue in understanding the relative risk conferred by early life adversity concerns the molecular mechanisms mediating altered HPA function as well as other pathways underlying vulnerability that respond in a manner that is both contingent upon the adversity and stable in the face of similar perturbations in later life. Epigenetic mechanisms include DNA methylation, histone modifications, and non-coding RNA. The methylation of cytosine in cytosine-guanine dinucleotides (CpGs) in the DNA itself (i.e., 5meC) is the best understood epigenetic mark and the focus of the majority of current investigations. However other modifications to DNA, including hydroxymethylation (5-hmC) and other recently identified DNA modifications, are attracting increasing interest as potential gene regulatory mechanisms (14). It should be noted that the conventional methods used for mapping 5-mC, such as bisulfite sequencing and methylation-sensitive restriction enzyme-based approaches, do not differentiate it from 5-hmC. As such, although I use the term "DNA methylation" in this review to be consistent with the majority of primary publications to date, the term "DNA modification" is a more accurate descriptor.

Variations in these modifications occur as a result of genetic, stochastic, and environmental factors, all of which drive the epigenetic regulation of gene expression. There is some debate as to the primacy of stochastic and environmental factors in epigenetic variation (15). It is clear that proper epigenetic regulation is essential for normal development and cell division, conferring cell-type identity in a stable manner that appears to a large degree unresponsive to early life adversity. There also is now compelling evidence of epigenetic regulation by environmental factors. Epigenetic regulation thus provides a potential mechanism for understanding well-defined environmental effects on phenotypes.

Elucidating which regions of the genome are labile in response to early life adversity, how rapidly changes can occur, and the ontological time-course of epigenetic changes remains a matter of active investigation. As I discuss below, these epigenetic responses likely depend on the genomic loci under consideration. Humans are exposed to a variety of stressors throughout life, however early life stress appears to exert an profound effects on HPA function that is pervasive throughout life in part by altering epigenetic mechanisms in a stable manner. I will illustrate this point by discussing several studies in rodents that have provided foundational knowledge applicable to investigations in humans.

15.3 ANIMAL MODELS OF EPIGENETIC MECHANISMS IN EARLY LIFE SHAPING THE RESPONSE TO STRESS IN ADULTHOOD

Animal models of maternal care and perinatal stress have helped to provide a mechanistic understanding of the impacts of early life adversity, allowing for control of genetic variation and a temporal dynamics of environmental exposures. Classic examples are experiments pioneered by Levine in the late 1960s and Meaney beginning in the late 1980s that indicated that laboratory rodents exposed to different levels of maternal care show behavioral alterations in fearfulness in response to novel environments and endocrine-mediated stress responses (16). These studies have documented sustained alterations in the expression genes regulating HPA function, such as the Glucocorticoid Receptor (GR), in brain areas mediating anxiety behavior and HPA circuitry, such as the prefrontal cortex, hippocampus, and hypothalamus. As adults, the offspring of rat mothers providing relatively high or relatively low levels of maternal care display life-long alterations in DNA methylation and Histone 3 lysine 9 (H3K9) acetylation of the untranslated 17 splice variant of the GR promoter in the hippocampus and of the promoter of the GAD67 gene in the prefrontal cortex (17, 18). Other groups have provided evidence that additional genes in neural pathways mediating the stress response are epigenetically regulated in association with early life stress, including arginine vasopressin in the hypothalamus (19), and BDNF in the prefrontal cortex and hippocampus (20). Interestingly, apparently stable changes in GR promoter methylation emerge within the first week of life as a function of naturally occurring variations in maternal care. However, a recent study found evidence of sex-specific DNA methylation changes in BDNF and reelin in the medial prefrontal cortex of offspring subjected to an adverse maternal environment that emerge in the transition between adolescence and adulthood (21). These data indicate a complex temporal relationship between environmental adversity and epigenetic variation in the medial prefrontal cortex, dependent upon unknown mediating factors. The data suggest that the temporal dynamics of the epigenetic response to early adversity may, at least to some extent, be loci- and tissue-specific.

15.4 HUMAN STUDIES OF EPIGENETIC MECHANISMS IN EARLY LIFE SHAPING THE RESPONSE TO STRESS IN ADULTHOOD

In light of findings in animal models, GR is an obvious candidate gene of interest in exploring the relationship between epigenetic regulation as a function of early life adversity and mental health outcomes in humans. Perhaps less clear is the choice of appropriate cohorts and cell types in humans to test these relationships. As mentioned, epigenetic mechanisms play an important role in conferring cell-type identity during development and cell division. As a result, it is perhaps reasonable to assume that the impact of environmental factors on epigenetic marks is likely to be to some extent cell-type specific, limiting analysis to appropriate tissues of interest. We used hippocampal samples from suicide completers with and without a history of childhood abuse, and examined DNA methylation of the GR1F promoter, a region highly syntenic with the rat GR17 splice variant. We found higher levels of DNA methylation of the GR promoter region among suicide victims with a history of abuse or severe neglect in childhood, but not among suicide victims who were not abused in childhood or among a control group who had died of causes unrelated to suicide (22). This hypermethylation was associated with increased transcript abundance of both GR1F splice variant and total abundance of GR transcript, and in vitro analysis indicated that regions hypermethyated in abused suicide victims inhibited the binding of the EGR1 transcription factor (also known as NGFI-A, Zif268, Krox24, and ZENK) to select nucleotides within the promoter. Another recent study has replicated the finding of enhanced DNA methylation at this splice variant and gone on to identify altered DNA methylation in additional splice variants of the GR promoter and show that this response to early adversity is brain region specific, not occurring in the anterior cingulate (23).

15.5 STUDYING EPIGENETIC MECHANISMS OF HPA REGULATION BY EARLY ADVERSITY IN PERIPHERAL TISSUES IN HUMANS

A second important consideration for studies of the epigenetic response to early life adversity in living humans is its impacts on peripheral tissues, essential for efforts to sample potential changes over time and after interventions in humans. Lymphocytes are well-known targets of glucocorticoids, and immune profiles are known to be sensitive to alterations in GR abundance (24). One study found that childhood adversity (as measured by parental loss, childhood maltreatment, and parental care) was associated with increased DNA methylation of several sites within the GR1F promoter region in lymphocytes in adulthood (25). These results and other analogous data are important because they indicate that epigenetic alterations as a result of childhood adversity persist in peripheral tissues and are detectable in mixed lymphocyte cell populations. A recent investigation in whole blood of FKBP5, a negative regulator of GR, links PTSD to both genetic variation and early adversity (26). The authors of this study had previously characterized several genetic polymorphisms associated with PTSD risk. In the recent study, they found evidence of DNA demethylation in an intronic region only in individuals subjected to abuse in childhood and only in those carrying the "risk" allele of the gene, with experiments in cultured cells indicating an effect shown to occur before and persist after differentiation in cultured hippocampal cells. In light of previous animal work showing that glucocorticoid exposure can drive DNA demethylation in mouse hippocampal dentate gyrus, indicating neural target tissues and in vivo conditions where glucocorticoid activity may modulate other HPA-responsive genes (27). These data investigating candidate genes demonstrate the capacity of the epigenetic machinery to respond to the psychosocial environment in early life in a manner that confers stable changes in stress pathways in lymphocytes – cells that evidently go through numerous cycles of cell division throughout life.

15.6 EPIGENOMIC REGULATION BY EARLY LIFE ADVERSITY IN GENE REGULATORY ELEMENTS AND BEYOND

A third consideration addressed by these studies is the need to identify genomic loci that are epigenetically labile in response to early life adversity. Studies to date have predominantly focused on epigenetic changes in gene regulatory elements (e.g., promoters) and defined candidate genomic loci. A study using a microarray approach combined with methylated DNA immunoprecipitation to interrogate promoter regions in all known protein-coding genes found that evidence of hypo- and hypermethylation among hundreds of genes in hippocampi from suicide completers with a history of early life abuse compared to non-abused controls (28). This study identified novel candidate genes (e.g., ALS2; involved in small GTPase regulation) and enriched candidate pathways (e.g., neuroplasticity) that may be epigenetically regulated in response to early life abuse and suicide. Another study of whole blood using the Illumina 450 K array, which examines the methylation status at single-nucleotide resolution in ~480,000 CpG sites, covering most known genes and regulatory elements, found evidence of predominantly hypermethylated DNA within exons and 3′ UTRs of differentially expressed genes in PTSD patients with a history of early abuse, with epigenetic differences showing general agreement with levels of transcription (29). This study indicated that changes in DNA methylation among PTSD patients were enhanced in a with a positive history of childhood abuse, suggesting a potentially distinct epigenetic profile in this subgroup.

We documented changes in DNA methylation, H3K9 acteylation and gene expression across a 7 Mb region flanking the GR gene hippocampus using a tiling microarray approach in rats (30). Differences in the amount of maternal care received during the first week of life were associated with epigenetic differences over large genomic regions (~100 kB) in hippocampi of adult animals. Differences in transcription occurred in the context of hyperacetylation and hypomethylation of promoters and hypermethylation of exons. Interestingly, hypermethylation within exons was the largest detect difference in DNA methylation as a response to higher levels of maternal care. Using this methodology, we identified a novel linkage between altered epigenetic status of a large protocadherin (PCDH) gene cluster of cell-adhesion molecules and maternal care. Previous studies have indicated that PCDH gene clusters regulate neuronal morphology and synaptic plasticity (31). It remains to be determined whether epigenetic alterations in these genes are linked to differences in neuroplasticity observed as a function of differences in maternal care (32). Nevertheless, as technologies for generating genome-wide epigenetic profiles become economically accessible to a wider array of researchers and bioinformatics tools for genomic analysis become more standardized, these approaches will likely provide powerful methods for hypothesis generation by consolidating multiple levels of biological information.

In a follow-up to this study, we analyzed the GR locus in hippocampi of adult suicide victims who were abused early in life compared to non-abused controls (33). Abused suicide victims showed broad statistical dependencies in DNA methylation differences in a manner akin to what was observed in the rat study described above (30). As in the previous study, the clustered PCDH gene cluster showed the largest alterations in DNA methylation within the locus examined. In humans, alterations in PCDH genes impair intellectual function, and mutations in PCDH genes are linked to autism (34). PCDH genes show evidence of distinct DNA methylation in whole blood from individuals with a childhood history of low socio-economic (35). The function of these epigenetic differences in PCDH remains unknown, however the data suggest that these genes are epigenetically labile in response to the early life social environment in both rodents and humans (33). Taken together, the data suggest that animal model of parental care may have broad applicability for understanding the consequences of epigenetic modification of PCDH gene pathways in humans.

An important caveat of these studies is that they often report data from mixed cell populations, potentially masking epigenetic differences in select cell types or skewing group differences due to cell admixture. Fluorescence-associated cell sorting followed by cell-type-specific epigenomic analysis is a potential solution. However, the relevant cell types are not often known, and cell types that are routinely extracted (e.g., CD4+ T-cells) can often be divided into functional classes that are dissociable by additional rounds of selection, making it difficult to know whether one has attained the necessary level of specificity. An additional method to address this problem is informatic. Data gathered by the Encyclopedia of DNA Elements (ENCODE) project and other large-scale genomics initiatives are providing multidimensional representations of epigenetic and functional genomic signatures from a large number of cell types (36). These data will serve as important information on regions that identify cell types that can be used to bioinformatically deconvelute the constituents of cell admixture in mixed tissue populations [e.g., peripheral blood; (37)]. The data will also provide a valuable method to identify epigenetically invariant genomic regions that can serve to reduce genomic complexity in genome-wide analysis of epigenetic signaling, and transcriptional "silent" regions in specified cell types unlikely to be responsive to environmental perturbations. These data, together with an accumulating array of published epigenomic analysis, should help move research on the impacts of early life adversity beyond candidate gene to "candidate pathway" and "candidate network" levels of analysis, which are finding utility in other areas of complex disease research [e.g., (38)].

15.7 PROSPECTIVE FOR PTSD RESEARCH

Early life trauma shapes resiliency to stress in later life and is a risk factor for the development of PTSD, itself characterized by a "transformational" change in the neurophysiological response to stress that occurs in some but not all individuals exposed to trauma (39). Inter-individual differences in PTSD susceptibility are modulated at least to some extent by early life adversity inasmuch as both are associated with HPA axis alterations – at least in a subset of PTSD patients. Both early life trauma or severe neglect and PTSD are generally associated with lower basal circulating cortisol levels and an attenuated response to acute stress challenge (10). These results have been proposed to explain a paradox of PTSD: namely that HPA dysfunction observed in PTSD appears distinct from that observed in chronic stress or major depression, conditions associated with elevated levels of cortisol. Because PTSD and major depression co-occur ~50% of the time, the results indicate a distinct profile of PTSD in patients with a past history of trauma or early life abuse (10). Likewise, not all who experience trauma develop PTSD. A few studies have identified epigenetic variation associated with PTSD [e.g., (40)], and patients with a history of early life adversity may show distinct epigenomic profiles (29). These contrasts have made it challenging to identify epigenetic mechanisms linking early adversity to PTSD risk, calling for a variety of approaches in appropriate animal models and human studies. The molecular and epigenetic mechanisms associated with PTSD with and without a history of early life adversity are beyond the scope of the present manuscript, however this topic has been the focus of a number of excellent reviews [e.g., (10, 41–43)] – including in this volume (44).

Questions that need to be addressed for a more complete understanding of the role of epigenetic mechanisms in conferring risk of PTSD via early life adversity, include: when, precisely, during development, do epigenetic changes related to early adversity emerge? In what contexts, genomic regions/pathways, and in cell types? These principles remain poorly understood. However, some interesting parallels have been identified between regions of the genome that are epigenetically responsive to psychosocial factors (e.g., maternal care) in rodents, and syntenic regions of the human genome that are epigenetically labile in conditions of early adversity [e.g., childhood abuse; (33)]. Studies in animal models have suggested that early life stress impairs neuroplasticity in brain regions such as the hippocampus and has a lasting impact on endocrine systems underlying the response to psychosocial stressors (45, 46).

Many animals, including rodents and humans, appear to have evolved to respond both to immediate threats to life and limb and to psychosocial stress associated with predation risk, including via the transfer of information about environmental conditions to the offspring via maternal factors. For example, a number of studies in wildlife ecology and comparative endocrinology over the past 20 years have indicated that the influence of predators on stress in free-living animals is long-lasting, resembling stress effects in laboratory animal models of PTSD (47). Response mechanisms mediating the adaptive processes responsible for this transmission implicate the HPA axis and pathways involved in neuroplasticity (48, 49). Epigenetic research in this area is in its infancy, but offers an important avenue to study the extent to which developmentally regulated epigenetic mechanisms and environmental stressors interact in the context in which they have evolved.

Elucidating the biological mechanisms underlying effects of early social experiences on later mental health is challenging in humans for reasons that include technical/analytic complexity and limited access to relevant biological material. New methods that offer the ability to examine DNA methylation at single-nucleotide resolution genome-wide are advancing rapidly and, in tandem, a vast array of analytical tools and statistical methods are now available to normalize known technical biases, visualize epigenetic modifications, and identify differences among subjects (50). Genome-wide changes with early adversity appear to occur in association with pathway or network-specific alterations of the epigenomic landscape. Thus, the selection of epigenetic modification(s) for study and identification of the impacted pathways, which rely on computationally predicted and biologically validated relationships, remain a challenge for future studies. The use of whole-genome screens to identify stable combinations of epigenetic modifications that distinguish cell- or tissue-specific functional effects may be useful in tissue-specific gene targeting of therapeutics while minimizing off-target effects (51). It may not be clear, however, which cell types are relevant to the question under study. Nevertheless, there is some indication that even buccal epithelial cells may index the response to early life adversity, though not via epigenetic changes in GR per se (52). Buccal cells share embryonic stem cell origin with neurons, and therefore may provide a valuable means of identifying the epigenetic signature of early life adversity in young children, where blood sampling is problematic. In addition, because changes in epigenetic patterns are often only measured at one time-point, the involvement of later life experiences in conferring epigenetic changes are difficult or impossible to rule out. Prospective research validating the use of peripheral markers of early life impacts (which can also be done in animal models) will offer critical insights into the dynamic nature of epigenetic regulation and its role as a mechanism for programing gene function in response to early life trauma.

REFERENCES

1. Davidson RJ, McEwen BS. Social influences on neuroplasticity: stress and interventions to promote well-being. Nat Neurosci (2012) 15:689–95. doi:10.1038/nn.3093
2. Vythilingam M, Heim C, Newport J, Miller AH, Anderson E, Bronen R, et al. Childhood trauma associated with smaller hippocampal volume in women with major depression. Am J Psychiatry (2002) 159:2072–80. doi:10.1176/appi.ajp.159.12.2072
3. De Bellis MD, Chrousos GP, Dorn LD, Burke L, Helmers K, Kling MA, et al. Hypothalamic-pituitary-adrenal axis dysregulation in sexually abused girls. J Clin Endocrinol Metab (1994) 78:249–55. doi:10.1210/jc.78.2.249
4. Heim C, Nemeroff CB. The role of childhood trauma in the neurobiology of mood and anxiety disorders: preclinical and clinical studies. Biol Psychiatry (2001) 49:1023–39. doi:10.1016/S0006-3223(01)01157-X
5. Fergusson DM, Horwood LJ, Lynskey MT. Childhood sexual abuse and psychiatric disorder in young adulthood: II. Psychiatric outcomes of childhood sexual abuse. J Am Acad Child Adolesc Psychiatry (1996) 35:1365–74. doi:10.1097/00004583-199610000-00023
6. Widom CS, Dumont K, Czaja SJ. A prospective investigation of major depressive disorder and comorbidity in abused and neglected children grown up. Arch Gen Psychiatry (2007) 64:49–56. doi:10.1001/archpsyc.64.1.49
7. Beckett C, Maughan B, Rutter M, Castle J, Colvert E, Groothues C, et al. Do the effects of early severe deprivation on cognition persist into early adolescence? Findings from the English and Romanian adoptees study. Child Dev (2006) 77:696–711. doi:10.1111/j.1467-8624.2006.00898.x
8. Mann JJ, Currier DM. Stress, genetics and epigenetic effects on the neurobiology of suicidal behavior and depression. Eur Psychiatry (2010) 25:268–71. doi:10.1016/j.eurpsy.2010.01.009
9. Turecki G, Ernst C, Jollant F, Labonte B, Mechawar N. The neurodevelopmental origins of suicidal behavior. Trends Neurosci (2012) 35:14–23. doi:10.1016/j.tins.2011.11.008
10. Yehuda R, Flory JD, Pratchett LC, Buxbaum J, Ising M, Holsboer F. Putative biological mechanisms for the association between early life adversity and the

subsequent development of PTSD. Psychopharmacology (Berl) (2010) 212:405–17. doi:10.1007/s00213-010-1969-6

11. Hackman DA, Farah MJ, Meaney MJ. Socioeconomic status and the brain: mechanistic insights from human and animal research. Nat Rev Neurosci (2010) 11:651–9. doi:10.1038/nrn2897
12. Hanson M, Godfrey KM, Lillycrop KA, Burdge GC, Gluckman PD. Developmental plasticity and developmental origins of non-communicable disease: theoretical considerations and epigenetic mechanisms. Prog Biophys Mol Biol (2010) 106:272–80. doi:10.1016/j.pbiomolbio.2010.12.008
13. Sasaki A, De Vega WC, McGowan PO. Biological embedding in mental health: an epigenomic perspective. Biochem Cell Biol (2013) 91:14–21. doi:10.1139/bcb-2012-0070
14. Labrie V, Pai S, Petronis A. Epigenetics of major psychosis: progress, problems and perspectives. Trends Genet (2012) 28:427–35. doi:10.1016/j.tig.2012.04.002
15. Petronis A. Epigenetics as a unifying principle in the aetiology of complex traits and diseases. Nature (2010) 465:721–7. doi:10.1038/nature09230
16. Meaney MJ. Maternal care, gene expression, and the transmission of individual differences in stress reactivity across generations. Annu Rev Neurosci (2001) 24:1161–92. doi:10.1146/annurev.neuro.24.1.1161
17. Weaver IC, Cervoni N, Champagne FA, D'Alessio AC, Sharma S, Seckl JR, et al. Epigenetic programming by maternal behavior. Nat Neurosci (2004) 7:847–54. doi:10.1038/nn1276
18. Zhang TY, Hellstrom IC, Bagot RC, Wen X, Diorio J, Meaney MJ. Maternal care and DNA methylation of a glutamic acid decarboxylase 1 promoter in rat hippocampus. J Neurosci (2010) 30:13130–7. doi:10.1523/JNEUROSCI.1039-10.2010
19. Murgatroyd C, Patchev AV, Wu Y, Micale V, Bockmuhl Y, Fischer D, et al. Dynamic DNA methylation programs persistent adverse effects of early-life stress. Nat Neurosci (2009) 12:1559–66. doi:10.1038/nn.2436
20. Roth TL, Lubin FD, Funk AJ, Sweatt JD. Lasting epigenetic influence of early-life adversity on the BDNF gene. Biol Psychiatry (2009) 65:760–9. doi:10.1016/j.biopsych.2008.11.028
21. Blaze J, Scheuing L, Roth TL. Differential methylation of genes in the medial prefrontal cortex of developing and adult rats following exposure to maltreatment or nurturing care during infancy. Dev Neurosci (2013) 35:306–16. doi:10.1159/000350716
22. McGowan PO, Sasaki A, D'Alessio AC, Dymov S, Labonte B, Szyf M, et al. Epigenetic regulation of the glucocorticoid receptor in human brain associates with childhood abuse. Nat Neurosci (2009) 12:342–8. doi:10.1038/nn.2270
23. Labonte B, Yerko V, Gross J, Mechawar N, Meaney MJ, Szyf M, et al. Differential glucocorticoid receptor exon 1(B), 1(C), and 1(H) expression and methylation in suicide completers with a history of childhood abuse. Biol Psychiatry (2012) 72(1):41–8. doi:10.1016/j.biopsych.2012.01.034
24. Baschant U, Tuckermann J. The role of the glucocorticoid receptor in inflammation and immunity. J Steroid Biochem Mol Biol (2010) 120:69–75. doi:10.1016/j.jsbmb.2010.03.058

25. Tyrka AR, Price LH, Marsit C, Walters OC, Carpenter LL. Childhood adversity and epigenetic modulation of the leukocyte glucocorticoid receptor: preliminary findings in healthy adults. PLoS ONE (2012) 7:e30148. doi:10.1371/journal.pone.0030148
26. Klengel T, Mehta D, Anacker C, Rex-Haffner M, Pruessner JC, Pariante CM, et al. Allele-specific FKBP5 DNA demethylation mediates gene-childhood trauma interactions. Nat Neurosci (2013) 16:33–41. doi:10.1038/nn.3275
27. Yang X, Ewald ER, Huo Y, Tamashiro KL, Salvatori R, Sawa A, et al. Glucocorticoid-induced loss of DNA methylation in non-neuronal cells and potential involvement of DNMT1 in epigenetic regulation of Fkbp5. Biochem Biophys Res Commun (2012) 420:570–5. doi:10.1016/j.bbrc.2012.03.035
28. Labonte B, Suderman M, Maussion G, Navaro L, Yerko V, Mahar I, et al. Genome-wide epigenetic regulation by early-life trauma. Arch Gen Psychiatry (2012) 69:722–31. doi:10.1001/archgenpsychiatry.2011.2287
29. Mehta D, Klengel T, Conneely KN, Smith AK, Altmann A, Pace TW, et al. Childhood maltreatment is associated with distinct genomic and epigenetic profiles in posttraumatic stress disorder. Proc Natl Acad Sci USA (2013) 110:8302–7. doi:10.1073/pnas.1217750110
30. McGowan PO, Suderman M, Sasaki A, Huang TC, Hallett M, Meaney MJ, et al. Broad epigenetic signature of maternal care in the brain of adult rats. PLoS ONE (2011) 6:e14739. doi:10.1371/journal.pone.0014739
31. Yagi T. Molecular codes for neuronal individuality and cell assembly in the brain. Front Mol Neurosci (2012) 5:45. doi:10.3389/fnmol.2012.00045
32. Bagot RC, Van Hasselt FN, Champagne DL, Meaney MJ, Krugers HJ, Joels M. Maternal care determines rapid effects of stress mediators on synaptic plasticity in adult rat hippocampal dentate gyrus. Neurobiol Learn Mem (2009) 92:292–300. doi:10.1016/j.nlm.2009.03.004
33. Suderman M, McGowan PO, Sasaki A, Huang TC, Hallett MT, Meaney MJ, et al. Conserved epigenetic sensitivity to early life experience in the rat and human hippocampus. Proc Natl Acad Sci USA (2012) 109(Suppl 2):17266–72. doi:10.1073/pnas.1121260109
34. Morrow EM, Yoo SY, Flavell SW, Kim TK, Lin Y, Hill RS, et al. Identifying autism loci and genes by tracing recent shared ancestry. Science (2008) 321:218–23. doi:10.1126/science.1157657
35. Borghol N, Suderman M, Mcardle W, Racine A, Hallett M, Pembrey M, et al. Associations with early-life socio-economic position in adult DNA methylation. Int J Epidemiol (2011) 41:62–74. doi:10.1093/ije/dyr147
36. Consortium EP, Dunham I, Kundaje A, Aldred SF, Collins PJ, Davis CA, et al. An integrated encyclopedia of DNA elements in the human genome. Nature (2012) 489:57–74. doi:10.1038/nature11247
37. Houseman EA, Accomando WP, Koestler DC, Christensen BC, Marsit CJ, Nelson HH, et al. DNA methylation arrays as surrogate measures of cell mixture distribution. BMC Bioinformatics (2012) 13:86. doi:10.1186/1471-2105-13-86
38. Broderick G, Craddock TJ. Systems biology of complex symptom profiles: capturing interactivity across behavior, brain and immune regulation. Brain Behav Immun (2013) 29:1–8. doi:10.1016/j.bbi.2012.09.008

39. Yehuda R, Bierer LM. The relevance of epigenetics to PTSD: implications for the DSM-V. J Trauma Stress (2009) 22:427–34. doi:10.1002/jts.20448
40. Uddin M, Aiello AE, Wildman DE, Koenen KC, Pawelec G, De Los Santos R, et al. Epigenetic and immune function profiles associated with posttraumatic stress disorder. Proc Natl Acad Sci USA (2010) 107:9470–5. doi:10.1073/pnas.0910794107
41. Seckl JR, Meaney MJ. Glucocorticoid "programming" and PTSD risk. Ann N Y Acad Sci (2006) 1071:351–78. doi:10.1196/annals.1364.027
42. Pratchett LC, Yehuda R. Foundations of posttraumatic stress disorder: does early life trauma lead to adult posttraumatic stress disorder? Dev Psychopathol (2011) 23:477–91. doi:10.1017/S0954579411000186
43. Skelton K, Ressler KJ, Norrholm SD, Jovanovic T, Bradley-Davino B. PTSD and gene variants: new pathways and new thinking. Neuropharmacology (2012) 62: 628–37. doi:10.1016/j.neuropharm.2011.02.013
44. Zovkic IB, Meadows JP, Kaas GA, Sweatt JD. Interindividual variability in stress susceptibility: a role for epigenetic mechanisms in PTSD. Front Psychiatry (2013) 4:60. doi:10.3389/fpsyt.2013.00060
45. Szyf M, McGowan P, Meaney MJ. The social environment and the epigenome. Environ Mol Mutagen (2008) 49:46–60. doi:10.1002/em.20357
46. McEwen BS. Brain on stress: how the social environment gets under the skin. Proc Natl Acad Sci USA (2012) 109(Suppl 2):17180–5. doi:10.1073/pnas.1121254109
47. Clinchy M, Schulkin J, Zanette LY, Sheriff MJ, Mcgowan PO, Boonstra R. The neurological ecology of fear: insights neuroscientists and ecologists have to offer one another. Front Behav Neurosci (2010) 4:21. doi:10.3389/fnbeh.2011.00021
48. Barker JM, Boonstra R, Wojtowicz JM. From pattern to purpose: how comparative studies contribute to understanding the function of adult neurogenesis. Eur J Neurosci (2011) 34: 963–77. doi:10.1111/j.1460-9568.2011.07823.x
49. Love OP, McGowan PO, Sheriff MJ. Maternal adversity and ecological stressors in natural populations: the role of stress axis programming in individuals, with implications for populations and communities. Funct Ecol (2013) 27(1):81–92. doi:10.1111/j.1365-2435.2012.02040.x
50. Bock C. Analysing and interpreting DNA methylation data. Nat Rev Genet (2012) 13:705–19. doi:10.1038/nrg3273
51. de Groote ML, Verschure PJ, Rots MG. Epigenetic editing: targeted rewriting of epigenetic marks to modulate expression of selected target genes. Nucleic Acids Res (2012) 40:10596–613. doi:10.1093/nar/gks863
52. Essex MJ, Thomas Boyce W, Hertzman C, Lam LL, Armstrong JM, Neumann SM, et al. Epigenetic vestiges of early developmental adversity: childhood stress exposure and DNA methylation in adolescence. Child Dev (2013) 84: 58–75. doi:10.1111/j.1467-8624.2011.01641.x

CHAPTER 16

Increased Frequency of Micronuclei in Adults with a History of Childhood Sexual Abuse: A Discordant Monozygotic Twin Study

TIMOTHY P. YORK, JENNI BRUMELLE, JANE JUUSOLA, KENNETH S. KENDLER, LINDON J. EAVES, ANANDA B. AMSTADTER, STEVEN H. AGGEN, KIMBERLY H. JONES, ANDREA FERREIRA-GONZALEZ, AND COLLEEN JACKSON-COOK

16.1 INTRODUCTION

Childhood sexual abuse (CSA) not only compromises well-being in childhood but is also associated with a broad range of psychopathology and morbidity in adulthood [1], [2], [3], [4]. However, little is known about the biological mechanisms involved in mediating the long-term pathogenic effect of early-life trauma. One possible means for CSA to be biologically "embedded" in a manner that could lead to a latent pathologic consequence would be if it resulted in a change in the individual's somatic cell DNA. Evidence shows childhood maltreatment predicts an increased risk of clinically relevant levels of inflammation in adulthood [5],[6], and inflammation-associated reactive oxygen/nitrogen species are known to cause DNA damage/chromosomal changes. Stress-related inflammation also leads to perturbations in the regulation/expression of several genes, including (but not limited to) nuclear factor-kappa B (NF-kβ), interleukin-1B, interleukin-6, and tumor necrosis factor-α [7], [8]. Additional evidence that early-life stress can lead to DNA-based alterations comes from reports of shortened telomeres in children exposed to adverse rearing settings [9], and in adults with a history of chronic or severe childhood illness [10] or childhood maltreatment [11], but the potential correlation between childhood maltreatment and telomere length is controversial [12].

Given that both telomere shortening and/or inflammation-related generation of oxygen and/or nitrogen species are phenomena that have been associated with an increased frequency of acquired chromosomal abnormalities [13], [14], [15], [16], [17], [18], [19], we hypothesize that an alternative or additional biological effect of stress could be the acquisition of somatic cell chromosomal instability. Moreover, since such damage can cause mutations and chromosomal abnormalities that disrupt cellular function and viability through aberrant gene expression and protein formation [20], [21], [22], the accumulation of chromosomal imbalances over time provides a plausible account by which CSA exposure could contribute to the development of later health and psychiatric symptoms observed in adults with a CSA history.

The cytokinesis-block micronucleus (CBMN) assay is an attractive biomarker for estimating chromosomal damage associated with environmental insults or exposures and is considered an acceptable alternative to data obtained from the assessment of metaphase chromosomal analyses [23], [24], since it is less labor intensive and less prone to producing artifacts than classical chromosomal studies [25]. Briefly, a micronucleus (MN) is a small chromatin-containing structure that can be visualized juxtaposed to the main daughter nuclei following the completion of mitosis (Figure 1). MN formation can occur spontaneously or in response to environmental exposures and can accumulate over several months or years [26]. MN form when whole chromosomes or chromosomal fragments fail to correctly migrate to spindle poles during mitosis [27], [28], [29]. The lagging chromosome(s) or fragment(s) are subsequently excluded from

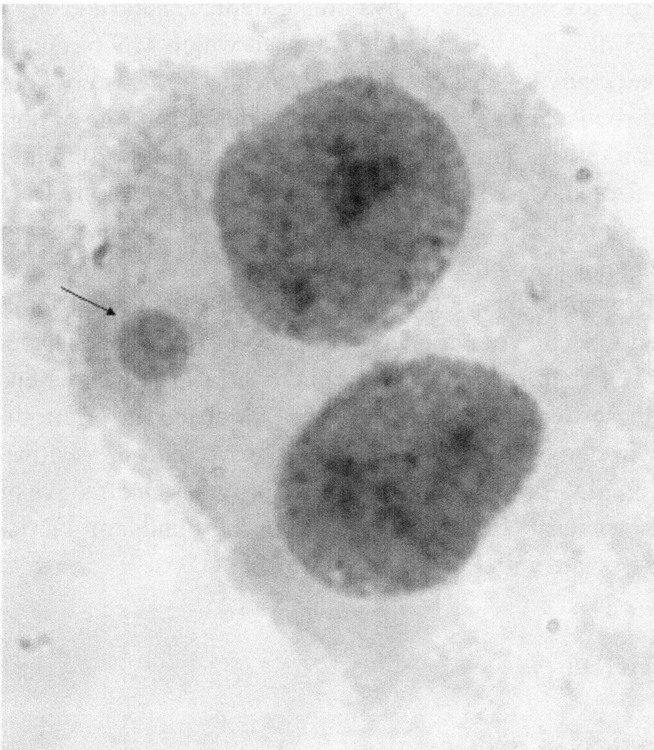

Figure 1. Giemsa stained micronucleus (MN) (arrow) and corresponding daughter binucleates. By definition, a MN is no larger than one-third the size of the parental nuclei and appears adjacent to the binucleate.

the daughter nuclei and are encased in their own nuclear envelope [27]. The exclusion of chromatin into a MN can result in alterations of cellular gene dosage, which, in turn, could result in abnormal gene expression and/or perturbations in cellular proliferation that could have a broad cascade of consequences on biological systems [30]. MN frequency is known to increase with age [23], [31], [32] and has been shown to be elevated in patients with several health conditions, including cancer [33], cardiovascular disease [34], [35], Alzheimer's disease and Parkinson's disease [36].

MN frequency is influenced by both heritable genetic and environmental factors [32], [37]. However, the extent to which MN frequency is impacted by exposure to a traumatic event, such as CSA, is not known. One of the most robust approaches to determine the causal role of non-genetic influences on trait variation is to study monozygotic (MZ) twins who are discordant for exposure histories. Theoretically, because the DNA of MZ twins differs only for induced changes, they provide a unique opportunity to study the long-term biological impact of childhood traumatic events.

In the present study we tested the hypothesis that adult females who experienced CSA have a higher frequency of spontaneously occurring leukocyte MN than their identical twins who did not experience CSA. Although these twin pairs are quite rare, we elected to use a discordant identical twin study design since it allows one to control for known genetic influences on MN formation [32], [37] and provides an effective means for separating the causal effects of CSA from background familial risk factors known to associate with CSA.

16.2 METHODS

16.2.1 ETHICS STATEMENT

Human subjects research was approved by the Virginia Commonwealth University IRB (#12407 and #179). Written informed consent was obtained from all research participants.

16.2.2 SAMPLE AND ASSESSMENT OF CHILDHOOD SEXUAL ABUSE

Female-female CSA discordant MZ twins were ascertained from the population based Virginia Adult Twin Study of Psychiatric and Substance Use Disorders [38] and the Mid-Atlantic Twin Registry (MATR) at Virginia Commonwealth University (VCU), with the details of ascertainment outlined elsewhere [39], [40], [41]. Briefly, the pairs derive from two related samples, born from 1934–1974, who were eligible to participate in the previous study [4] if both members responded to a mailed questionnaire (response rate was about 64%). Eighty-eight percent of the participants in the original study were first interviewed face to face in 1987–1989 (at which time their mean [SD] age was 30.1 [7.6] years [range, 17.0–55.0 years]). They were subsequently interviewed three additional times by telephone with at least a one year interval between follow-ups. The remaining 12% were first interviewed face-to-face in 1992–1994 and assessed a second time (with the same interview given to the rest of the sample during the fourth wave) by telephone in 1996–1997. During the second-wave interview, twins were queried about their willingness to respond to questions about CSA and their preferred method of assessment. Most preferred a mailed self-report questionnaire, which was employed using items developed by Martin et al. [42]. The initial item was:

> "Before you were 16, did any adult, or any other person older than yourself, involve you in any unwanted incidents like (i) inviting or requesting you to do something sexual, (ii) kissing or hugging you in a sexual way, (iii) touching or fondling your private parts, (iv) showing their sex organs to you, (v) making you touch them in a sexual way or (vi) attempting or having sexual intercourse?"

Of the 1411 individuals completing this portion of the interview, there were 326 MZ twin pairs where both twins provided information about CSA exposure, of which 74 pairs were classified as discordant for CSA. For the present study, specimens were collected from 17 of these discordant MZ twin pairs (Table 1) in which one twin endorsed none of the CSA items and the other twin fell into one of three exclusive, hierarchical exposure categories: (1) non-genital (N = 3 pairs) [numbers (i), (ii) and (iv)], (2) genital (N = 8 pairs) [numbers (iii) and (v)] and (3) intercourse (N = 6 pairs) [number (vi)]. The mean age at the time of the first CSA incident was 10.7 years-old (s.d. = 3.9) and ranged from 5 to 16 years of age. These CSA discordant MZ twin pairs were invited to complete a health history questionnaire and submit blood samples (VCU IRB #12407). After providing their informed consent, blood samples were obtained by a health care provider of the participants' choosing and shipped to our cytogenetics laboratory (overnight delivery carrier) at room temperature per standard procedures. A random sample of age-matched female MZ twins (7 pairs plus 3 individuals without a cotwin [N = 17]) was also obtained from the MATR to serve as an unselected reference sample (VCU IRB #179), with health history questionnaire completion and blood specimen processing occurring using the identical protocol. The mean current age of the discordant MZ twin pairs (Mean = 48.8, SD = 9.7) was not significantly different from that of the reference sample (Mean = 53.7, SD = 9.4) (t-test, $t29$ = 1.47, P = 0.154).

16.2.3 ASSESSMENT OF ADULT PSYCHOPATHOLOGY

A number of psychiatric and substance use disorders were assessed multiple times in the discordant twins using DSM-IIIR [43] or DSM-IV [44] criteria. Lifetime diagnosis of major depression, generalized anxiety disorder and alcohol and other drug dependence was assessed at the fourth interview by trained interviewers [35]. Lifetime panic disorder was assessed at earlier interviews only (waves 1 and 3). Further details of the diagnostic algorithms and diagnostic reliability can be found in Kendler et al. [38].

16.2.4 DNA ISOLATION AND ZYGOSITY DETERMINATION

Twin zygosity status was confirmed, using genomic DNA that was isolated from whole blood using the Puregene DNA Isolation Kit (Qiagen), based on the patterns of 13 highly polymorphic short tandem repeat sequences (AmpFlSTR® Profiler Plus® and Cofiler® kits, Applied Biosystems, Foster City, CA).

16.2.5 CELL CULTURE

To ensure that erythrocytes did not confound the recognition and scoring of MN, leukocytes were isolated using Histopaque-1077 (Sigma) and then established in culture according to standard procedures (RPMI 1640 media supplemented with 15% fetal calf serum and the mitogen

TABLE 1. Prevalence and Adjusted Relative Risk of Smoking by ACE Exposure Among Non-Hispanic White Adults in Nebraska, Behavioral Risk Factor Surveillance System, 2011.

Childhood sexual abuse	%	Perpetrator status	%
CSA type		Female	0.06
Sexual invitation (i)*	75.0	Multiple individuals	18.8
Sexual kissing (ii)	62.5	Forced or threatened you	47.1
Fondling (iii)	70.6	Age of perpetrator(s)	
Exposing (iv)	60.0	<15 y	15.0
Sexual touching (v)	26.7	15–18 y	35.0
Intercourse (vi)	37.5	19–24 y	20.0
		25–49 y	15.0
After these incidents:		>50 y	15.0
I told no one	81.3		
I told someone and was believed and supported	17.6	Relationship with perpetrator	
		Relative living at home	17.6
I told someone and was believed but not supported	0.06	Non-relative living at home	0.0
		Relative not living at home	6.0
I told someone and was not believed, blame, or punished	0.0	Family friend or other important adult not living at home	29.4
Telling someone put an end to the abuse	100.0	Acquaintance or neighbor	41.2
		Stranger	17.6

*Type as listed in Methods sub-section, 'Sample and Assessment of Childhood Sexual Abuse'. 70.6% of affected individuals experienced more than one CSA type. Participants were classified into three exclusive, hierarchical exposure categories: (1) non-genital (N = 3 pairs) [numbers (i), (ii) and (iv)], (2) genital (N = 8 pairs) [numbers (iii) and (v)] and (3) intercourse (N = 6 pairs) [number (vi)].

phytohemagglutinin) [45]. Forty-four hours after initiation of the cultures, cytochalasin-B was added (3 μg/ml final concentration). Cells were harvested at 72 hours using standard techniques, including a 10-minute incubation in hypotonic solution (0.075 M KCl), and serial fixation (three times in 3:1 methanol: acetic acid solution) [45]. Slides were made following standard procedures [46].

16.2.6 CBMN ASSAY

MN were visualized following Giemsa staining (4% Harleco Giemsa solution) and identified according to the criteria established by Fenech et al. [47] (Figure 1). The frequencies of MN observed in the cytochalasin-B blocked binucleated cells of the twins were calculated by averaging the values obtained from two replicate scores (1000 binucleates were evaluated from two independent areas of the slide for a total of 2000 binucleates per study participant). Given that differences in nuclear proliferation could impact observed MN frequencies, the nuclear division cytotoxicity index (NDCI) was calculated using Fenech's adaptation of the protocol of Eastmond and Tucker [45], [48], as follows: NDCI = [Ap+Nec+M1+2(M2) +3(M3) +4(M4)]/N, where Ap = the number of apoptotic cells; Nec = the number of necrotic cells; M1; M2; M3; and M4 = the number of cells having 1, 2, 3, or 4 nuclei, respectively; and N = total number of cells scored (viable as well as non-viable). The cytogeneticists were blinded to twin pair membership and CSA exposure status.

16.2.7 STATISTICAL ANALYSIS

Differences in MN rates and NDCI values in the CSA exposed twins versus their nonexposed cotwins were assessed by a paired Student's t-test. A general effect of CSA, not differentiated by severity of exposure, was examined in all tests since this was deemed appropriate based on the current literature [1], [3], [4]. A variance stabilizing square root transformation was applied to the MN frequency data for pairwise analyses, given that it was reasonable to assume the distribution of MN scores follow a Poisson distribution. The Wilcoxon signed rank test was also used as a nonparametric equivalent to the paired t-test since data transformations were not required and it provided an additional safeguard against biases sometimes encountered with modest sample sizes. Two-sided P-values were reported for all pairwise comparisons and exact P-values were calculated for non-parametric tests.

One could speculate that the nonexposed twin of pairs discordant for CSA could have elevated MN levels because of exposure to other shared adverse family factors not directly related to CSA or potentially from stress arising from knowledge that her cotwin was abused. To further test whether an effect of CSA on MN levels was restricted only to the abused twin a population sample of age-matched MZ female twins was incorporated in the analyses to serve as a reference group. Tests were performed using generalized mixed-effect models [49] with Poisson error distribution adjusting for covariance within families and the effect of age. Two fixed effect terms were included to specify the relevant contrasts among the different twin exposure classes. A CSA exposure term was coded positive for CSA exposed twins and negative for CSA nonexposed and reference sample twins. An additional term to indicate exposure to adverse familial environment was created where discordant pairs were coded as positive and reference sample twins as negative. Evidence for a CSA related family adversity effect beyond that of direct CSA exposure would be indicated by a significant coefficient for the second term while controlling for any influence of the first term. These models were also used for additional tests exploring differences in the rate of MN formation by age between CSA exposed and nonexposed twins. All analyses were performed using the R statistical programming language [50].

16.3 RESULTS

16.3.1 PAIR-WISE COMPARISONS

MZ twins exposed to CSA exhibited on average a 1.63-fold increase in the occurrence of MN compared to their nonexposed cotwin. The absolute MN frequency values were greater in the CSA exposed twins for 12 of the 17 discordant twin pairs (Figure 2A). Furthermore, the slope of the comparison line was near zero for 3 of the 5 pairs where their MN level was nominally higher in the CSA nonexposed twins. To determine if there might be differential levels of cellular proliferation/viability between the cotwins, their NDCI values were compared using a paired t-test, but showed no significant difference ($t16 = 0.66$, $P = 0.518$) (Figure 2B). In contrast, a paired t-test comparison indicated a significantly higher frequency of MN formation in the CSA exposed twins ($t16 = 2.65$, $P = 0.017$) and resulted in a significant Wilcoxon rank sum test ($W = 124$, $P = 0.023$). We then tested if these results were largely influenced by the discordant twin pair having the largest difference in MN level (the steepest slope in Figure 2A) by removal of this pair and repeating the analysis. This repeat assessment also showed a significant increase in MN frequency in the twins exposed to CSA ($t15 = 2.38$, $P = 0.031$). CSA discordant cotwins did not differ on measured diet and lifestyle factors and no significant differences were found for rates of adult disease (Table 2). It should be clarified that the present sample was not designed to replicate the modest odds ratios reported by Kendler et al. between CSA exposure and the presence of adult psychiatric and substance disorders [4]. The goal of performing these latter tests was to examine whether the presence of adult health/behavioral conditions might confound the association between CSA status and MN formation.

16.3.2 GROUP COMPARISONS

The overall mean [SD] MN frequency in CSA exposed twins was 22.0 [11.3] compared to 14.9 [5.6] per 1000 cells in their nonexposed cotwins (Figure 3). The mean MN level in the unselected reference twins (14.2 [9.4]) was not significantly different from that of the CSA nonexposed set. While CSA exposure status was highly significant in this combined sample ($P<0.001$), there was no indication of an additional effect attributable to the familial environment ($P = 0.406$) based on results from generalized mixed-effect models. Removal of the most extreme value in the reference sample (greater than 3 standard deviations from the mean) resulted in a reduction of the mean MN level to12.3 and a more similar estimate of variability as the CSA nonexposed sample ($SD = 5.4$), but still yielded similar modeling results as the full sample.

Not surprisingly, the clearly established association of age with MN that has been shown by our lab and several previous investigators was

A.

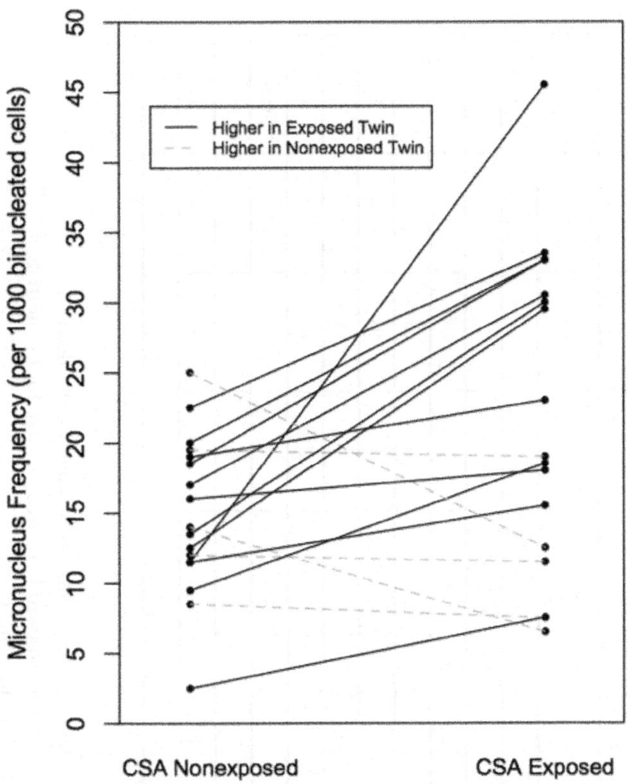

Figure 2. Pairwise comparison of (A) MN frequencies (t_{16} = 2.65, P = 0.017) and (B) nuclear division cytotoxicity index (t_{16} = 0.66, P = 0.518) in CSA discordant MZ twin pairs (t_{16} = 2.65, P = 0.017).

not identified in this study, as estimated using mixed-effect models (P = 0.661), since the twins selected for study were from a narrow age range. However, the difference in MN frequencies between discordant cotwins showed a significant interaction with age, with the divergence increasing over time (coefficient [SE] = 0.030 [0.009], P = 0.0006) (Figure 4). Separate tests of age on each group indicated the interaction between age and

TABLE 2. Lifestyle characteristics and adult psychiatric and substance use disorders in CSA discordant MZ twin pairs.

	CSA Exposed[1]	CSA Nonexposed[2]	Both Endorsed	Neither Endorsed	Odds Ratio[3]	P*
Medication Use[4]	1	3	7	5	0.3	0.63
Green, Leafy Vegetable Intake (5 days per week)	1	6	4	5	0.2	0.13
Smoking Status						
Lifetime (>50 cigarettes)	1	1	5	5	1.0	0.50
Last 30 days (>15 days)	2	0	0	10	$-\infty$	0.50
Heart Disease	1	1	0	13		1.0
High Blood Pressure	2	2	1	10		1.0
Cancer Diagnosis	0	2	0	13	$+\infty$	0.50
Alcohol Dependence	2	1	0	14	2.0	1.0
Any Drug Abuse or Dependence	2	0	0	15	$+\infty$	0.50
Lifetime Depression	5	2	5	5	2.5	0.45
Lifetime Generalized Anxiety Disorder	1	0	0	16	$+\infty$	1.0
Panic Disorder	2	0	0	12	$+\infty$	0.50

1 indicates pairs discordant for CSA and item where the exposed twin was positive for the item (n_{21}).
2 indicates pairs discordant for CSA and item where the nonexposed twin was positive for the item (n_{12}).
3 odds ratio for twin pairs doubly discordant for CSA and item (n_{21}/n_{12}).
4 prescription and non-prescription use for more than 1 year excluding birth control.
$+/-\infty$, value is positive/negative and infinite due to a null value in at least one category.
*two-sided P value from exact binomial test.

CSA exposure was driven primarily by a significant increase of the level of MN in the CSA exposed group (coefficient [SE] = 0.017 [0.005], P = 0.001) rather than a decrease in MN level for the CSA nonexposed group (coefficient [SE] = −0.012 [0.007], P = 0.072). There was no increase in MN frequency with age over the limited age-matched range evaluated for the reference group (P = 0.361).

16.4 DISCUSSION

The present study yielded three main findings. Firstly, female twins exposed to CSA had an increased frequency of acquired somatic chromosomal changes (measured using MN), compared to their nonexposed, genetically identical (MZ) cotwins. Secondly, our analyses ruled out the hypothesis that the higher MN level was due to an indirect association through other shared familial risk factors. Thirdly, evidence was found for an increase in MN level with age in the CSA exposed twins that was not observed in their genetically identical nonexposed cotwins. This latter finding suggests that there may be a cumulative effect of CSA exposure on the frequency of acquired MN in lymphocytes.

16.4.1 CSA IS ASSOCIATED WITH MN FORMATION

The short- and long-term negative sequelae of CSA have been extensively documented. Kendler, et al. [51], who recently reported that the impact of environmental experiences, including traumatic event exposure, contributes substantially to stable and predictable inter-individual differences in symptoms of depression and anxiety that are observed by middle adult life. Although a number of possibilities exist, the biological mechanisms whereby childhood adversity "gets under the skin" to result in latent adult health/behavior consequences have not been well established [52], [53]. For example, there is ample support for the association of chronic psychological stress with persistent sensitizations of the hypothalamic-pituitary-adrenal axis and autonomic stress response [6], [53], [54]. The atypical development of stress reactivity could bring forth direct changes leading

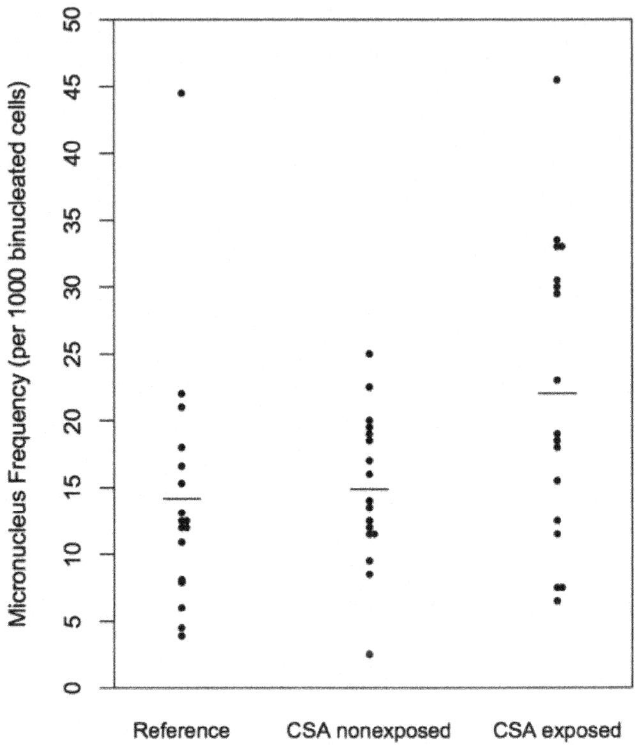

Figure 3. MN frequencies for discordant MZ twin pairs and age-matched controls. The mean level is indicated by a horizontal bar for controls (mean [SD] 14.2 [9.4]), CSA nonexposed (14.9 [5.6]) and CSA exposed (22.0 [11.3]) twins. CSA exposure status was significant in this combined sample (P<0.001), while there was no indication of an additional effect attributable to the familial environment (P = 0.406) based on results from generalized mixed-effect models.

to acquired chromosomal abnormalities in lymphocytes through the induction of inflammatory factors known to influence MN formation, such as IL-6 [55]. Investigators have also shown that an increase in inflammatory activity can elicit the formation of reactive oxygen species, through the deleterious effects of chronically elevated glucocorticoid levels [55]. The resulting oxidative stress may lead to DNA or telomere damage/chromosomal aberrations, resulting in MN formation. Alternatively, epigenetic

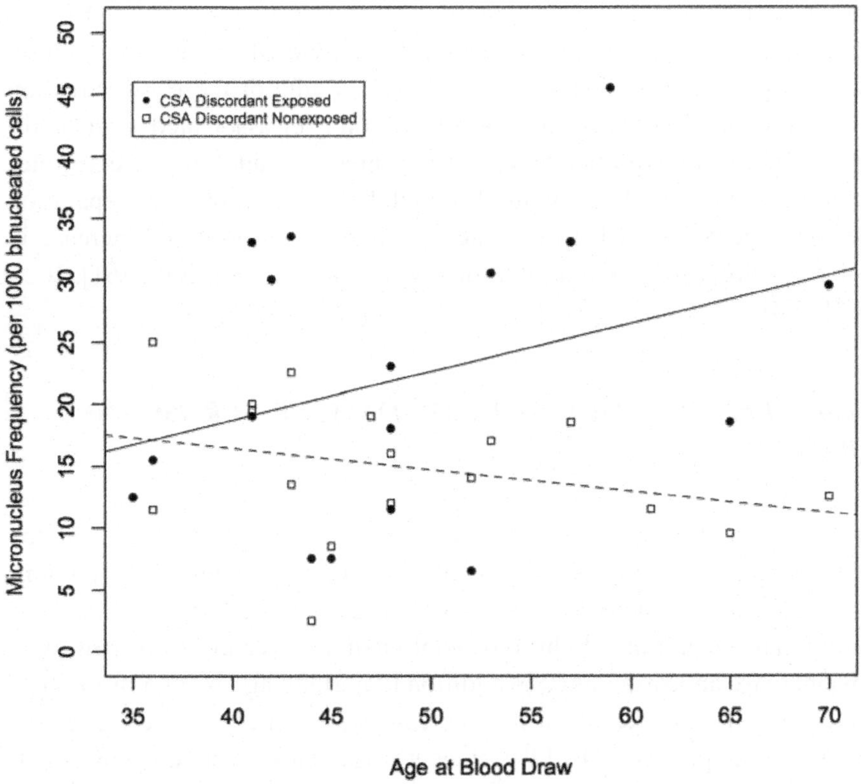

Figure 4. Relationship between MN frequency and age for CSA exposed and nonexposed twins. A significant interaction effect was observed (coefficient [SE] = 0.030 [0.009], P = 0.0006) with the MN level in CSA exposed twins increasing with age while the MN level remained constant across the limited age range evaluated in CSA nonexposed twins.

changes in genes associated with the cascade of biological responses to stress may lead to perturbations in mitotic apparatus formation, chromosomal alignment and/or DNA synthesis, which could subsequently lead to chromosomal malsegregation [55], [56], [57], [58], [59]. Evidence that methylation changes influence acquired chromosomal abnormality frequencies comes from studies of hypomethylated cells obtained following either: (1) in vitro induction (primarily using 5-azacytidine); or (2) as a result of mutation (cells from patients having immunonodeficiency, centromeric heterochromatin instability, and facial anomalies [ICF] syndrome, which is a condition in which the individuals have a mutation in the DNA methyltransferase 3b gene). The results of these investigation have shown increases in the rate of micronuclei associated with methylation alterations (particularly chromosomes 1, 9, and 16 in the samples from people having ICF), with observed delays in centromere separation being suggested as at least one means whereby the observed increase in somatic chromosomal abnormalities was acquired [59], [60], [61], [62], [63], [64].

16.4.2 THE ACCUMULATION OF DAMAGE ACROSS THE LIFESPAN

Interestingly, we observed a significant statistical interaction whereby only twins exposed to CSA displayed an increased MN level over the limited age range evaluated in this study. This association suggests that these individuals accumulated chromosomal changes over their lifespan, with this increase appearing to be in addition to normal, age-related or stochastic events. It is unlikely that this increase was limited to an effect of the normal aging process [21], [29], since it was not also seen in identical cotwins who were not exposed to CSA; nor was it seen in the negative control reference group. Extrapolating from data collected in our previous study of MN frequencies in healthy individuals [32], the "biological age" of the CSA exposed twins was inferred to be 9.9 years older, on average (95% CI, 2.8–17.1), than their CSA nonexposed cotwins. The accumulation of chromosomal instability acquired over the lifespan provides one plausible explanation for the non-specific adverse health effects of child maltreatment and suggests a framework for general susceptibility to a wide variety of adult illnesses and mental health outcomes. Alternatively, rather than chromosomal instability being causally related to the latent health problems observed in adults experiencing CSA, its presence could serve as an accessible and easily measured proxy for recognizing other biologically relevant changes that have occurred and could place the individual at an increased health risk.

16.4.3 METHODOLOGICAL STRENGTHS AND LIMITATIONS

In this study, the relationship between CSA and MN formation was tested using a powerful model; the discordant MZ twin design. Perhaps the most significant advantage of this approach is its ability to address issues related to direction of causality within cross-sectional data. Given that CSA has been shown to correlate with multiple family background risk factors, nearly all of which are shared by twins (such as interpersonal loss, family discord, and economic adversity), the discordant MZ twin design was effective for controlling for the effect of these influences. Without sufficient control in epidemiological samples, which necessitates the measurement of all confounding factors (some of which are unknown) the clustering of childhood adversities would likely serve to overestimate the association between CSA and MN formation. Similarly, the use of MZ discordant twins served as a control for factors related to MN formation that could be shared by twins, including but not limited to, inherited defects in genome maintenance [56], [57]. Another strength of this study design was our sampling of discordant twins who are currently in mid to late adulthood, thereby allowing an appreciable time for the accumulation of stress-related cellular damage to arise from an early life trauma (CSA occurred before 16 years of age). Aspects of this study that are novel include: (1) the conjecture that chromosomal instability could serve as a candidate system for the dysregulation of biological systems that could be "remembered" and accumulated through multiple cell divisions over time and; (2) the use of MN frequency as a potential biomarker for acquired biological changes that have accrued following CSA.

Although our discordant MZ twin study design provided a powerful test of our primary hypothesis, this investigation had methodological limitations. For instance, since we studied lymphocytes, the observation of an increased frequency of acquired chromosomal changes in twins experiencing CSA might have the greatest relevance to health problems associated with the cascade of biological effects mediated through the inflammatory system and may or may not be directly applicable to the acquisition of adult psychopathology. Indeed, this tissue sampling limitation may explain, at least in part, the lack of a clear relationship between MN frequency and the presence of adult psychopathology/morbidity for the limited number of conditions evaluated in our sample. However, it is of interest to note that chromosomal changes, primarily aneuploidy, are acquired in many tissues, normal brain and nerve cells, throughout development and that the brain and other somatic cells from individuals having a variety of health and/or psychiatric conditions show higher levels of acquired chromosomal abnormalities than controls [20], [65], [66], [67].

16.5 SUMMARY

In summary, our study results showed increases in acquired chromosomal instability in female twins exposed to CSA, with the effect appearing to be cumulative with age, and independent of the family environment. Improvements in our understanding of this and other biological changes associated with CSA could lead to the development of biomarker panels for identifying individuals who are most at risk for acquiring health problems. In addition, these persisting biological alterations underscore the gravity of sexual abuse in children.

REFERENCES

1. Nelson EC, Heath AC, Madden PA, Cooper ML, Dinwiddie SH, et al. (2002) Association between self-reported childhood sexual abuse and adverse psychosocial outcomes: results from a twin study. Archives of General Psychiatry 59: 139–145. doi: 10.1001/archpsyc.59.2.139
2. Bulik CM, Prescott CA, Kendler KS (2001) Features of childhood sexual abuse and the development of psychiatric and substance use disorders. Br J Psychiatry 179: 444–449. doi: 10.1192/bjp.179.5.444
3. Dinwiddie S, Heath AC, Dunne MP, Bucholz KK, Madden PA, et al. (2000) Early sexual abuse and lifetime psychopathology: a co-twin-control study. Psychological Medicine 30: 41–52. doi: 10.1017/s0033291799001373
4. Kendler KS, Bulik CM, Silberg J, Hettema JM, Myers J, et al. (2000) Childhood sexual abuse and adult psychiatric and substance use disorders in women: an epidemiological and cotwin control analysis. Arch Gen Psychiatry 57: 953–959. doi: 10.1001/archpsyc.57.10.953

5. Danese A, Pariante CM, Caspi A, Taylor A, Poulton R (2007) Childhood maltreatment predicts adult inflammation in a life-course study. Proceedings of the National Academy of Sciences of the United States of America 104: 1319–1324. doi: 10.1073/pnas.0610362104
6. Heim C, Newport DJ, Miller AH, Nemeroff CB (2000) Long-term neuroendocrine effects of childhood maltreatment. JAMA : the journal of the American Medical Association 284: 2321. doi: 10.1001/jama.284.18.2321
7. Bartsch H, Nair J (2006) Chronic inflammation and oxidative stress in the genesis and perpetuation of cancer: role of lipid peroxidation, DNA damage, and repair. Langenbeck's archives of surgery/Deutsche Gesellschaft fur Chirurgie 391: 499–510. doi: 10.1007/s00423-006-0073-1
8. Miller GE, Chen E, Parker KJ (2011) Psychological stress in childhood and susceptibility to the chronic diseases of aging: moving toward a model of behavioral and biological mechanisms. Psychological Bulletin 137: 959–997. doi: 10.1037/a0024768
9. Drury SS, Theall K, Gleason MM, Smyke AT, De Vivo I, et al.. (2011) Telomere length and early severe social deprivation: linking early adversity and cellular aging. Molecular Psychiatry.
10. Kananen L, Surakka I, Pirkola S, Suvisaari J, Lonnqvist J, et al. (2010) Childhood adversities are associated with shorter telomere length at adult age both in individuals with an anxiety disorder and controls. PLoS ONE 5: e10826. doi: 10.1371/journal.pone.0010826
11. Tyrka AR, Price LH, Kao HT, Porton B, Marsella SA, et al. (2010) Childhood maltreatment and telomere shortening: preliminary support for an effect of early stress on cellular aging. Biological Psychiatry 67: 531–534. doi: 10.1016/j.biopsych.2009.08.014
12. Glass D, Parts L, Knowles D, Aviv A, Spector TD (2010) No correlation between childhood maltreatment and telomere length. Biological Psychiatry 68: e21–22; author reply e23–24.
13. Harley CB (1991) Telomere loss: mitotic clock or genetic time bomb? Mutation Research 256: 271–282. doi: 10.1016/0921-8734(91)90018-7
14. Counter CM, Avilion AA, LeFeuvre CE, Stewart NG, Greider CW, et al. (1992) Telomere shortening associated with chromosome instability is arrested in immortal cells which express telomerase activity. The EMBO journal 11: 1921–1929.
15. Day JP, Limoli CL, Morgan WF (1998) Recombination involving interstitial telomere repeat-like sequences promotes chromosomal instability in Chinese hamster cells. Carcinogenesis 19: 259–265. doi: 10.1093/carcin/19.2.259
16. Filatov L, Golubovskaya V, Hurt JC, Byrd LL, Phillips JM, et al. (1998) Chromosomal instability is correlated with telomere erosion and inactivation of G2 checkpoint function in human fibroblasts expressing human papillomavirus type 16 E6 oncoprotein. Oncogene 16: 1825–1838. doi: 10.1038/sj.onc.1201711
17. Samper E, Goytisolo FA, Menissier-de Murcia J, Gonzalez-Suarez E, Cigudosa JC, et al. (2001) Normal telomere length and chromosomal end capping in poly(ADP-ribose) polymerase-deficient mice and primary cells despite increased chromosomal instability. The Journal of Cell Biology 154: 49–60. doi: 10.1083/jcb.200103049

18. Schwartz JL, Jordan R, Liber H, Murnane JP, Evans HH (2001) TP53-dependent chromosome instability is associated with transient reductions in telomere length in immortal telomerase-positive cell lines. Genes, chromosomes & cancer 30: 236–244. doi: 10.1002/1098-2264(2000)9999:9999<::aid-gcc1085>3.0.co;2-g
19. Leach NT, Rehder C, Jensen K, Holt S, Jackson-Cook C (2004) Human chromosomes with shorter telomeres and large heterochromatin regions have a higher frequency of acquired somatic cell aneuploidy. Mechanisms of ageing and development 125: 563–573. doi: 10.1016/j.mad.2004.06.006
20. Iourov IY, Vorsanova SG, Yurov YB (2008) Chromosomal mosaicism goes global. Molecular Cytogenetics 1: 26. doi: 10.1186/1755-8166-1-26
21. De S (2011) Somatic mosaicism in healthy human tissues. Trends in genetics : TIG 27: 217–223. doi: 10.1016/j.tig.2011.03.002
22. Chen M, Huang JD, Deng HK, Dong S, Deng W, et al. (2011) Overexpression of eIF-5A2 in mice causes accelerated organismal aging by increasing chromosome instability. BMC Cancer 11: 199. doi: 10.1186/1471-2407-11-199
23. Bonassi S, Fenech M, Lando C, Lin YP, Ceppi M, et al. (2001) HUman MicroNucleus project: international database comparison for results with the cytokinesis-block micronucleus assay in human lymphocytes: I. Effect of laboratory protocol, scoring criteria, and host factors on the frequency of micronuclei. Environmental and molecular mutagenesis 37: 31–45. doi: 10.1002/1098-2280(2001)37:1<31::aid-em1004>3.3.co;2-g
24. Mateuca R, Lombaert N, Aka PV, Decordier I, Kirsch-Volders M (2006) Chromosomal changes: induction, detection methods and applicability in human biomonitoring. Biochimie 88: 1515–1531. doi: 10.1016/j.biochi.2006.07.004
25. Battershill JM, Burnett K, Bull S (2008) Factors affecting the incidence of genotoxicity biomarkers in peripheral blood lymphocytes: impact on design of biomonitoring studies. Mutagenesis 23: 423–437. doi: 10.1093/mutage/gen040
26. Kirsch-Volders M, Plas G, Elhajouji A, Lukamowicz M, Gonzalez L, et al. (2011) The in vitro MN assay in 2011: origin and fate, biological significance, protocols, high throughput methodologies and toxicological relevance. Archives of Toxicology 85: 873–899. doi: 10.1007/s00204-011-0691-4
27. Fenech M, Morley AA (1985) The effect of donor age on spontaneous and induced micronuclei. Mutation Research 148: 99–105. doi: 10.1016/0027-5107(85)90212-x
28. Lindberg HK, Wang X, Jarventaus H, Falck GC, Norppa H, et al. (2007) Origin of nuclear buds and micronuclei in normal and folate-deprived human lymphocytes. Mutation research 617: 33–45. doi: 10.1016/j.mrfmmm.2006.12.002
29. Fenech M, Kirsch-Volders M, Natarajan AT, Surralles J, Crott JW, et al. (2011) Molecular mechanisms of micronucleus, nucleoplasmic bridge and nuclear bud formation in mammalian and human cells. Mutagenesis 26: 125–132. doi: 10.1093/mutage/geq052
30. Fenech M (2011) Micronuclei and their association with sperm abnormalities, infertility, pregnancy loss, pre-eclampsia and intra-uterine growth restriction in humans. Mutagenesis 26: 63–67. doi: 10.1093/mutage/geq084
31. Miller B, Potter-Locher F, Seelbach A, Stopper H, Utesch D, et al. (1998) Evaluation of the in vitro micronucleus test as an alternative to the in vitro chromosomal aberration assay: position of the GUM Working Group on the in vitro micronucleus test.

Gesellschaft fur Umwelt-Mutations-forschung. Mutation Research 410: 81–116. doi: 10.1016/s1383-5742(97)00030-6

32. Jones KH, York TP, Juusola J, Ferreira-Gonzalez A, Maes HH, et al. (2011) Genetic and environmental influences on spontaneous micronuclei frequencies in children and adults: a twin study. Mutagenesis 26: 745–752. doi: 10.1093/mutage/ger042
33. Bonassi S, Znaor A, Ceppi M, Lando C, Chang WP, et al. (2007) An increased micronucleus frequency in peripheral blood lymphocytes predicts the risk of cancer in humans. Carcinogenesis 28: 625–631. doi: 10.1093/carcin/bgl177
34. Murgia E, Maggini V, Barale R, Rossi AM (2007) Micronuclei, genetic polymorphisms and cardiovascular disease mortality in a nested case-control study in Italy. Mutation research 621: 113–118. doi: 10.1016/j.mrfmmm.2007.02.015
35. Federici C, Botto N, Manfredi S, Rizza A, Del Fiandra M, et al. (2008) Relation of increased chromosomal damage to future adverse cardiac events in patients with known coronary artery disease. The American journal of cardiology 102: 1296–1300. doi: 10.1016/j.amjcard.2008.07.024
36. Petrozzi L, Lucetti C, Scarpato R, Gambaccini G, Trippi F, et al. (2002) Cytogenetic alterations in lymphocytes of Alzheimer's disease and Parkinson's disease patients. Neurological sciences : official journal of the Italian Neurological Society and of the Italian Society of Clinical Neurophysiology 23 Suppl 2S97–98. doi: 10.1007/s100720200087
37. Surowy H, Rinckleb A, Luedeke M, Stuber M, Wecker A, et al. (2011) Heritability of baseline and induced micronucleus frequencies. Mutagenesis 26: 111–117. doi: 10.1093/mutage/geq059
38. Kendler KS, Prescott CA (2006) Understanding the Causes of Psychiatric and Substance Use Disorders. New York: Guilford Press.
39. Kendler KS, Neale MC, Kessler RC, Heath AC, Eaves LJ (1992) A population-based twin study of major depression in women. The impact of varying definitions of illness. Arch Gen Psychiatry 49: 257–266. doi: 10.1001/archpsyc.1992.01820040009001
40. Kendler KS, Prescott CA (1998) Cannabis use, abuse, and dependence in a population-based sample of female twins. Am J Psychiatry 155: 1016–1022. doi: 10.1192/bjp.173.4.345
41. Kendler KS, Prescott CA (1999) A population-based twin study of lifetime major depression in men and women. Arch Gen Psychiatry 56: 39–44. doi: 10.1001/archpsyc.56.1.39
42. Martin J, Anderson J, Romans S, Mullen P, O'Shea M (1993) Asking about child sexual abuse: methodological implications of a two stage survey. Child Abuse and Neglect 17: 383–392. doi: 10.1016/0145-2134(93)90061-9
43. American Psychiatric Association (1987) Diagnostic and Statistical Manual of Mental Disorders, Revised Third Edition. Washington, DC: American Psychiatric Association.
44. American Psychiatric Association (1994) Diagnostic and Statistical Manual of Mental Disorders, Fourth Edition. Washington, DC: American Psychiatric Association.
45. Fenech M (2000) The in vitro micronucleus technique. Mutation research 455: 81–95. doi: 10.1016/s0027-5107(00)00065-8
46. Leach NT, Jackson-Cook C (2001) The application of spectral karyotyping (SKY) and fluorescent in situ hybridization (FISH) technology to determine

the chromosomal content(s) of micronuclei. Mutation research 495: 11–19. doi: 10.1016/s1383-5718(01)00194-2

47. Fenech M, Chang WP, Kirsch-Volders M, Holland N, Bonassi S, et al. (2003) HUMN project: detailed description of the scoring criteria for the cytokinesis-block micronucleus assay using isolated human lymphocyte cultures. Mutation research 534: 65–75. doi: 10.1016/s1383-5718(02)00249-8
48. Eastmond DA, Tucker JD (1989) Identification of aneuploidy-inducing agents using cytokinesis-blocked human lymphocytes and an antikinetochore antibody. Environmental and Molecular Mutagenesis 13: 34–43. doi: 10.1002/em.2850130104
49. Faraway JJ (2006) Extending the Linear Model with R: generalized linear, mixed effects and nonparametric regression models. New York: Chapman & Hall/CRC.
50. R Development Core Team (2010) R: A language and environment for statistical computing. Vienna, Austria: R Foundation for Statistical Computing.
51. Kendler K, Eaves L, Loken E, Pedersen N, Middledop C, et al.. (2011) The impact of environmental experiences across the lifespan on symptoms of anxiety and depression. Psychological Science.
52. Scott J, Varghese D, McGrath J (2010) As the twig is bent, the tree inclines: adult mental health consequences of childhood adversity. Archives of general psychiatry 67: 111–112. doi: 10.1001/archgenpsychiatry.2009.188
53. McCrory E, De Brito SA, Viding E (2011) The impact of childhood maltreatment: a review of neurobiological and genetic factors. Frontiers in psychiatry/Frontiers Research Foundation 2: 48. doi: 10.3389/fpsyt.2011.00048
54. Miller GE, Chen E, Zhou ES (2007) If it goes up, must it come down? Chronic stress and the hypothalamic-pituitary-adrenocortical axis in humans. Psychological Bulletin 133: 25–45. doi: 10.1037/0033-2909.133.1.25
55. Yan B, Peng Y, Li CY (2009) Molecular analysis of genetic instability caused by chronic inflammation. Methods in molecular biology 512: 15–28. doi: 10.1007/978-1-60327-530-9_2
56. Samanta S, Dey P (2010) Micronucleus and its applications. Diagnostic cytopathology.
57. van Leeuwen DM, Pedersen M, Knudsen LE, Bonassi S, Fenech M, et al. (2011) Transcriptomic network analysis of micronuclei-related genes: a case study. Mutagenesis 26: 27–32. doi: 10.1093/mutage/geq074
58. Drazen JM, Yandava CN, Dube L, Szczerback N, Hippensteel R, et al. (1999) Pharmacogenetic association between ALOX5 promoter genotype and the response to anti-asthma treatment. NatGenet 22: 168–170.
59. Herrera LA, Prada D, Andonegui MA, Duenas-Gonzalez A (2008) The epigenetic origin of aneuploidy. Current genomics 9: 43–50. doi: 10.2174/138920208783884883
60. Fauth E, Scherthan H, Zankl H (1998) Frequencies of occurrence of all human chromosomes in micronuclei from normal and 5-azacytidine-treated lymphocytes as revealed by chromosome painting. Mutagenesis 13: 235–241. doi: 10.1093/mutage/13.3.235
61. Hernandez R, Frady A, Zhang XY, Varela M, Ehrlich M (1997) Preferential induction of chromosome 1 multibranched figures and whole-arm deletions in a human pro-B cell line treated with 5-azacytidine or 5-azadeoxycytidine. Cytogenet Cell Genet 76: 196–201. doi: 10.1159/000134548

62. Rodriguez MJ, Lopez MA, Garcia-Orad A, Vig BK (2001) Sequence of centromere separation: effect of 5-azacytidine-induced epigenetic alteration. Mutagenesis 16: 109–114. doi: 10.1093/mutage/16.2.109
63. Stacey M, Bennett MS, Hulten M (1995) FISH analysis on spontaneously arising micronuclei in the ICF syndrome. J Med Genet 32: 502–508. doi: 10.1136/jmg.32.7.502
64. Schmid M, Grunert D, Haaf T, Engel W (1983) A direct demonstration of somatically paired heterochromatin of human chromosomes. Cytogenet Cell Genet 36: 554–561. doi: 10.1159/000131972
65. Faggioli F, Vijg J, Montagna C (2011) Chromosomal aneuploidy in the aging brain. Mechanisms of Ageing and Development 132: 429–436. doi: 10.1016/j.mad.2011.04.008
66. Iourov IY, Vorsanova SG, Yurov YB (2008) Molecular cytogenetics and cytogenomics of brain diseases. Current genomics 9: 452–465. doi: 10.2174/138920208786241216
67. Kingsbury MA, Friedman B, McConnell MJ, Rehen SK, Yang AH, et al. (2005) Aneuploid neurons are functionally active and integrated into brain circuitry. Proceedings of the National Academy of Sciences of the United States of America 102: 6143–6147. doi: 10.1073/pnas.0408171102

PART III

CONCLUSION

CHAPTER 17

Lessons Learned from Child Sexual Abuse Research: Prevalence, Outcomes, and Preventive Strategies (continued)

DELPHINE COLLIN-VÉZINA, ISABELLE DAIGNEAULT, AND MARTINE HÉBERT

17.1 PREVENTIVE STRATEGIES: HOW CAN WE PREVENT CSA FROM HAPPENING IN THE FIRST PLACE?

In light of the high prevalence of CSA and the wealth of deleterious outcomes associated with this abusive experience, it stands to reason that research attention must turn toward preventing CSA. Two widespread forms of sexual assault prevention efforts have been extensively studied and disseminated, namely, offender "management" and educational programs delivered, for the most part, in school settings. Offender management is the approach that aims to control known offenders, for example, registries, background employment checks, longer prison sentences and various intervention programs. It is a tertiary prevention initiative that acts mostly in the individual sphere and, as such, presents certain inherent limitations in regards to preventing CSA from happening in the first place [107]. Indeed, although the public generally approves of so-called punitive legal practices, such as longer sentences, they are based on a misconception of sexual abusers as pedophiles, "guileful strangers" who prey on children in public places, when in actual fact the child sex offender population is more varied, includes individuals known to the victim and is comprised of juveniles in almost a third of cases [107].

The second most frequent approach, primary prevention, involves universal educational programs generally delivered in schools and aimed at potential victims. In the majority of cases, these universal programs also intervene in the individual preventive sphere and more infrequently in the family or societal sphere. Regarding children attending elementary school, meta-analyses by Zwi and colleagues [108], covering 15 studies, and by Davis and Gydicz [109], covering 27 studies, revealed that programs are effective at building children's knowledge about sexual abuse and their preventive skills. The second of those two meta-analyses further demonstrated that programs are more effective if they are longer in duration (four sessions or more), if they repeat important concepts, if they provide children with multiple opportunities to actively practice the taught notions and skills, and if they are based on concrete concepts (what is forbidden) rather than abstract notions (rights or feelings). Some programs have proven effective for building knowledge and skills among children in an average socio-economic environment [110], but presented mitigated results in a multi-ethnic and underprivileged urban environment, indicating that the program may need to be adapted in order to optimize its effects with specific clientele [111]. As per adolescents or young adults attending high school or college, a meta-analysis of 69 studies involving close to 20,000 participants revealed that programs are effective for improving participants' knowledge and attitudes [112]. However, changes in terms of behaviours or intentions to act were too low to be clinically significant. Also, factors related to the clientele, the facilitator, the setting and the format of the program have all been shown to impact the effectiveness of sexual violence prevention programs in college or university settings [113]. For some of the above programs, data are available to suggest that they are associated with a reduction of the incidence of child sexual assault [114] and sexual victimization in teenage romantic relationships [115]. However, too few studies are available to draw a firm conclusion as to the efficacy of prevention efforts, introduced since the 1970s, to reduce the true incidence of CSA observed by authorities in some countries, most notably the US [116-119].

The advantages of the universal approach are numerous: these programs can be offered at low cost, they are fairly easy to implement widely, and they allow to reach a maximum number of children while avoiding the stigmatization of a particular population. Yet, this approach has also been criticized since it places the responsibility of prevention in the hands of children. Consequently, this approach should not be considered as the only answer to a social problem as complex as CSA. A multi-factorial approach may indeed constitute a more promising solution to solve the problem of sexual abuse. A multi-factorial conceptualization of sexual assault suggests that only the development of global preventive approaches, targeting personal, family as well as societal norms that influence the risk of assault, may substantially reduce incidence and prevalence rates [119,120]. Those actions may take a variety of forms, such as awareness campaigns, efforts to provide the proper training to all persons who may work with children and adolescents, including sexual abuse and trauma themes in academic programs of future practitioners, or even the development of up to date and comprehensive kits to help the media provide information free of sexism, prejudices and sensationalism when reporting on sexual assault cases. In addition, parents' participation is a fundamental element for a successful prevention initiative as this may increase the acquisition of preventive abilities in children [110], thus, future endeavors will need to tackle the challenges to foster a greater participation of parents. While most prevention initiatives have favoured a universal approach, targeting at-risk groups may also ensure optimal efficacy of prevention efforts. Integrating new technologies and using social medias (web site, applications for cell phones, online interactive games) may be particularly relevant for prevention efforts targeting teenagers. If such approaches were implemented and coordinated on a broad scale, they may have a greater impact on the number of sexual assault victims.

17.2 CONCLUSION

The sexual abuse of children is a form of maltreatment that provokes reactions of indignation and incomprehensibility in all cultures. Yet, CSA is, unfortunately, a widespread problem that affects more than 1 out of 5 women and one out of 10 men worldwide. This alarming rate clearly calls for extensive and powerful policy and practice efforts. While the effects of CSA may not always be initially visible, survivors of CSA still carry the threat to their well-being. The traumatic experience of CSA is one major risk factor in the development of mental health problems affecting both the current and future well-being of victims. Considering that many victims continue to be undetected, the roots of these mental health problems may also be unrecognized. In an effort to provide effective services to all victims, we should prioritize the development of strategies to address the barriers to disclosure and reporting. Although the taboo of CSA might not be as prominent as a few decades ago when CSA was rarely spoken of, veiled issues may still prevent victims from reaching out to authorities to reveal the abuse they suffer. To effectively prevent CSA, global preventive approaches, targeting personal, family and societal conditions, need to be explored and validated so to protect the next generations of children and youth from sexual victimization.

REFERENCES

107. Finkelhor D: The prevention of childhood sexual abuse. Future Child 2009, 19:169–194.
108. Zwi K, Woolfenden S, Wheeler D, O'Brien T, Tait P, Williams K: School-based education programmes for the prevention of child sexual abuse. Cochrane Database Syst Rev 2007, 3:1–37.
109. Davis M, Gidycz CA: Child sexual abuse prevention programs: A metaanalysis. J Clin Child Psychol 2000, 29:257–265.
110. Hébert M, Lavoie F, Piché C, Poitras M: Proximate effects of a child sexual abuse prevention program in elementary school children. Child Abuse Negl 2001, 25:505–522.
111. Daigneault I, Hébert M, McDuff P, Frappier J-Y: Evaluation of a sexual abuse prevention workshop in a multicultural, impoverished urban area. J Child Sex Abus 2012, 21:521–542.
112. Anderson LA, Whiston SC: Sexual assault education programs: A meta-analytic examination of their effectiveness. Psychol Women Q 2005, 29:374–388.

113. Vladitu CJ, Martine SL, Macy RJ: College- or University-based sexual assault prevention programs: A review of program outcomes, characteristics, and recommendations. Trauma Violence Abuse 2011, 12:67–86.
114. Gibson LE, Leitenberg H: Child sexual abuse prevention programs: Do they decrease the occurrence of child sexual abuse? Child Abuse Negl 2000, 24:1115–1125.
115. Foshee VA, Bauman KE, Ennett ST, Suchindran C, Benefield T, Linder G: Assessing the Effects of the Dating Violence Prevention Program "Safe Dates" Using Random Coefficient Regression Modeling. Prev Sci 2005, 6:245–258.
116. Breitenbecher KH: Sexual assault on college campuses: Is an ounce of prevention enough? Appl Prev Psychol 2000, 9:23–52.
117. Hickman LJ, Jaycox LH, Aronoff J: Dating violence among adolescents: Prevalence, gender distribution, and prevention program effectiveness. Trauma Violence Abuse 2004, 5:23–142.
118. Rothman E, Silverman J: The Effect of a College Sexual Assault Prevention Program on First-year Students' Victimization Rates. J Am Coll Health 2007, 55:283–290.
119. Wurtele SK: Preventing Sexual Abuse of Children in the Twenty-First Century: Preparing for Challenges and Opportunities. J Child Sex Abus 2009, 18:1–18.
120. Wurtele SK: School-based child sexual abuse prevention. In Preventing violence in relationships: Interventions across the life span. Edited by Schewe PA. Washington, DC: American Psychological Association; 2002:9–25.

AUTHOR NOTES

CHAPTER 1, 6, and 17

Acknowledgments

The Article processing charge (APC) of this manuscript has been funded by the Deutsche Forschungsgemeinschaft (DFG)

Author Contributions

The project was initiated by Prof. Dr. Collin-Vézina who wrote the sections on prevalence and mental health outcomes of CSA. Prof. Dr. Daigneault and Prof. Dr. Hébert led the writing on CSA prevention strategies. All authors read and approved the final manuscript.

Competing Interests

The authors declare that they have no competing interests.

CHAPTER 2

Acknowledgments

First and foremost, the authors are grateful to the *Bundesministerium für Familie, Senioren, Frauen und Jugend* (BMFSFJ) for having provided funding for the study, and thus allowing this important issue to be analyzed and the results to be published. Special thanks go to Almut Hornschild-Rentsch and her team who accompanied the development of the study.

We thank Anna Herboly for her excellent work on editing the manuscript.

Last but not least, we would like to thank the library of *Asklepios Medical School GmbH* in Hamburg, namely Sabrina Juhst, Birgit Scherpe and Verena Reiser, for their straightforward support by providing the literature needed.

Author Contributions

JMF and JW conceived the idea of the study, reviewed the manuscript and gave final approval of the version to be published. JMF obtained funding for the study. JW advised SH on the study design. SH conceived the calculation model and drafted the manuscript. SB gave methodological support and coordinated external and internal affairs. All authors have read and approved the final manuscript.

Competing Interests

The authors declare that they have no competing interests.

CHAPTER 5

Author Contributions

Conceived and designed the experiments: GF CG GD AT. Performed the experiments: GF ES. Analyzed the data: GF VC GD AT. Wrote the paper: GF CG AT. Other: Collected the psychometric data: GD. Collected the psychometric data: LP. Project Manager: AS.

CHAPTER 7

Acknowledgments

The authors thank the families whose generous donation of time made this project possible and the research staff responsible for data collection.

Contributors

MBE designed the study, with collaboration of the coauthors as described below, and was largely responsible for the writing of the manuscript. BE designed the parent study, directed data collection and contributed to the study design and editing of the manuscript. EAB helped to design the study's analyticstrategy, ran the statistical analyses and contributed to the interpretation of the data and the writing of the Methods and Results sections. ROW and RJW contributed to the study design and writing of the Introduction and Discussion sections. Each of the authors has reviewed the manuscript and made edits as appropriate. MBE, BE and EAB had access to the data presented in the manuscript and take responsibility for the integrity of the data and accuracy of the data analyses. There are no other individuals who fulfil the criteria for authorship.

Competing Interests
None.

Funding
The research was supported by grants to BE from the Maternal and Child Health Service (MCR-270416), the William T Grant Foundation, New York, and the National Institute of Mental Health (MH-40864). During preparation of this manuscript, the authors were supported by K08MH074588 (MBE), R01HD054850 (BE), R01ES013744 (ROW) and R01 MD006086 (RJW). The content is solely the responsibility of the authors and does not necessarily represent the official views of the National Institutes of Health.

CHAPTER 8

Acknowledgments
This study would not have been possible without the support of many colleagues in the local NHS and in voluntary sector and other community support organizations. We are grateful for their advice and time. We are grateful to Cheryl McElroy for the support received in study development and implementation. The study relied heavily on the continued efforts of Charlie Gibbons, Georgina Bellis, Olivia Sharples, Katherine Hardcastle, Mark O'Keefe, Phil McHale, Clare Perkins, Paul Duffy, Jim McVeigh and Neil Potter. We are also grateful to Howard Spivak and Lynn Jenkins at the Centers for Disease Control and Prevention for sharing their insight into US ACE studies. Finally, we are indebted to all those individuals who took time to participate in this survey. We were overwhelmed not only with their enthusiasm for the survey but often with the hospitality they showed researchers visiting their homes.

Funding

This work was supported by Liverpool John Moores University and National Health Service Research and Development Funds.

CHAPTER 9

Acknowledgments

The authors have no funding sources to report.

CHAPTER 10

Competing Interests

The authors declare that they have no competing interests.

Authors' Contributions

TWS developed the research question, conducted the statistical analysis, conducted the literature review, and wrote the initial draft of the manuscript.VJE, SRD and SD assisted with the statistical analysis. MW, AWP, SR, VJE, and JBC assisted with subject matter content. All authors read and approved the final manuscript.

CHAPTER 11

Competing Interests

The authors declare that they have no competing interests.

Authors' Contributions

DC, JC, YL all have made substantial contributions to the conception, design, and acquisition of data. AW, DC, JC, GP, LPC, VE all has made substantial contributions to the analysis and interpretation of data. DC, JC, YL have been involved in drafting the manuscript; AW, DC, GP, JC, LPC, VE have been involved in critically revising the manuscript for important intellectual content. All co-authors have read and approved this manuscript.

Sources of Support

AGW received support from a fellowship through a cooperative agreement (award number 3U50CD300860) between the Association for Prevention

Teaching and Research and the Centers for Disease Control and Prevention. This project was supported, in part, by cooperative agreement U58/CCU324336-05 between the National Association of Chronic Disease Directors and the Centers for Disease Control and Prevention.

CHAPTER 12

Competing Interests

The authors have declared that no competing interests exist.

Author Contributions

Conceived and designed the experiments: MPB EJ SAA. Performed the experiments: SAA PSK. Analyzed the data: MPB. Contributed reagents/materials/analysis tools: MPB EJ SAA PSK. Wrote the paper: MPB EJ AK. Approved the manuscript: MPB EJ AK SAA PSK.

Acknowledgments

We would like to thank all the adolescents for their participation in this study. At the time of the study conduct Dr. Sonia Alemagno and Ms. Peggy Shaffer-King were at University of Akron, Akron, Ohio.

CHAPTER 14

Competing Interests

The authors declare that they have no competing interests.

Author Contributions

Study was designed by CP, CH and MS. Participants were selected by CP and CH. Methylation analysis was completed by NB and JP. Bioinformatic analysis was performed by MS. The entire process was overseen by MS. JP, NB, CH, MP, SPP, CP, MS and MS all contributed to writing the manuscript. All authors read and approved the final manuscript.

Acknowledgments

We dedicate this work to the memory of our recently deceased co-author Clyde Hertzman, who played a central role in conceiving of this study and inspiring its completion. Grants from the Canadian Institute of Health

Research; MOP-42411 the Sackler program in Psychobiology and Epigenetics at McGill University (to M.S.); fellowship from the Canadian Institute of Health Research and the Fragile X Research Foundation of Canada (to N.B.); the UK Medical Research Council (MRC) (grant G0000934 to the clinical examination and DNA banking of the 1958 cohort); and funding received for the MRC Centre of Epidemiology for Child Health (Grant G0400546) (for SPP). Work undertaken at Great Ormond Street Hospital/University College London, Institute of Child Health is in part supported by funding from the Department of Health's National Institute of Health Research ('Biomedical Research Centres' funding). Laboratory work in the Department of Social Medicine, University of Bristol was supported in part by a grant to MP from the Welcome Trust.

CHAPTER 15

Conflict of Interest Statement

The author declares that the research was conducted in the absence of any commercial or financial relationships that could be construed as a potential conflict of interest.

Acknowledgments

Work in Dr. McGowan's laboratory is supported by operating grants from the Natural Sciences and Engineering Research Council of Canada (NSERC), the Chronic Fatigue and Immune Dysfunction Association of America (CFIDS), and the Canadian Institutes of Health Research (CIHR).

CHAPTER 16

Competing Interests

Dr. Kimberly H. Jones is an employee of Neodiagnostix, Inc. This does not alter the authors' adherence to the PLOS ONE policies on sharing data and materials. The other authors declare no competing interests.

Funding

This work was supported by grants from the National Institute on Aging [R01AG037986 (CJC, TPY)] and the National Institute of Environmental

Health Sciences [R01 ES12074 (CJC)]. The funders had no role in study design, data collection and analysis, decision to publish, or preparation of the manuscript.

Author Contributions

Conceived and designed the experiments: TPY CJC. Performed the experiments: CJC JB JJ KSK KHJ AFG TPY. Analyzed the data: TPY CJC KSK LJE SHA JB. Contributed reagents/materials/analysis tools: TPY CJC KSK LJE ABA AFG. Wrote the paper: TPY CJC.

INDEX

A

B

N

O

P

R

S

T

U